P9-ANY-060

Congenital and Acquired Color Vision Defects

Current Ophthalmology Monographs

Series Consultant
Robert D. Reinecke, M.D.
Professor and Chairman
Department of Ophthalmology
The Albany Medical College
Albany, New York

Other books in this series

Vitrectomy: A Pars Plana Approach
Robert Machemer, M.D.
First Edition

Ocular Histoplasmosis
T. F. Schlaegel, Jr., M.D.

The Pathogenesis of Nerve Damage in Glaucoma:
Contributions in Fluorescein Angiography
George L. Spaeth, M.D.

Ocular Toxoplasmosis and Pars Planitis
T. F. Schlaegel, Jr., M.D.

Immunology of Uveitis and Ocular Tumors
Devron H. Char, M.D.

Vitrectomy
Robert Machemer, M.D., Thomas M. Aaberg, M.D.
Second Edition

Intraocular Lens Implants in Children
David A. Hiles, M.D.
In Press

Congenital and Acquired Color Vision Defects

Joel Pokorny, Ph.D.
Professor of Ophthalmology and Behavioral Sciences
The University of Chicago

Vivianne C. Smith, Ph.D.
Professor of Ophthalmology
The University of Chicago

Guy Verriest, M.D.
Associate Professor of Ophthalmology
State University of Ghent, Belgium

A. J. L. G. Pinckers, M.D.
Lecturer in Ophthalmology
University of Nijmegen, Netherlands

EDITORS

GRUNE & STRATTON
A Subsidiary of Harcourt Brace Jovanovich, Publishers
New York   London   Toronto   Sydney   San Francisco

RE
921
C72

© 1979 by Grune & Stratton, Inc.
All rights reserved. No part of this publication
may be reproduced or transmitted in any form or by
any means, electronic or mechanical, including
photocopy, recording, or any information storage
and retrieval system, without permission in
writing from the publisher.

Grune & Stratton, Inc.
111 Fifth Avenue
New York, New York 10003

Distributed in the United Kingdom by
Academic Press, Inc. (London) Ltd.
24/28 Oval Road, London NW 1

Library of Congress Catalog Number 79-2974
International Standard Book Number 0-8089-1203-8
Printed in the United States of America

Contents

Acknowledgments

The final manuscript and bibliography were edited and typed at the University of Chicago. We thank colleagues for substantive and stylistic suggestions. In particular, the following individuals provided editorial help: Ian Chisholm (Chapter 8), Paul Kinnear (Chapters 6 and 9), Jean-Jacques de Laey (Chapter 8), Dennis Lund (Chapters 1–4), Steven Shevell (Chapters 6–7), and Richard Wallstein (Chapters 5–8). Danuta Sawicki typed the manuscript and bibliography. The index was prepared by Richard Wallstein. Contributions of Joel Pokorny and Vivianne C. Smith were supported in part by USPH NEI Grants EY 00901, EY 01876, and EY 70652.

Joel Pokorny
Vivianne C. Smith

Foreword

It is always a pleasure to be invited to write a foreword to a book your friends have written, although this can cause qualms if the book is of dubious quality. No such qualms here, though! I would judge this book to be quite first class, with excellent introductory chapters followed by detailed descriptions of many different color vision tests and testing methods. The heart of the book, the massive Chapters 7 and 8, includes well-documented accounts of experimental studies that have been made, many by the authors themselves, on congenital and acquired color vision defects. These chapters are full of factual material and underline the enormous depth and breadth of the subject.

It could not have been easy to harmonize the contributions from the eight different authors, but there is no obvious disparity in the treatment of the various sections. The book appeals to me especially because it is not slanted towards one theory rather than another. In fact, it strikes a decidedly cautious note in Chapter 3. It is also delightfully practical, as when it refers to the embarrassment that elderly and arthritic patients may experience should they drop or find difficulty in manipulating the discs in the Farnsworth-Munsell 100-Hue Test.

I do have just one quarrel with the authors, namely their retention of the misleading description of the tritan-type color defect as a "blue–yellow" defect. This occurs in Chapters 4 and 7 and many times in Chapter 8 in connection with acquired defects. The truth is that the tritan defect is due to a loss of blue sensitivity, a loss that leads to blue–green and yellow–violet color confusions, but never, so far as I know, to confusions on the blue–yellow axis. What a marvelous opportunity this would have been to correct an error that has been around in the literature for far too long.

In my estimation, however, *Congenital and Acquired Color Vision Defects* is destined to become the definitive handbook on defective color vision for a good many years to come. It derives much of its authority from the fact that the contributors span continental Europe, Great Britain, and the United States. This implies a tremendous advantage so far as literature coverage is concerned. Altogether, a bold and successful venture on the part of the four editors.

W. D. Wright, D.Sc., A.R.C.S., D.I.C.
Emeritus Professor of Applied Optics
Imperial College
University of London

Preface

Abnormalities of color perception have been recognized for more than three centuries. The study of congenital color vision defects proceeded simultaneously in the great ophthalmology clinics of continental Europe as well as in physics, biology, and psychology departments in Europe and the United States. The clinicians were known for their painstaking pedigree analyses and development of practical color vision tests; their work is little known in Great Britain and the United States, where the dominant interest has been on precise studies of congenital color defects and development of color vision theory. The growth of clinical testing of congenital color defective observers in both Europe and the United States is usually attributed to the development of mass transport with the accompanying mandate to screen color defective observers from sensitive occupations in the industry. The study of acquired dyschromatopsias developed almost entirely in Europe within the ophthalmology clinic.

Recognition of the need for this book arose in conversations among contributors at the Third Symposium of the International Research Group on Color Vision Deficiencies in Amsterdam. The International Research Group on Color Vision Deficiencies was founded in order to study both congenital and acquired color vision disorders in an interdisciplinary way. The growing membership of the Society and increased paper submissions to the symposia are evidence of a wide and expanding interest in color vision research, both from clinicians seeking to apply advanced research techniques and from psychologists and biologists seeking to apply their basic knowledge to the evaluation of the patient in the clinic. At the time of the Amsterdam meeting, there was no modern textbook that gave a systematic review of the study of acquired dyschromatopsias. The major recent literature is found in the collections of symposia papers of the International Research Group on Color Vision Deficiencies. There is wide textbook coverage of congenital color defects, but few texts make a deliberate effort to incorporate the divergent traditions of research in Europe and the United States. No textbook introduces the clinician to precise psychophysical techniques, and none introduces the psychophysicist or physiologist to the clinical field. After the Amsterdam meeting, possible contributors were approached; as a result, the contributors to this volume represent not only a wide geographical expanse but also varied backgrounds, including both clinicians and basic researchers.

The book is designed to fulfill a variety of needs for people of varied backgrounds. Its major goal is to provide a comprehensive review of the current status of research in congenital and acquired color vision defects. Secondarily, it aims to present a body of practical information concerning techniques of basic research and of clinical color vision evaluation.

Chapters 1 and 2 present some fundamental methods of producing, specifying, and measuring a color stimulus within the framework of normal color vision. Chapter 3 presents a review of the physiological basis of color vision and its relation to modern color theory. This chapter is designed to render a conceptual framework within which color vision defects may be viewed. Chapter 4 reviews the various classification systems for defective color vision. Chapters 5 and 6 describe clinical and specialized psychophysical techniques available for evaluating abnormalities of color vision. Chapter 7 is a review of congenital color vision defects, and Chapter 8 reviews the occurrence of color vision defects acquired in different disease states. Finally, Chapter 9 reviews some practical implications and consequences of color defects in our society. Chapters 1 through 4 and 7 were jointly written; for Chapters 5, 6, and 8, the contributions were independently written and then subjected to overall editing. Contributors are listed alphabetically.

We hope that this book will fulfill its aim—to provide a review of the current status of the field and act as a handbook to guide the clinician and researcher into a fascinating and fruitful field.

The Editors

Contributors

Jennifer Birch, M. Phil., F.B.O.A.
Department of Optometry and Visual Sciences
City University
London, England

Ian A. Chisholm, M.D., F.R.C.S.
Associate Professor of Ophthalmology
Department of Ophthalmology
University of Saskatchewan
Saskatchewan, Canada

Paul Kinnear, Ph.D.
Senior Lecturer in Psychology
University of Aberdeen
King's College
Aberdeen, Scotland

Marion Marré, Doz. Dr. Sc. Med.
Augenabteilung der Poliklinik
Der Medizinischen Akademie "Carl Gustav Carus"
Dresden, German Democratic Republic

A. J. Pinckers, M.D.
Lecturer in Ophthalmology
Institute of Ophthalmology
University of Nijmegen
Nijmegen, The Netherlands

Joel Pokorny, Ph.D.
Professor of Ophthalmology and Behavioral Sciences
The University of Chicago
Chicago, Illinois

Vivianne C. Smith, Ph.D.
Professor of Ophthalmology
The University of Chicago
Chicago, Illinois

Guy Verriest, M.D.
Associate Professor of Ophthalmology
Department of Ophthalmology
State University of Ghent
Ghent, Belgium

Joel Pokorny, Ph.D.
Vivianne C. Smith, Ph.D.
Guy Verriest, M.D.

1

Production and Specification of the Stimulus

In this chapter we describe how to produce a color stimulus for visual research and how the physical characteristics of such stimuli are usually specified. Much of this material may seem rather specialized for the general reader interested in an introduction to color vision defects; the chapter is primarily intended to introduce some of the technical terms used in the study of color vision deficiency.

BASIC TERMINOLOGY

Electromagnetic Radiation

Light is electromagnetic radiation that we see Like other electromagnetic radiation, light propagates through space and is recognized to have a dual, wave–particle nature. When light is reflected or refracted, its wave properties are important, and wave principles, assuming straight-line propagation, are used to trace rays through optical systems. When light is absorbed (or emitted), it acts as though its energy were contained in discrete particles, which are termed quanta. Since radiation must be absorbed to initiate vision, the quantal nature of light is important in discussions of the absolute threshold for vision or the behavior of visual photoreceptors. Electromagnetic wave motion is characterized by its speed *in vacuo,* the constant c (approximately 3×10^8 m/sec, and by its frequency, the variable v.

Frequency and Wavelength

In the study of vision, it is usual to specify visible electromagnetic radiation by its wavelength ($\lambda = c/v$) expressed in nanometers (10^{-9} meters, abbreviated nm). The terms millimicron (equivalent to nm) and angstrom (10^{-10} m) are no longer used in visual

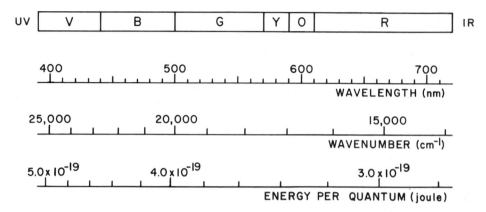

Fig. 1.1. Schematic diagram of the visible spectrum (banded by ultraviolet [UV] and infrared [IR]), showing the perceived hues (V, violet; B, blue; G, green; Y, yellow; O, orange; R, red), the wavelength, the wave number, and the energy per quantum for monochromatic radiations.

research. For most observers and available light sources, the visible spectrum extends from about 380 to 780 nm.

When electromagnetic radiation enters a medium, such as glass or the eye, its speed is reduced. The reduction is expressed by the refractive index (n), which is the ratio of the velocity* (v) of light in air to that in the medium, $n = v_{air}/v_{medium}$. The difference in the speed of light in vacuum, c, and in air is very small; relative to air, the index of refraction, n, is given by $v_{air}/c \cong 0.9998$. In a given medium the frequency of light remains constant; the wavelength (v/ν), however, changes with speed and is given approximately by $c/\nu n$, where c/n approximates the speed of light in the medium. This relation has led researchers to point out that frequency (ν) is the preferable form for expressing radiation. An alternative specification is the wave number, given by ν/c (alternatively $10^7/\lambda$). Wave number is widely used in certain research areas; however, the use of wavelength remains widespread in color specification. The relation between wavelength and wave number is depicted in Fig. 1.1.

When electromagnetic radiation occurs at a single wavelength, it is called a monochromatic radiation. Radiation occurring within a narrow band of wavelengths is also termed monochromatic (alternatively narrow-band or spectral) radiation. Monochromatic radiations are associated with a characteristic color appearance to the normal observer, as indicated in Fig. 1.1. When electromagnetic radiation occurs at several wavelengths, it is called a complex radiation (often termed broad-band radiation). An example of a source containing complex radiations is sunlight, which includes energy at all visible wavelengths.

Energy and Quanta

Each quantum has a characteristic energy proportional to its frequency, ν, given by the equation

---

*It is common practice in dealing nontechnically with light (such as in the study of vision) rather than with its physical properties to use the terms "speed" and "velocity" interchangeably; in a strictly mathematical sense it is "speed" that is always meant ("velocity" is technically the *speed* of something in a given *direction*).

$$E = h\nu = hc/\lambda, \tag{1.1}$$

where h is the Planck constant (approximately 6.624940×10^{-34} joule sec) and λ is the wavelength in meters. The energy per quantum, expressed in joules, varies inversely with wavelength, as shown in Fig. 1.1.

PRODUCTION OF SPECTRALLY SELECTIVE STIMULI

Chromatic stimuli are produced when various portions of the electromagnetic spectrum are isolated. We may differentiate between methods using optical principles (such as dispersion, diffraction, interference, or absorption) to isolate specific portions of the electromagnetic spectrum from a continuous (white) light source, and methods using light sources (such as gas discharge lamps or lasers) whose output is concentrated in specific portions of the spectrum or in a set of spectral lines.

Selective Filters

Color filters transmit a selected portion of the spectrum. Several types are available, each having advantages in terms of performance and/or cost. A color filter is specified by its transmission characteristics. The measurement of transmission is further described below.

Description of the transmission characteristics of a filter showing a single peak in the visible spectrum includes (1) the wavelength and peak transmission at maximum output and (2) the half-width (also called half-height bandwidth or half-height bandpass). This specification may be supplemented by other characteristics (Scharf, 1965). The half-width is obtained by finding the wavelength difference between the two wavelengths having half the maximum output. In Fig. 1.2a the wavelength maximum is 649.3 nm and the half-width is 11.5 nm.

If the filter transmits only at one end of the spectrum, it is known as a pass, cut-on, or cut-off filter. Such filters are specified by (1) the cut-on wavelength, usually the wavelength having 5 percent transmission, and (2) the slope, calculated as the difference in nanometers between the cut-on wavelength and the wavelength of 70 percent transmission (Scharf, 1965). In Fig. 1.2b the cut-on wavelength is 607 nm and the 70 percent transmission wavelength is 628 nm, giving a slope of 21 nm. Other values of transmission may be used to specify the cut-on wavelength and to calculate the slope; furthermore, the slope may be expressed as a percentage of the wavelength difference relative to the cut-on wavelength. Thus it is important to check the manufacturer's conventions for specification (Scharf, 1965).

Gelatin and color glass filters obtain selectivity by absorption. Typically, these filters have broad transmission characteristics (with half-widths of 50–100 nm). Also, efficient cut-on gelatin filters passing long wavelengths (long-pass filters) are available with maximal transmission values near 100 percent. Although the measured transmittance of a filter is unaffected by the type of illuminant (see below), it should be noted that the transmitted spectral distribution and hence color appearance depends upon both the energy distribution of the source and the transmission characteristic of the filters. Advantages of color filters include high efficiency, high stability, ready availability, and low cost.

Interference filters typically transmit only a very narrow band of wavelengths; the

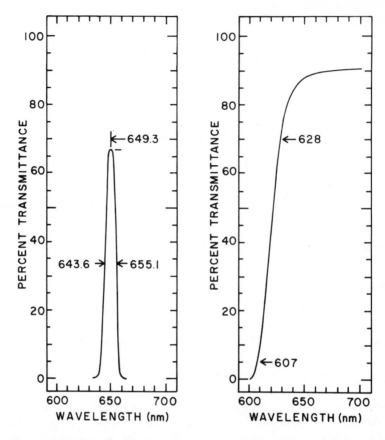

Fig. 1.2. (left) Specification of a band-pass filter includes the wavelength of maximal output and calculation of half-height bandwidth. The peak wavelength is 649.3 nm and has maximal transmittance of 67 percent. The two wavelengths in the band that have half the maximum output, or 33.5 percent transmittance, are found (643.6 and 655.1 nm), and the difference between these, 11.5 nm, is the half-height bandwidth.   (right) Specification of a long-pass filter includes the cut-on wavelength and slope. The cut-on wavelength occurs at 5 percent transmittance (607 nm). The slope may be calculated as the wavelength difference between the cut-on wavelength and the wavelength of 70 percent transmittance (628 nm), giving a value of 21 nm.

remainder of the light is reflected off the filter. Frequently, such filters have multiple transmission peaks, and blocking filters (glass or gelatin) are required to yield a single-peaked transmission characteristic. Interference filters used for visual research typically have half-widths ranging from 3 to 20 nm (although broad-band interference filters are available). Interference filter specifications are based upon test conditions in which collimated light passes to the filter orthogonal to the surface of the filter. If the filter is rotated, maximal transmission shifts to shorter wavelengths. Similarly, when an interference filter is placed in a converging or diverging beam of light, the bandpass widens asymmetrically and the peak transmission shifts to shorter wavelengths.

Many selective filters have transmission in the infrared. It is important to control this transmission when making relative energy measurements (see below) or in studies using high light levels. Infrared absorbing or reflecting filters can be used in conjunction with selective filters to avoid delivering large quantities of infrared radiation to the eye.

Monochromators

An instrument that allows selection of narrow portions of the spectrum is called a monochromator. Monochromators can be made using prisms in which the entering light is separated into its spectrum by dispersion (Fig. 1.3). A spectroradiometer (see below) is used to measure the relative spectral output at the selected wavelengths. A band of wavelengths may then be specified by the wavelength of maximal output and the half-width, just as described for filters. The operator has control of both the mean wavelength (by rotation of the prism) and the width of the wavelength band (by varying the widths of the entrance and exit slits). Other types of monochromators make use of interference wedges or diffraction gratings to separate the entering white light. The diffraction grating monochromator has the advantages that the peak wavelength is a linear

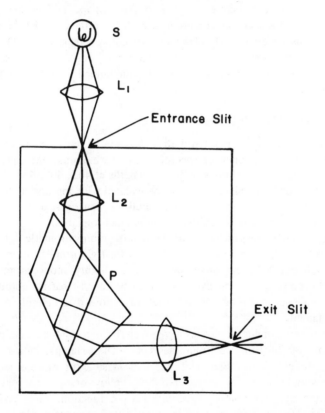

Fig. 1.3. Schematic diagram of a monochromator employing a constant-deviation (Pellica-Broca) prism. An image of the source (S) is produced on the entrance slit of the monochromator by lens L₁. Light is then collimated by lens L₂ and passes to the prism P. Light exiting from the prism at a 90° angle is collected by lens L₃ and imaged on the exit slit. The wavelength composition of the exiting light depends upon the angle of rotation of the prism. [From Pokorny, J. & Smith, V. C. Color vision of normal observers. In A. M. Potts (Ed.), *The assessment of visual function.* St. Louis: The C. V. Mosby Company, 1972 (reproduced by permission of The C. V. Mosby Company).]

function of the angle of rotation of the grating and that the width of the wavelength band does not change with wavelength.

Colored Paper

A third method of obtaining spectrally selected stimuli from white light is the use of colored papers. A physical description of a colored paper is its spectral reflectance. (Measurement of reflectance is described below.) Colored papers form the basis of many tests of color defect and are among the most widely used of all colored stimuli; however, papers can rarely be obtained whose spectral reflectance lies within a narrow band of wavelengths.

There are several precautions that should be observed when using colored papers. As with broadband filters, the color appearance will change as illumination is changed. The color depends on both the reflective characteristics of the paper and the energy distribution of the illumination. Adequate specification of both the reflectance of the paper and the illumination is thus necessary. Disadvantages of colored papers are (1) the ease with which their appearance may be changed by fingerprints, dust, and other superficial dirt, (2) the limited range of reflective values, and (3) the tendency of dyes to fade with time and exposure to light.

Chromatic Light Sources

Another way of obtaining color stimuli is through the use of a source whose output may be concentrated in one or more spectral lines. For example, the cadmium-mercury gas lamp has principal spectral lines with wavelengths at 405, 408, 436, 468, 480, 509, 546, 578, 635, and 644 nm. Single lines can be isolated with appropriate blocking filters. Such lamps provide highly monochromatic stimuli for visual research. Furthermore, the lamps have an important use in the calibration of monochromators.

The laser is another class of light source providing monochromatic light of extremely high energy levels. (The term laser is an acronym for *l*ight *a*mplification by *s*timulated *e*mission of *r*adiation.) Lasers have one or more highly monochromatic emission wavelengths. Recently developed dye lasers may be tuned (that is, output wavelength varied) over a wide spectral region with the use of various dyes. Highly monochromatic light can be obtained.

Advances in semiconductor physics have given rise to a solid-state lamp that operates on the principle of junction electroluminescence. These lamps, called light-emitting diodes (LEDs), directly convert electrical energy into visible (or infrared) radiation. LEDs that emit wavelengths appearing greenish-yellow, yellow-orange, and red are available and are specified by their relative spectral emission function. They typically have a half-width of 25–50 nm. They respond very quickly to changes in electrical input (rise and fall times on the order of 10^{-7}–10^{-8} sec) and do not require much input power. Disadvantages include relatively low light output and peak wavelengths limited to wavelengths longer than 560 nm.

SPECIFICATION OF SPECTRALLY SELECTIVE STIMULI

Chromatic light sources are characterized by their relative spectral emission function. The color properties of a transparent object such as a glass filter are determined primarily by its spectral transmittance; the color properties of an opaque object such as colored paper are primarily determined by its spectral reflectance.

Measurement of Spectral Emittance

Light sources are characterized by their relative spectral energy in the visible range. The relative spectral energy is measured by a device called a spectroradiometer, which samples the energy output at successive narrow monochromatic bands. A spectroradiometer consists of a monochromator, which selects the wavelength and width of the sampling band, and a photodetector, which converts electromagnetic energy into electrical energy. The output will depend on the size of the band sampled. A spectroradiometer is usually used to give the relative spectral emittance of the unknown source in comparison with the emittance of a known reference source. Absolute calibration in terms of watts cm^{-2} is rarely used and requires a supplementary measurement, for example, the use of a thermopile to give the total irradiance of the source (see below). Wyszecki and Stiles (1967) describe some techniques to derive absolute measurements of spectral emittance.

Transmittance

When light is incident on a liquid or glass filter, it is customary to measure spectral transmittance (using a device called a spectrophotometer). Spectral transmittance, $\tau(\lambda)$, is the ratio of transmitted (t) to incident (i) light as a function of wavelength. The spectrophotometer is similar to a spectroradiometer in that it uses a photodetector to measure selected narrow wavelength bands. The measurement differs from spectroradiometry in that it involves a comparison of incident and transmitted flux:

$$\tau(\lambda) = \frac{\Phi_t(\lambda)}{\Phi_i(\lambda)}, \tag{1.2}$$

where $\Phi_i(\lambda)$ is the flux incident on the filter and $\Phi_t(\lambda)$ is the flux transmitted by the filter at wavelength λ (Fig. 1.4). According to Bouguer's law, for a glass filter deriving its properties from absorption

$$\tau(\lambda) = 10^{-lm(\lambda)}, \tag{1.3}$$

where l is the pathlength of the beam through the absorbing medium of the filter and $m(\lambda)$ is the spectral absorptivity of the filter. The product $lm(\lambda)$ is called the absorbance. When incident light is normal to the surface, l is identical to the thickness of the filter, and $\tau(\lambda)$ may be called the internal spectral transmittance.

Another way of expressing transmittance is in the form of optical density $d(\lambda)$, given by the negative decadic logarithm of transmittance:

$$d(\lambda) = -\log \frac{\Phi_t(\lambda)}{\Phi_i(\lambda)} = -\log[\tau(\lambda)]. \tag{1.4}$$

Transmittance through multiple filters, say glass A and glass B, separated by air may be calculated in succession (Fig. 1.4). The flux incident on glass B is that transmitted from glass A,

$$\Phi_i(\lambda)_B = \Phi_t(\lambda)_A. \tag{1.4a}$$

(a)

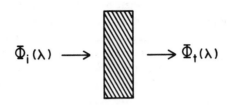

(b)

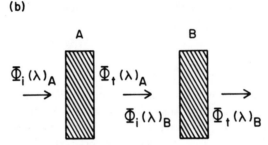

Fig. 1.4. Measurement of transmittance. (a) The radiant flux $\Phi_i(\lambda)$ is incident normal to the surface and the transmitted flux $\Phi_t(\lambda)$ is measured. (b) A schematic diagram of light passing through two filters, A and B. See text for further explanation.

The total transmittance through A and B is

$$\tau(\lambda)_{AB} = \frac{\Phi_t(\lambda)_B}{\Phi_i(\lambda)_A} = \frac{\Phi_t(\lambda)_A}{\Phi_i(\lambda)_A} \times \frac{\Phi_t(\lambda)_B}{\Phi_i(\lambda)_B}. \tag{1.5}$$

Transmittance through multiple filters is thus given by the product of the separate transmittances, at each wavelength.

The optical density $d(\lambda)_{AB}$ will be given by the sum of separate optical densities, $d(\lambda)_A + d(\lambda)_B$, since the logarithm of the product of the separate transmittances is equal to the sum of the logarithms of the transmittances. Figure 1.5 gives a graphical example of the spectral transmittance of two colored glass filters and their products.

If a filter transmits an approximately equivalent amount of light at each wavelength, it is called a neutral-density filter. Such a filter may be characterized by a single number representing its overall transmittance or density.

Reflectance

Reflectance is measured using a spectrophotometer to compare incident and reflected flux. The measure of reflectance of a pigmentary object is far more complicated than the measurement of transmittance of a glass filter (Judd & Wyszecki, 1975). For a perfectly reflecting surface, approximated by a high-quality mirror, reflection is specular, the angle of incidence being equal to the angle of reflection (Fig. 1.6a); for a perfectly diffusing

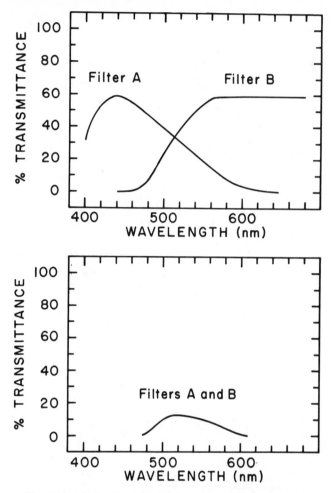

Fig. 1.5. Spectral transmittance of two filters, A and B, compared with spectral transmittance for the pair of filters.

surface, approximated by a block of smoked magnesium oxide, reflectance encompasses all possible angles, with equal flux at each reflected angle (Fig. 1.6b). For a real surface (Fig. 1.6c), flux is reflected at many angles, but some angles are more efficient than others, causing a phenomenon called gloss. Gloss refers to the capacity of a surface to produce specular reflection. Many papers have some degree of gloss and look shiny or dull depending on the angle of view. The measurement of reflectance of sample objects therefore varies with the particular geometry of the measurement. Factors that must be specified include the angles of direction of incident and reflected flux, as well as the size, specified by the solid angle ω (defined below and in Fig. 1.11) of the cone of reflected flux.

It is customary to define reflectance relative to a standard opaque object whose reflectance is measured under identical conditions (Fig. 1.7) (Judd & Wyszecki, 1975). For many years the standard was a block of smoked magnesium oxide with spectral reflectance of unity in the visible spectrum. In 1969, the Commission Internationale d'Eclairage (CIE) adopted as a standard a perfectly diffusing and reflecting surface (as in

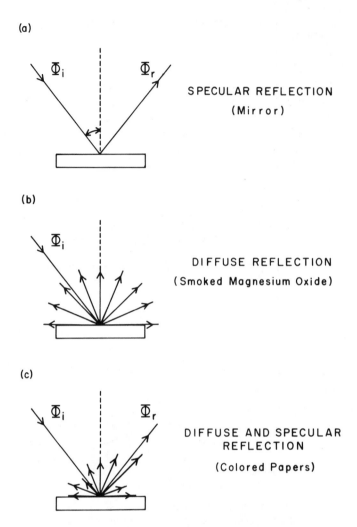

Fig. 1.6. Three types of reflection. (a) Specular reflection is produced by a highly polished surface such as a mirror. (b) Diffuse reflection is produced by a diffusing surface such as smoked magnesium oxide. (c) A mixture of diffuse and specular reflection is produced by objects such as most colored papers.

Fig. 1.6b). The CIE standard is not a physical standard but it is closely approximated by magnesium oxide. In practice, magnesium oxide may be used and data corrected to those of the CIE standard. The most common measurement technique is to make successive measurements for the standard and the sample object. Under these conditions the spectral reflectance factor $\beta(\lambda)$ is given by the ratio of flux reflected in a solid angle ω by the sample, $\Phi_r(\lambda)\omega$, to that reflected in a solid angle ω by the standard, $\Phi_D(\lambda)\omega$:

$$\beta (\lambda) = \Phi_r (\lambda)\, \omega/\Phi_D (\lambda)\, \omega. \tag{1.6}$$

There are two subtypes of reflectance measurement, differing in the size of the solid angle sampled in the measurement. The spectral radiance factor is measured when ω approaches

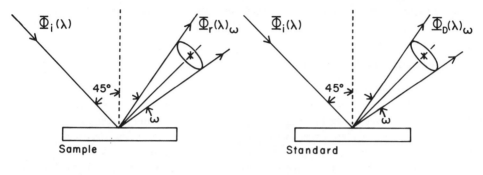

SPECTRAL REFLECTANCE FACTOR:

$$\beta(\lambda) = \Phi_r(\lambda)_\omega \; / \; \Phi_D(\lambda)_\omega$$

Fig. 1.7.   Measurement of the spectral reflectance factor. The radiant flux $\Phi_i(\lambda)$ is incident at 45° to the normal. A reflected cone $\Phi_r(\lambda)_\omega$ of solid angle ω is measured at 45° to the normal beam. The spectral reflectance factor is the ratio of flux reflected from the sample, $\Phi_r(\lambda)_\omega$, to that reflected from the standard, $\Phi_D(\lambda)_\omega$.

zero; the spectral reflectance given by $\rho(\lambda)$ is measured when ω is 2π. Spectral reflectance, $\rho(\lambda)$, is measured using an integrating sphere.

PRODUCTION OF SPECTRALLY NONSELECTIVE STIMULI

There are many physical stimuli that are correlated with the sensation white, some involving the mixture of as few as two wavelengths. Common white stimuli such as sunlight or light from a tungsten lamp have continuous spectra; some energy is present at all visible wavelengths. Fluorescent lamps have line spectra superimposed on a continuous spectrum. The major white light sources include the sun, incandescent lamps (carbon, platinum, and tungsten), and electrical discharge lamps (xenon, mercury, and zirconium arc lamps and fluorescent tubes). Such light sources may be characterized by their relative spectral energy in the visible range (see above) using a spectroradiometer. An equal-energy source has unit radiant energy output at all wavelengths. An alternative means of specification of achromatic sources uses the concept of color temperature (described below).

Incandescent Sources

Incandescent sources use substances (carbon, platinum, tungsten filaments) that may be heated to high temperatures so that they emit radiation. The filaments are heated in vacuo or in an inert gas. The most commonly available incandescent source is the tungsten lamp. The relative spectral output of the tungsten depends both on the emissivity of the tungsten and on the operating temperature.

In recent years, tungsten-halogen lamps have been developed. A small amount of a halogen (usually iodine) is included with the inert gas. When tungsten evaporates off the heated filament, it combines with the halogen in a regenerative cycle and is continually redeposited on the filament. Tungsten-halogen lamps maintain virtually all their original light output throughout life. Tungsten-halogen lamps should be operated near their rated input voltage, since the halogen cycle does not occur at lower voltages and lamp life is reduced.

Electrical Discharge Lamps

Discharge lamps emit radiant energy when electrical energy is passed through a gas or vapor. These lamps emit line spectra superimposed on a continuous output spectrum. The line spectra vary for different lamp types; they are dependent principally on the vapor but also on other characteristics of the lamp. The most important electrical discharge lamps in visual research include arc lamps and fluorescent tubes.

Arc lamps are widely used in specialized optical systems for psychophysical research in color vision. Some of the most useful are the xenon and zirconium arc lamps. The xenon high-pressure arc has a high level of radiant energy output that is almost constant across the visible spectrum (Fig. 1.8a). The size of the arc is usually small (<3 mm) and can be easily used in most optical systems. In the zirconium lamp, the source size is a function of the power rating of the lamp; a low-power (2 W) lamp may be regarded as a point source. The lamp has a continuous spectral output increasing with wavelength and showing occasional line spectra (Fig. 1.8b).

Fluorescent lamps emit line spectra superimposed on a continuous spectrum (Fig. 1.8c). There is wide variability in the color appearance of different fluorescent lamps, reflecting both differences in the continuous spectrum as well as different energy outputs of the major line spectra. There is a corresponding variability in color appearance of surfaces viewed under fluorescent lamps. A number of fluorescent lamps have been devised especially for use in color vision research (Chapter 5).

SPECIFICATION OF SPECTRALLY NONSELECTIVE STIMULI

Color Temperature

The usual method of specifying an incandescent light source is by means of color temperature. As the source is heated (for example, the voltage on a tungsten lamp is increased), the radiant energy emitted by the body extends over an increasingly wide band of wavelengths. At low temperatures the rate of radiation is low and the radiation is chiefly of relatively long wavelength. At 800 K the source emits enough radiant energy to be self-luminous and appears "red-hot."

The manner of specification of the spectral output of emission is in terms of temperature, but since different sources have different outputs when heated to the same temperature, all sources are referred to a theoretical standard called a "blackbody" or ideal radiator. A blackbody is a theoretical surface that absorbs all the energy that impinges upon it. It also emits all this energy and has a characteristic spectral output, determined by Planck's law, that depends only on its temperature (Fig. 1.9). Available sources, such as tungsten or carbon, have different spectral outputs at a given temperature, but it is possible to specify them in terms of the temperature of a blackbody with nearly equivalent spectral response. The color temperature of a specimen lamp is the operating temperature of an ideal radiator whose spectral output matches that of the specimen lamp. Tabulations of relative spectral output as a function of temperature are given by Moon (1961).

The concept of color temperature may also be extended to specification of the

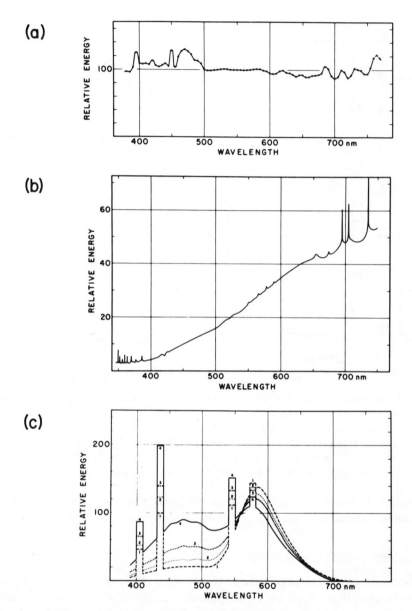

Fig. 1.8. Spectral energy distribution of some electrical discharge lights. (a) High-pressure xenon. (b) Zirconium. (c) Conventional fluorescent lamps. [From Wyszecki, G., & Stiles, W. S. *Color science*. New York: John Wiley & Sons, 1967 (reproduced by permission of John Wiley & Sons, Inc.).]

appearance of discontinuous or filtered continuous light sources whose spectral output does not conform to that of a blackbody but whose appearance is close to that of a blackbody source. It is possible, for example, to specify various fluorescent lamps by stating the color temperature correlated with their spectral appearance. When color temperature is applied to nonblackbody radiation it is called the "correlated color temperature." Fluorescent lamps usually have higher correlated color temperatures than

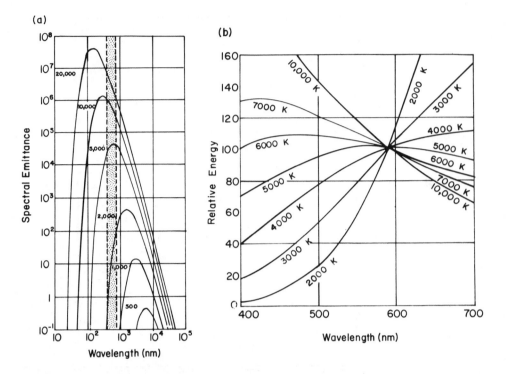

Fig. 1.9. (a) Spectral energy distribution of a blackbody as a function of temperature. The band indicates the range of visible radiation. (b) The relative energy in the visible region of the spectrum as a function of color temperature. The heights of the curves have been adjusted so that the energy at 590 nm is equal to 100. [From Pokorny, J. & Smith, V. C. Color vision of normal observers. In A. M. Potts (Ed.), *The assessment of visual function*. St. Louis: The C. V. Mosby Company, 1972 (reproduced by permission of The C. V. Mosby Company).]

incandescent lamps, indicating that their energy is more concentrated at shorter wavelengths. This phenomenon may have practical importance to the ophthalmologist.

Reciprocal Color Temperature

The reciprocal color temperature R (expressed in reciprocal megakelvins) is an alternative specification of color temperature. In the past, the term "mired" (*microreciprocal degree*) has been used for R. Reciprocal color temperature has two important properties: a given ΔR is approximately an equal perceptible step for a wide range of color temperatures, and a given color temperature conversion filter will cause the same change in R over a wide range of actual color temperatures. The color temperature conversion filters (or color-correcting filters) are a special class of selective filters designed to alter the color temperature of a blackbody source while maintaining its conformation to a blackbody radiator. Many filter manufactuers specify a color temperature conversion filter in terms of its R shift value (still called mired shift in many catalogues). The color temperature achieved by use of such a filter with a blackbody source is predicted by

$$K_{\text{source + filter}} = \cfrac{1}{R_{\text{source}} + \Delta R_{\text{filter}}} \times 10^6. \qquad (1.7)$$

Yellow-appearing filters, which lower color temperature, have positive R shifts; blue-appearing filters, which raise color temperature, have negative R shifts.

Standard Illuminants

Several practical working standards for white lights have been specified by the CIE and are called standard illuminants. The relative spectral distribution of three such standards are shown in Fig. 1.10. They are representative of the following types of radiant energy distribution:

Standard illuminant A: incandescent lamp light at color temperature of 2854 K.

Standard illuminant B: direct sunlight with a correlated color temperature of 4874 K.

Standard illuminant C: light of the overcast sky (northern for northern hemisphere) with a correlated color temperature of 6774 K.

Standard illuminant D_{65}: daylight with a correlated color temperature of 6504 K.

Source A is realized directly by operating an incandescent lamp at a color temperature of 2854 K. Sources B and C are obtained by modifying the spectral distribution of source A with precisely specified liquid filters. Source D_{65} is one of a group of sources that represent various phases of daylight; each is characterized by the letter D and a subscript representing the first two digits of the color temperature. Illuminants D are specified for

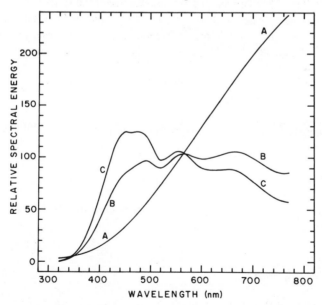

Fig. 1.10. Specified illuminants. Spectral energy distribution of the CIE illuminants A, B, and C. (Based on data tabulations of Wyszecki, G., & Stiles, W. S. *Color science*. New York, John Wiley & Sons, 1967.)

near ultraviolet as well as visible light and have important application in analysis of fluorescent materials.

RADIOMETRY

Measurement of the quantity of radiant energy (radiometry) is achieved by determining the temperature rise of a blackened surface as it absorbs radiation. Practical instruments for radiation measurement include thermopiles and bolometers. Such devices measure the total energy emitted at all wavelengths. In the case of a complex radiation, it is often convenient to consider this as the sum of several monochromatic radiations.

There are three fundamental types of energy measurement: the total energy emitted from a source in a given direction (radiant intensity), the energy incident on a surface at some distance from a source (irradiance), and the energy emitted from a unit area of a surface (radiance) (see Table 1.1).

Radiant Intensity

When electrical power is supplied to a lamp, radiation is emitted. The radiant energy emitted per unit of time is called flux, P_e (watts). Not all of the electrical power is converted into radiant flux; some is lost by heat conduction, heat convection, and absorption.

A set of lines radiating from a point defines a solid angle at that point (Fig. 1.11a). With this point as center and with any distance R as radius, a spherical surface may be constructed. The set of lines emanating from the center of the sphere defines an area A on the surface of the sphere. The steradian measure of the solid angle ω is the ratio $\omega = A/R^2$. If $A = R^2$, then the solid angle is one steradian (sr). Since the total area of a sphere is $4\pi R^2$, the total solid angle subtended at the point is

$$\omega_{(total)} = \frac{4\pi R^2}{R^2} = 4\pi \text{ sr.} \qquad (1.8)$$

The radiant intensity I_e of a point source with radiant flux P_e is the radiant flux per solid angle,

$$I_e = P_e/\omega, \qquad (1.9)$$

expressed in units of W/sr. A point source rated at 5 watts will have a radiant intensity of $5/(4\pi)$ W/sr, or approximately 0.4 W/sr.

Table 1.1
Specification of Radiometric Units

Term	Symbol	Units
Radiant flux	P_e	watts (W)
Radiant intensity	I_e	W sr^{-1}
Irradiance	E_e	W m^{-2}
Radiance	L_e	W m^{-2} sr^{-1}

Irradiance

When radiant flux is incident on a surface, the surface is said to be irradiated. Let P_e be the radiant flux incident on the interior surface of a sphere of radius R. The total area of the sphere is $4\pi R^2$. The irradiance E_e is the radiant flux from a point source falling on a unit area of this surface:

$$E_e = P_e / \omega R^2. \tag{1.10}$$

Irradiance is radiant flux incident per unit area, expressed in watts per square meter.

The irradiance E_e is usually expressed in terms of the radiant intensity I_e by substituting $P_e = \omega I_e$ into Eq. (1.10). Irradiance is related to radiant intensity I_e by the expression

$$E_e = I_e / R^2 \tag{1.11}$$

Thus a point source rated at 5 watts will have an irradiance on the interior surface of a sphere of 100 cm radius of approximately 0.4×10^2 W/m^2.

The radiant flux emitted by a point source falls on a successively greater area as the distance from the source increases (Fig. 1.11b). As noted in Eq. (1.11) the irradiance E_e varies inversely with the square of the distance R from the source P_e. This relation is called the inverse square law.

Suppose the surface is a flat screen rather than a spherical surface (Fig. 1.12a). Two important changes occur as α, the angle from the normal, increases. First, the distance to the surface, C, is greater than R by the factor $1/\cos\alpha$, and in accord with the inverse square law the irradiance will be reduced by a factor of $\cos^2\alpha$. Second, since the area of the surface is irradiated at angle α rather than perpendicularly, the radiant flux contained in a narrow solid angle ω will be spread over a larger area. For example, in Fig. 1.12a the object lies in plane C and is thus at angle α to the normal plane A; the irradiated area in plane C is $1/\cos\alpha$ times the area at A with perpendicular irradiance. The irradiance is therefore reduced by a factor of $\cos\alpha$ in comparison to perpendicular incidence. The total irradiance on C at angle α is given by

$$E_e = \frac{I_e \cos^2\alpha}{R^2} \cos\alpha = \frac{I_e \cos^3\alpha}{R^2}. \tag{1.12}$$

Thus on a flat surface irradiance from a point source decreases with the $\cos^3$ of the angle from the normal.

The definition of irradiance and the operation of the inverse square law are valid only for a point source of light. Few physical light sources approximate a point source. Examples of natural point sources are stars as seen from earth. For practical purposes of measurement, the inverse square law will operate with error less than 1 percent provided the maximal dimension of the source is one-tenth the distance at which irradiance is measured (Teele, 1965).

Radiance

The majority of light sources do have finite dimensions and are called extended sources. Radiance, L_e, is used to describe the radiant flux per unit of solid angle of an extended source measured in a given direction per unit area of the source when projected

(a)

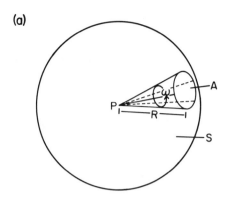

(b)

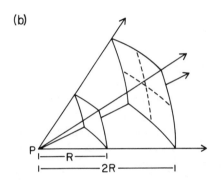

Fig. 1.11. Definition of solid angle ω and the inverse square law. (a) Point P lies at the center of sphere S with radius R. A set of lines of radius R emanating from P defines an area A on the surface of S. The steradian measure of solid angle ω is the ratio $\omega = A/R^2$. (b) The radiant flux emitted by point source P irradiates a larger area as the distance R from the source increases. The irradiance varies inversely with the square of the distance R. Thus at distance $2R$ the irradiance is $1/4$ that at distance R.

in that direction. Radiance refers to the areal density of radiant intensity either leaving or arriving at the surface of a source or object. In the measurement of radiance (Fig. 1.12b) of an extended source in a direction normal to the surface, L_e is given by I_e/A, where A is the area of an infinitesimal surface element of the source. With measurement at angle θ to the normal, only the projected surface A' of A is sampled. The projected area A' is given by $A \cos\theta$. Radiance is expressed as

$$L_e = \frac{I_e}{A \, \cos\theta} = \frac{P_e}{\omega A \, \cos\theta} \tag{1.13}$$

in watts per steradian per square meter, where A is the area of the surface of the source and θ is the angle between the normal from the surface and the direction of measurement.

Many extended sources have emission characteristics which follow or approximate Lambert's law,

$$I_\theta = I_0 \, \cos\theta, \tag{1.14}$$

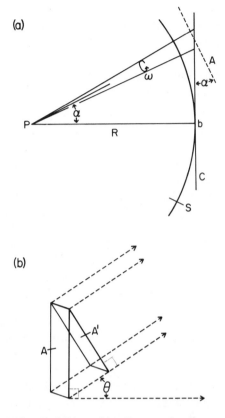

Fig. 1.12. Definition of irradiance and radiance at an angle. (a) The irradiated surface C is a flat screen tangent to sphere S only at point b. As α, the angle from the normal to C, increases, the distance from source P to the surface of C increases by the factor $1/\cos\alpha$. In addition, since the irradiating beam striking C deviates from the perpendicular by angle α, the radiant flux contained in a narrow solid angle ω incident perpendicularly on surface A will cover a larger area on surface C (by a factor of $1/\cos\alpha$). (b) The horizontal dashed line shows the perpendicular measurement of the radiance of surface element A of an extended source. If the direction of measurement varies from the perpendicular by angle θ, only the projected area A' is sampled, and the area of A' is less than that of A by a factor of $\cos\theta$.

in which the radiant intensity in watts per steradian decreases as the angle θ from the normal to the surface of the source increases. Thus L_e decreases by the factor $\cos\theta$, but since measurements of radiance are made in a plane normal to the direction of radiation and since the area of the projected surface of the source, A', also decreases exactly with $\cos\theta$ (Fig. 1.12b), the measured radiance of a Lambertian emitter remains constant. Further, radiance is independent of the distance of measurement. Surfaces appear equally radiant no matter from which angle or distance they are viewed.

For a perfect Lambertian emitter it is possible to derive the radiant flux per unit area by calculating the total power radiated into a hemisphere by a Lambertian emitter. It is found that for a perfect Lambertian emitter of surface area A and radiant intensity I watts per steradian, the total power radiated into the hemisphere is πIA watts. Thus radiation per unit area of source into the hemisphere is πI W/m^2.

Practical Aspects of Radiometric or Spectroradiometric Calibration

Absolute radiometric measurements are rarely performed in the color vision laboratory, nor for that matter are they usually required. Relative energy measurement and/or photometric calibration (Chapter 2) is usually adequate. A major experimental endeavor in a color vision laboratory requiring precise absolute spectral radiometric calibration has been the measurement of the Stiles two-color threshold (Chapter 6). Absolute radiometric calibration has been used for other purposes, including colorimetry and modern color perimetry. The calculation of absolute energy is also required in procedures investigating photic damage to the retina.

Measurement of absolute spectral radiant energy may be made with a thermal detector, such as a thermocouple. It is important to match the acceptance angle of the detector to the aperture of the optical system at the point of measurement to ensure sufficient sensitivity of the detector. This may be especially important for measurements at short wavelengths.

Measurements of relative spectral radiant output of narrow-band radiations obtained by use of monochromators or filters are a common requirement of the color vision laboratory. This type of measurement is quite easily accomplished today using a calibrated photodiode available from many commercial laboratories. The photodiode gives a summated response to the full wavelength band transmitted by the monochromator or filter. The actual sensitivity of the photodiode may extend well into the infrared. Therefore when calibrating colored glass or interference filters (above) it is important to use blocking filters. Spectroradiometry of continuous sources is a much rarer requirement, since these sources are usually specified by means of color temperature. Such measurement does require a spectroradiometer. Spectrophotometric measurements of filters are sometimes available (for a fee) from the manufacturer.

CONTROL OF THE LEVEL OF RADIANCE OR IRRADIANCE

In many experimental procedures, it is necessary to control or vary the total radiance of a chromatic or achromatic source. Methods include varying the power applied to an incandescent source or LED, neutral-density and polarizing filters, and variable apertures (sector discs, slits, or diaphragms). Irradiance of a surface may be controlled by varying the distance of a lamp from the viewed surface.

Variation of Voltage

The spectral energy output of an incandescent source increases with increase in applied voltage; however, the color temperature (and color appearance) also vary. A tungsten source with a bandpass filter will change color as the voltage is changed. For these reasons, although voltage variation was used to control radiant energy levels in the 19th century, it is rarely used today. However, when dealing with the narrow-band output of interference filters or monochromators, it is an appropriate technique. Current variation may be used to control the energy output of a light-emitting diode (LED).

Neutral Filters

In visual research using optical systems, manipulation of light level is often accomplished by means of neutral-density filters. These filters, which appear visually gray, have approximately uniform transmittance for all visible wavelengths. They may be obtained in sets with optical densities ranging up to four log units (0.0001 transmittance). Theoretically, the optical densities of multiple neutral filters, separated by air, are additive; in practice, deviations may arise caused by multiple reflections off the various surfaces. Neutral-density wedges offer continuous variation of light level. Optical systems using neutral-density wedges should be designed so that a gradient does not appear across the viewing field.

Neutral-density filters that derive their properties by absorption are made by sandwiching dyed gelatin or carbon particles in glass or by batch-dyeing glass. Such filters often show significant deviation from uniform absorption across the spectrum, and at high densities the transmitted light appears tinged with color. As indicated in Eq. (1.3), absorption is dependent on path length through the absorbing medium. Deviations from light paths orthogonal to the surface of the filter result in longer path lengths. For example, light incident at an angle of 45° results in an increase in optical density of 1.4 (ignoring differential reflection at the surfaces). Modern alternatives to the dyed filters are neutral-density filters made by vacuum deposition of tiny metal particles. These filters are quite neutral—deviations average less than 5 percent in the visible spectrum. The optical density is determined by the thickness of the deposition. High-density filters are highly reflective, reflecting most of the light they do not transmit. When they are used in optical systems, this reflectance characteristic must be remembered to avoid allowing reflected light back into the optical system. The filters may be placed at a slight angle to the optical axis so that the reflected light passes out of the system.

Inverse Square Law

When colored papers are viewed under an illuminant, a convenient way of varying the irradiance is by varying the distance between source and object. No other sources of light should be present. This technique uses the inverse square law (see above). For a source of fixed radiant intensity I_e, the irradiance E_e decreases as the distance from the source to object increases [Eq. (1.11)].

Bibliographic Note

The majority of the material in this chapter is available in greater detail in works by Wyszecki and Stiles (1967, sec. 1) or Judd and Wyszecki (1975). The former contains many useful tabulations of physical data that are necessary to the visual scientist. Kingslake (1965) lists data on light sources and filters. Boynton (1966) has described instrumentation used for visual research.

Joel Pokorny, Ph.D.
Vivianne C. Smith, Ph.D.
Guy Verriest, M.D.

2
Specification of Light and Color

Chromatic and achromatic stimuli are defined not only by their physical characteristics but also by their visual effects. The measurement of light is called photometry. There are two approaches to specification of color. Colors may be specified by a color-ordering system; in this chapter we consider two systems that order or classify colors according to their visual appearances. Alternatively, colors may be specified by considering conditions under which colored surfaces are visually identical. This is the discipline of colorimetry. As with Chapter 1, much of this material may seem rather technical for the reader interested in an introduction to color vision defects; however, the concepts of photometry and colorimetry are constantly used in the research literature and are necessary for specification of visual stimuli.

SPECIFICATION OF LIGHT

Photometry is the measurement of light. When electrical power is supplied to a lamp, radiant flux P_e(watts) is emitted, but only a fraction lies within the wavelength interval (380–780 nm) that evokes the visual sensation in the normal eye. Luminous flux is defined as the radiant flux weighted by the spectral luminous efficiency function of the eye.

Measurement of the Spectral Luminous Efficiency Function

The human eye is not equally sensitive to all wavelengths of light. The spectral sensitivity function describes the relative sensitivity of the eye to different wavelengths.

The spectral sensitivity function varies with the retinal area stimulated as well as with the psychophysical technique. Basic aspects of the anatomy of the retina are described in many texts. The existence of two receptor classes, rods and cones, is well recognized. Rods, numbering about 120 million per eye, are distributed throughout the periphery and parafovea of the retina but are absent at the fovea. Cones, numbering about 6–7 million, are distributed throughout the retina, with the greatest density at the fovea.

In terms of visual sensitivity, we distinguish two functional systems, one active under daylight conditions, mediated by cones, and one active under dim light conditions, mediated by rods. Vision is said to be photopic if the eye is adapted to daylight levels of light and scotopic if it is adapted to nocturnal conditions. Photopic vision usually refers to central vision and occurs at luminance levels above 3 cd m^{-2} (see the technical report of the CIE, TC 1.4, 1977). The photometric quantity cd m^{-2} is defined below. At intermediate levels of light adaptation (twilight conditions), where both rods and cones play a role in vision, the adaptation state is called mesopic. Mesopic vision occurs at luminance levels of 0.001–3.0 cd m^{-2}. Dark-adapted, scotopic vision for all but the long wavelengths will involve only rods. Scotopic vision occurs at luminance levels below 0.001 cd m^{-2}, typically with extrafoveal fixation. Photopic and mesopic vision give rise simultaneously to brightness sensations and to color sensations, whereas scotopic vision gives rise only to brightness sensations. The relative spectral luminous efficiency functions for the cones and rods differ. Thus a system of photometry may be defined for photopic vision, applicable to central fixation and high light levels, as well as for scotopic vision, applicable to low light conditions and eccentric fixation.

There are many psychophysical techniques to derive a spectral sensitivity function. For example, the absolute threshold is the least energy at which the presence of a monochromatic test light is detectable on a criterion percentage of trials. The energy required to elicit a response at the cone-mediated foveal visual threshold is greatest in the shortwave and longwave ends of the spectrum and is at a minimum at about 550 nm (Hsia & Graham, 1952). In contrast, in the parafovea and periphery, absolute thresholds are rod mediated; energy is at a minimum at about 507 nm. Other psychophysical techniques include constant-criterion techniques (e.g., equal visual acuity) and matching techniques (e.g., brightness matching).

The scotopic spectral sensitivity function does not vary with the psychophysical technique of measurement. The absolute threshold response gives an adequate definition of the scotopic spectral luminous efficiency function. In photopic vision, the relative spectral sensitivity function varies according to the psychophysical technique. The techniques that proved important in development of photometry for photopic levels are heterochromatic matching techniques, in which spectral lights are matched to a reference light presented at a fixed radiance well above the visual threshold. The methods include heterochromatic side-by-side brightness matching, heterochromatic flicker photometry, and minimally distinct border. The obtained functions are called spectral efficiency functions (luminosity functions). In these methods, a comparison stimulus is present and the data are often expressed relative to the peak sensitivity of the observer.

BRIGHTNESS MATCHING

In brightness matching, two test lights are presented side by side—one is of fixed wavelength, or white light, and the other is of variable wavelength. The observer matches the two test lights in brightness, disregarding hue differences. If the two fields are identical in hue—homochromatic matching—the match is made with high precision. If the two fields are of different hue—heterochromatic matching—observers may have difficulty abstracting the concept of brightness, and matches consequently show less precision.

A variation of heterochromatic side-by-side matching is the cascade (or step-by-step) technique. The experimenter starts with a standard wavelength (e.g., 550 nm) and a variable wavelength, (e.g., 560 nm)—a heterochromatic match with small hue difference. The observer matches the variable wavelength in luminance to the standard wavelength and the value is noted. Then the experimenter sets the standard wavelength equal to the variable wavelength (both are now at 560 nm), and the observer makes a homochromatic brightness match between the spectrally identical fields. The variable wavelength is then set at 570 nm (further toward the yellow) and the observer is then ready to make a new heterochromatic match. Thus in this technique the standard wavelength is constantly changed so that the hue difference between standard and variable wavelength is never very great. Any small errors in matching, however, are successively compounded. In both side-by-side and cascade matching techniques, the spectral sensitivity function is plotted as the relative reciprocal energy at the brightness match for each wavelength. An example of brightness matching functions obtained with the two techniques by Wagner and Boynton (1972) is shown in Fig. 2.1.

HETEROCHROMATIC FLICKER PHOTOMETRY (HFP)

The second and most common method of obtaining spectral luminosity functions is the method of heterochromatic flicker photometry (HFP). In this method, the white light or standard light is set at a standard level above absolute threshold. A test wavelength is alternated with the standard at a relatively slow rate (10–18 Hz). Under these conditions, no color alternation is perceived. When the luminance difference between the test and the standard is great, there is a sensation of brightness flicker, which becomes less apparent as the luminance of the test wavelength approaches that of the standard. When the test is equal in luminance to the standard, the sensation of flicker is at a minimum and may be

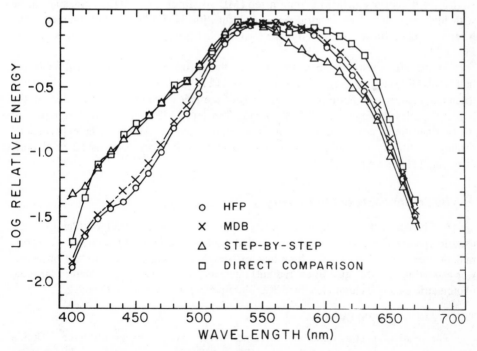

Fig. 2.1. Mean foveal spectral sensitivities for normal observers. [From Wagner and Boynton: *Journal of the Optical Society of America*, 1972, 65, 1508; plotted from tabulations supplied by the authors.]

eliminated by an increase in the alternation rate. At slightly higher rates of alternation, the appearance of flicker is eliminated not only at the luminance match but also in a narrow range of luminances close to the match, and the flicker sensation occurs only when a large luminance mismatch exists. Thus the observer's task consists of adjusting the test wavelength luminance in order to eliminate or minimize the sensation of flicker. The alternation rate at which flicker is eliminated varies with the spectral composition of the standard and test lights. For lights of similar appearance, the flicker rate will be lower than for more dissimilar lights. A good technique involves adjustment of the flicker rate for each standard-comparison pair until some narrow defined range, absent of flicker, is obtained. By convention, the reciprocal of the relative energy values obtained at a number of wavelengths define the spectral sensitivity function. The Wagner and Boynton (1972) HFP data are shown in Fig. 2.1.

THE MINIMALLY DISTINCT BORDER (MDB)

The minimally distinct border (MDB) is a relatively recent technique for measurement of spectral sensitivity developed by Boynton and his co-workers (reviewed by Boynton, 1973). The subject views a bipartite field whose borders are precisely juxtaposed. If the half-fields are homochromatic, containing identical spectral radiations, the distinctness of the border will depend only on the radiance difference between the fields. If the two half-fields are of different colors, containing dissimilar spectral radiation, the border cannot be made to disappear; however, it can be minimized. The task in the minimally distinct border experiment is to set the radiance of the variable half-field so that the border distinctness is minimized (MDB setting). The MDB settings are made with high precision. The spectral sensitivity function is similar to that obtained using heterochromatic flicker photometry; the Wagner and Boynton (1972) data are shown in Fig. 2.1.

At the MDB setting, the distinctness of the border varies with the colors in the half-fields (Kaiser, Herzberg, & Boynton, 1971). The greater the difference in computed tritanopic colorimetric purity (see Chapter 7) of the pair of colors, the more distinct the border (Tansley & Boynton, 1976; Valberg & Tansley, 1977). Further, the brightness of the two half-fields at the MDB setting is generally unequal. Although the experimental display is virtually identical to brightness matching, the observer is asked to abstract different qualities from the field.

Basic Concepts of Photometry

In Chapter 1, the units used to specify radiant energy were described. Parallel units used to specify the mount of light are called photometric units. Photometric energy is radiant energy modified by the luminous efficiency function of the standard observer. Corresponding to the quantities radiant intensity, irradiance, and radiance are the photometric quantities luminous intensity, illuminance, and luminance (Table 2.1.).

THE STANDARD OBSERVER

The relative spectral luminous efficiency curve varies between observers. Thus a match of luminous intensity made using HFP or MDB by one observer might not agree with the match made by another, although both viewed a standard source of equivalent radiance. The concept of the standard observer was devised by the Commission

Table 2.1
Radiometric and Photometric Terms Compared

Term	Radiometric Symbol	Unit	Term	Photometric Symbol	Unit
Radiant flux	P_e	W	Luminous flux	F_v	lumen (lm)
Radiant intensity	I_e	$W\ sr^{-1}$	Luminous intensity	I_v	candela (cd, $lm\ sr^{-1}$)
Irradiance	E_e	$W\ m^{-2}$	Illuminance	E_v	lux ($lm\ m^{-2}$)
Radiance	L_e	$W\ m^{-2}\ sr^{-1}$	Luminance	L_v	candela ($cd\ m^{-2}$, $lm\ m^{-2}\ sr^{-1}$); candela per square meter ($cd\ m^{-2}$; also called nit or meter candle

Internationale de L'Eclairage (CIE) in order to standardize a photopic spectral sensitivity function for use in photometry. Figure 2.2 shows the function accepted by the CIE in 1924, called the CIE relative photopic luminous efficiency function, $V(\lambda)$; this function represents average data from seven laboratories with a total of more than 300 observers. Some of the data are based on the cascade technique of side-by-side heterochromatic brightness matching and some on the flicker technique of heterochromatic photometry. More recent work suggests that the luminosities in the blue were underestimated. In 1951, Judd proposed a revision of the luminosity curve. The Judd (1951) revision has been used by color theorists, but the 1924 CIE $V(\lambda)$ function remains the standard function defined for purposes of photometry. In 1951, the CIE adopted a standard relative spectral luminous efficiency function for scotopic photometry. The 1951 CIE scotopic spectral efficiency function for young eyes, $V'(\lambda)$, is based on brightness matching and absolute threshold data. Both $V(\lambda)$ and $V'(\lambda)$ have been assigned a value of unity at their maxima.

ABNEY'S LAW

Radiant energy is measured as the increase in temperature of a blackened surface as it absorbs radiation. The temperature rise caused by a complex radiation is equivalent to the summed effects of the component monochromatic radiations. In defining photometry, this principle of additivity is required and is formalized as Abney's law. Abney's law states that the total luminance contributed by a complex radiation is equal to the sum of the luminances of the component monochromatic radiations.

The development of suprathreshold techniques was important in the derivation of a standard spectral luminous efficiency function for use in photometry. Abney's law requires that the standard spectral luminous efficiency function is additive. Luminances

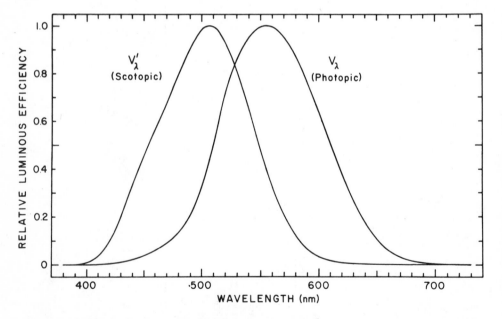

Fig. 2.2. Log relative spectral luminous efficiency for the rods and cones. The curve to the right is the 1924 CIE photopic luminosity $V(\lambda)$ function for the standard observer. The curve to the left is the 1951 CIE scotopic luminosity $V'(\lambda)$ function for young eyes. The curves are adjusted so that maximum sensitivity for each is set at unity.

estimated by heterochromatic flicker photometry and minimally distinct border are additive, at least for the usual conditions of measurement where the standard field is a specified white 2° field of approximately 100 tds retinal illuminance. A formal demonstration of additivity for lights measured by HFP was made by Sperling (1961) and for MDB by Wagner and Boynton (1972). The spectral sensitivity functions obtained by HFP and MDB techniques give very similar results (Fig. 2.1).

In comparison, brightness matching is not additive. Observers not experienced with brightness matching frequently make matches that deviate from Abney's law by more than 50 percent. The spectral sensitivity function derived from brightness matching shows reliable differences from the sensitivity functions obtained using heterochromatic flicker photometry or minimally distinct border (Fig. 2.1). Brightness matching is a commonly used photometric technique, and it is interesting to note that some experienced researchers trained themselves to abstract some quality in the bipartite field that allowed them to make matches that were consistent with Abney's law.

The aim of practical photometry using visual comparison is to produce a measurement that closely approximates the theoretical value that would be obtained by the standard observer. Estimates of equivalent luminance for chromatic stimuli should therefore be based on techniques of heterochromatic flicker photometry or minimally distinct border.

THE PHOTOMETRIC UNITS

With defined luminous efficiency functions $V(\lambda)$ and $V'(\lambda)$ for the standard observer, the luminous flux F_v (lumens) is related to the radiant flux by two equations:

$$F_v = K_m \int P_e (\lambda) V (\lambda) \, d\lambda, \qquad (2.1)$$

$$F'_v = K'_m \int P_e (\lambda) V' (\lambda) \, d\lambda, \qquad (2.2)$$

where K_m and K'_m are constants that relate (photopic, scotopic) lumens to watts. Equation (2.1) is applicable for photopic conditions of vision, Eq. (2.2) for scotopic levels of vision.

The unit of luminous intensity I_v (lumens per steradian, lm sr^{-1}) is called the candela (cd), that of illuminance E_v (lm m^{-2}), the lux, and that of luminance L_v (lm m^{-2} sr^{-1}, cd m^{-2}), the candela per meter squared (previously termed nit or meter-candle). Table 2.1 summarizes the relations between these radiometric and photometric quantities.

THE PRIMARY STANDARD FOR LIGHT

Since 1948 the primary standard for light has been defined as the luminance of a blackbody radiator at the temperature of freezing platinum (2042° K). Photometrists of the CIE and Bureau International des Poids et Mesures (BIPM) agreed that the photopic luminance of the primary standard should be 60 cd cm^{-2}. Using the Planckian formula an exact value may be calculated for K_m and is given as 680 lm W^{-1}. In a similar way, a scotopic standard for photometry was established. The scotopic luminance of a blackbody radiator at the temperature of freezing platinum is assigned the value of 60 scotopic cd cm^{-2} and K'_m assumes the value 1745 scotopic lm W^{-1}.

In a recent revision, the Consultative Committee for Photometry and Radiometry (CCPR) recommended a new standard that defines the photometric unit of the Système

Internationale to be the lumen, given by the luminous flux of a monochromatic radiation of 540.0154×10^{12} Hz (555 nm in air) whose radiant flux is 1/683 W. This new definition gives a value for K_m of 683 photopic lm W^{-1} and for K'_m of 1669 scotopic lm W^{-1}. This recommendation may be adopted within the next few years.

THE CONCEPT OF RETINAL ILLUMINANCE

Light is defined as electromagnetic radiation that we see. The photometric units are derived by weighting the radiant units by the standard luminous efficiency function. However, the amount of light arriving at the retina of a human observer is dependent not only on the luminance of the viewed object but also on characteristics of the observer, such as the diameter of the pupil.

The concept of retinal illuminance was introduced to take account of the effective illumination on the retina. The troland T (td) is the unit of retinal illuminance:

$$T = L_v A, \tag{2.3}$$

where L_v is the luminance in cd m^{-2} and A is the area of the pupil in mm^2. For example, a 100 cd m^{-2} surface viewed through a 2-mm diameter pupil would have a retinal illuminance of 314 td. Frequently, an artificial pupil is placed in front of a subject's eye to maintain a constant specifiable retinal illuminance. In some optical systems (Maxwellian view) other techniques may be used to limit the size of the entrance pupil. When the natural pupil is used, an approximate value for retinal illuminance can be made by estimating the size of the pupil for the luminance level employed.

Another factor affecting the total effective retinal illuminance, is the Stiles-Crawford effect (Chapter 6). According to the Stiles-Crawford effect, the luminous efficiency of a light beam is reduced by 50 percent when the light rays are directed through the pupillary aperture at ±2.5 mm from the optic axis. The calculation of retinal illuminance by Eq. (2.3) is thus in error for pupil sizes greater than 2 mm. Equations to calculate effective retinal illuminance, called the effective troland, for large natural or dilated pupils have been derived (deGroot & Gebhard, 1952; Le Grand, 1968).

OBSOLETE UNITS

The need for photometry developed simultaneously in a variety of disciplines and in a number of nations. Photometric quantities in England and the United States were defined using the foot as the unit of measurement for distance. In continental Europe, photometric quantities were based on both the centimeter and the meter.

A further complication was that some units of luminance (e.g., the meter-candle [nit] and stilb) were derived in terms of candelas per unit area and other units of luminance (e.g., the lambert, millilambert, footlambert, and apostilb) were defined in terms of lumens per unit area. Conversion to lumens per unit area was obtained using the concept of the perfect Lambertian emitter (Chapter 1). As we pointed out in Chapter 1, it is possible to calculate the flux per unit area of a perfect Lambertian emitter of known intensity. A perfect Lambertian emitter with a luminous intensity of I candelas will have a luminous flux of πI lumens. The lambert, millilambert, footlambert, and apostilb all contain the factor $1/\pi$ in their definitions.

Given the consideration that luminance is the areal density of luminous intensity, the unit of candelas per square meter (lumens per steradian per square meter) is the one that parallels luminous intensity of a point source measured in lumens per steradian (Teele,

1965). The rationale for the conversion to the form of lumens per square meter was to relate illuminance to luminance (Teele, 1965). A perfectly diffusing and transmitting surface having an illumination of 1 lux will have a luminance of $1/\pi$ cd m^{-2} (or 1 apostilb in the old notation). Similarly, a perfectly diffusing and transmitting surface having an illuminance of 1 footcandle will have a luminance of $1/\pi$ cd f^{-2} (or 1 footlambert in the old notation).

An array of terms for expressing luminance was developed, and photometric instruments were calibrated in these units. Despite acceptance of the SI (Système Internationale) units, many researchers still report photometric units measured in obsolete units. Table 2.2 gives some conversion factors to convert from obsolete to accepted SI units.

PRACTICAL ASPECTS OF PHOTOMETRY

In color vision research, the stimulus is usually specified in terms either of its luminance or illuminance.

Light arriving at an observer from an object (extended source) as in an optical system should be specified in units of luminance. Light impinging on an object (colored paper, etc.) should be specified in units of illuminance. There are thus two common ways of specifying the photometric quantity of light for visual research, by directly measuring the luminance (referenced to the observer) or by specifying the illuminance falling on the object, the reflectance of the object, and the viewing geometry. When dealing with materials of known reflectivity (e.g., Munsell papers, below) it is customary to specify the illuminance falling on the material. Measurements of luminance may be converted to retinal illuminance. Photometric techniques are not standardized for some stimuli of interest in color vision—for example, brief flashes.

Physical photometry may be performed using a spectroradiometer with absolute calibration (Chapter 1) and discrete approximation to Eq. (2.1). Photometric measurements are more typically accomplished using devices called photometers. A historical review of instruments and methods used in photometry was given by Walsh (1958).

One class of photometers use visual comparison. The instrument contains a comparison field, and measurement is accomplished by making a direct brightness match between the comparison and the field to be measured. For measurement of illuminance, the match is made to a test plate of known spectral reflectance. For precise measurements, the comparison light is itself calibrated against a working standard traceable to a national standards laboratory (e.g., in the U.S., the National Bureau of Standards). The comparison light contained within the photometer is usually an incandescent lamp run at specified current. Its appearance is yellowish-white but in some instruments may be modified by color filters. When two photometric fields are identical in spectral emittance and thus in visual appearance (homochromatic), a visual match may be made with accuracy better than 1 percent. As discussed above, accuracy of brightness matching deteriorates for fields of differing color appearance (heterochromatic matching).

In practical terms, a normal observer can make a reasonable photometric match by visual comparison between two "white" fields whose visual appearance is similar; however, a visual photometer should probably not be used to estimate luminance of a spectral field. A technique for evaluating the luminance of a spectral field involves first the match by HFP or MDB to a white field, followed by photometric measurement of the white field. In general, it is not appropriate for color-defective observers to use a visual

Table 2.2
Conversion Factors to Obtain SI Units

Conversion Factors for Illuminance

Unit	Geometry	Conversion Factor to Give Lux: Multiply Column Units By
Lux	1 lm m^{-2}	1
Phot	1 lm cm^{-2}	10,000
Milliphot	10^{-3} lm cm^{-2}	10
Footcandle	1 lm ft^{-2}	10.76

Conversion Factors for Luminance*

Unit	Geometry	Conversion Factor to Give cd m^{-2}: Multiply Column Units By
Candela per meter squared (nit or meter-candle)	1 cd m^{-2}	1
Lambert	$(1/\pi)$ cd cm^{-2}	3183
Millilambert	$10^{-3}(1/\pi)$ cd cm^{-2}	3.183
Stilb	1 cd cm^{-2}	10,000
Apostilb	$(1/\pi)$ cd m^{-2}	0.3183
Footlambert	$(1/\pi)$ cd ft^{-2}	3.4258

*Note: To derive the conversion factors for two luminance units: $3.4258 \times$ footlambert = 1 nit = $3.1827 \times$ millilambert; 1 millilambert = $3.426/3.183 \times$ footlambert = $1.076 \times$ footlambert.

comparison photometer to estimate luminances or illuminances, since their relative spectral luminous efficiency functions may differ significantly from that of the standard observer.

Photoelectric photometers for measurement of luminance and illuminance are also available. They offer the promise of greater accuracy but are more expensive. In a photoelectric device, current is generated when light is incident on a photosensitive surface. The spectral response of the photosensitive surface is corrected (by combinations of filters) to approximate that of the CIE standard observer. A word of caution is in order. Most photoelectric photometers have spectral response characteristics in which the integrated area across wavelength provides a close approximation to the CIE standard luminous efficiency function; however, there is often a slight shift of the entire function along the wavelength axis. This does not affect the accuracy of photometric measurement for white lights of widely varying color temperatures but can yield significant errors in the measurement of spectral radiations.

As a final remark, it can be said that rather few measurements of luminance or illuminance in the color vision literature can be considered precise (accuracy within 1 percent). Most photometric techniques available in the vision laboratory are not comparable to those of a standards laboratory. Errors of estimation may be as high as 50 percent. Fortunately, although such errors would seem terrible to a physicist working in a standards laboratory, the error is less serious with the visual system, with its dynamic range factor of 10^{12}.

A modern laboratory should have either a good visual photometer whose comparison light is traceable to a working standard or a high-quality photoelectric photometer. In either case, measurements should probably be restricted to white lights. The luminance of a chromatic stimulus can be derived using first a match to a white light (either using HFP or MDB techniques) and then measurement of the white with a photometer. The Macbeth illuminometer is a good example of a general purpose visual photometer of high quality. There are many excellent photoelectric photometers for measurements of illuminance and luminance. The exact instrument should be chosen to match the specific requirements of the laboratory (stimulus size and luminance, optical design), since these instruments are highly specialized.

SPECIFICATION OF COLOR—COLOR-ORDERING SYSTEMS

A color-ordering system represents a systematic attempt to classify color. The system consists of a set of standard colors formulated and arranged according to a set of rules. There have been many such color-ordering systems. The color-ordering systems that have been important in color vision research are color-appearance systems that depend on perceptual properties of color.

Perceptual Properties of Film or Aperture Colors

When a monochromatic radiation from a primary light source is directly presented to an observer, the observer sees a self-luminous color with no attributes of texture or surface. Such colors are called film or aperture colors and have three properties: hue, saturation, and brightness.

HUE

The electromagnetic spectrum is visible between about 380 and 780 nm. When various portions of this section of the electromagnetic spectrum are isolated, as in the rainbow, the normal observer sees an array of hues—violet, blue, green, yellow, orange, and red. An experiment in which observers assign color names to isolated spectral radiations is called color naming or hue estimation. The procedures and data of such experiments are further described in Chapter 6.

Observers can describe their color sensations arising from isolated spectral radiations by combinations of four hue names: blue, green, yellow, and red. The four percepts are often called unique colors or psychological primaries. An important property of the four unique colors is that they enjoy a natural organization of two opposing pairs, red–green and blue–yellow. Hues do not appear "reddish–green" or "yellowish–blue." The qualities of red and green are in opposition, as are the qualities of blue and yellow (i.e., they cannot co-occur perceptually). Complex hue percepts, however, (i.e., red–yellow, yellow–green, blue–green, red–blue), are all common experiences. A person with normal color vision can distinguish about 150–200 variations of hue in the spectrum. Discrimination varies with spectral region. The size of the wavelength difference at which the observer reports a hue difference is called the "wavelength discrimination step," $\Delta\lambda$. Wavelength discrimination is further described in Chapter 6.

There are also nonspectral hues. Purple (as opposed to spectral violet) cannot be produced by the presentation of a single wavelength. Purple is obtained when light from the long- and short-wavelength portions of the spectrum (red and blue) are simultaneously present. When all spectral wavelengths are simultaneously present—as in sunlight—we see a white, sometimes called an achromatic color (colorless color).

SATURATION

Colors vary in the amount of color saturation. A saturation scale is one in which colors vary in paleness or their white content. The spectral hues are called saturated colors, whereas white is called an unsaturated color. The spectral colors are not themselves seen as being equal in saturation: spectral blues and reds appear more saturated than spectral greens and yellows. An unsaturated color may be specified as a mixture of a spectral color and white. The term colorimetric purity, p, has been defined for such mixtures as the ratio $p = L\lambda/(L\lambda + Lw)$, where $L\lambda$ is the luminance of the spectral component and Lw is the luminance of the white component. Saturation discrimination usually refers to the measurement of least colorimetric purity (Δp) or the minimal amount of spectral wavelength that allows a mixture of colorimetric purity p to be distinguished from a spectral white. Colorimetric purity discrimination is further described in Chapter 6.

BRIGHTNESS

Brightness is the third perceptual correlate of color. A color appears brighter as radiant energy is increased. Discrimination of hue and saturation is optimal over a moderate range of photopic levels (above 3.0 cd m^{-2}). With reduction to mesopic levels (between 0.001 and 3.0 cd m^{-2}) there is discrimination loss for the blueness–yellowness content of colors. At low mesopic (0.001–0.01 cd m^{-2}) and scotopic (less than 0.001 cd m^{-2}) levels discrimination deteriorates further, fixation is eccentric, and both rod and cone systems may be involved in visual perception.

SURFACE OR OBJECT COLORS

Colors are commonly perceived when light is reflected from objects: that is, a blue coat is not self-luminous but is seen only when incident energy (sunlight, lamplight) is reflected from the material. Such percepts are called object or surface colors. Object colors have attributes of hue, saturation, and lightness. These properties are determined by both the nature of the incident radiation (e.g., sunlight) and the spectral reflective properties of the pigments in the object. An object color may appear of different color in sunlight than in artificial light. The physical correlates of hue, saturation, and lightness are similar to those for hue, saturation, and brightness of aperture colors. Hues arise for objects and illuminants that are more reflective in one spectral region than another. If the illuminant and the object reflect evenly in all spectral regions, the object will appear achromatic (white, gray or black).

Color Appearance Systems

The Munsell color system is an example of a color appearance system for specification of pigment color samples. The system is based on the three dimensions of color space—hue, saturtion, and lightness—and has colorimetric specification (see below). The Munsell system has seen particular application in color vision research (reviewed by Nickerson, 1976). Munsell colors have been used for a number of tests for defective color vision. A new color appearance system is the Uniform Color Scales system of the Optical Society of America (OSA), a color-ordering system in which color samples are separated by equal perceptual steps.

MUNSELL SYSTEM

Munsell devised a system of specifying object colors according to their appearance. Colors are classified with a unique notation according to hue, value, and chroma (Fig. 2.3). Hue refers to the color appearance and has a number and letter code; the letter codes for hue are R (red), Y (yellow), G (green), B (blue), P (purple), and intermediaries designated RP, PB, BG, GY, and YR. In front of the single- or double-letter code is a number varying from 0 to 10 to allow further subdivision of the hues.

Value is a compressive function of the reflectance of the sample (Judd & Wyszecki, 1975) and is thus related to its lightness. Values range from 0/ to 10/. A low-value sample has low reflectance and will be dark. A sample with high value will appear light.

Chroma refers to the extent to which the spectral reflectance of a given hue can be diluted by interspersed addition of pigments—black, white, and gray—that reflect equally at all wavelengths; it is related to the saturation of the sample. Chroma is identified by a number on a scale of /0 to /14. Chroma noted as /10 to /14 will appear to have maximal color saturation; a /0 chroma will be achromatic.

The samples are made to exacting standards with accurate control of their appearance under standard illuminant C using mixtures of chromatic with white and black pigments. The number of steps of chroma and value vary with the hue. The color gamut is the boundary enclosing all possible chroma steps at each value and depends on the dyes used to obtain the chromatic color in the colorant mixture of colorant and white and black pigments. The samples are available as the Munsell Book of Color. The samples may be arranged in charts of equal hue (the most common arrangement in the pocket edition), in charts of equal value, or in charts of equal chroma. Figure 2.4 shows an example of

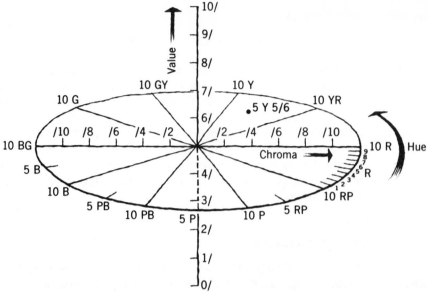

Fig. 2.3. Diagram of the Munsell color order system. Colors are arranged by hue in a hue circle, by value or lightness from top to bottom and by chroma or saturation according to distance out from the scale of grays making up the center column. [From Billmeyer and Saltzman: *Principles of color technology*. New York: John Wiley & Sons, 1966 (reproduced by permission of John Wiley & Sons, Inc.).]

arrangement for a chart of constant hue, 5R. The figure includes color names assigned by the ISCC-NBS (Kelly &Judd, 1955) to colors of Munsell's hues between 4R and 6R. A red sample of fixed medium value (5/) will range from reddish gray (5R 5/1) to strong red (5R 5/12) as chroma is increased from /1 to /12. A red sample (5R) of fixed medium chroma (/4) ranges from very dark red (5R 3/4) to light pink (5R 8/4) as value is increased from 3/ to 8/.

Samples should be viewed under northern daylight illumination in the northern hemisphere (standard illuminant C). Samples of constant chroma are intended to appear equally saturated; samples of constant value are intended to appear equally light. However, most observers will find this concept a difficult one and confuse lightness and saturation. More saturated colors (high chroma) tend to appear lighter than less saturated colors (low chroma). Similarly, dark colors (low value) tend to appear more saturated than light colors (high value).

The Munsell renotation system (sponsored by the OSA) is a modification of the original system (Nickerson, 1976). Renotation consisted of revising all three dimensions—hue, value, and chroma. Colors were given new Munsell notation on the revised dimensions and were additionally specified by their CIE x and y coordinates (see below), calculated for standard illuminant C. If Munsell colors are used in visual research, specification by and use of their CIE coordinates is appropriate only if the colors are actually viewed under standard illuminant C.

THE UNIFORM COLOR SPACE

A color system such as the Munsell system does not have the properties of perceptual color space, even though one aim of renotation was to make the colors more evenly separated in perceptual space. For example, two colors of equivalent high value but

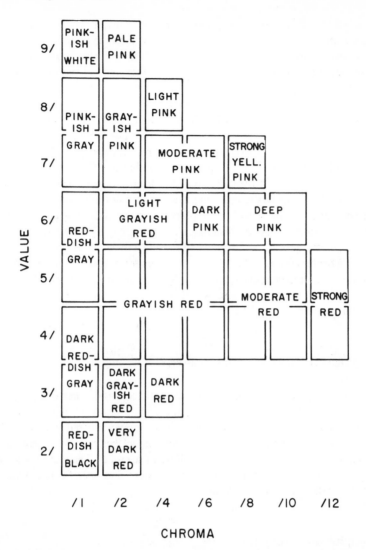

Fig. 2.4. Organization of the colors of constant Munsell hue (5R) with Munsell value on the ordinate and Munsell chroma on the abscissa. Color names from the ISCC-NBS Dictionary of Color Names (Kelly & Judd, 1955) are those assigned to colors with Munsell hues between 4R and 6R of various Munsell values and chromas.

separated by one chroma step will appear more different from each other than a corresponding pair of colors of equivalent low value. Since the late 1940s researchers again working under the aegis of the OSA have been developing a uniform perceptual color space (Nickerson, 1977). The colored papers have now been described; sets of the papers are available from the executive offices of the OSA. The properties of the color samples are described by MacAdam (1974).

The color samples are described by a notation according to lightness (L), yellowness (j), and greenness, (g). A color sample is specified by its coordinates (L, j, g), and $L, j,$ and g may have positive or negative values. A lightness L of zero is perceptually equivalent to a gray of 30 percent reflectance under CIE standard illuminant D_{65}. L values range from $+5$ to -7. The scales of j and g are hue scales, and neutral grays occur when coordinates j and g are zero. The j and g scale values range from $+10$ to -10. The yellowness scale is for yellowness for positive values and blueness for negative values. The greenness scale is for greenness for positive values and redness (actually red-purples) for negative values.

The result is a rhombohedral lattice in which each interior sample has 12 nearest neighbors (only 6 neighbors are possible in Munsell space). Even values of j and g occur for even values of L, odd values for odd values of L. The j and g planes are color planes with even L values at $j = 0$, $g = 0$ representing a reflectance scale of grays. The distance of an odd j, g plane from an even j, g plane is such that the distance between 2 neighbors in an odd (or even) plane is equivalent to the distance between the nearest neighbors where one lies in an odd and one lies in an even plane. Each color thus has 12 neighbors, 4 in its own plane (odd or even) and 4 each in the planes (even or odd) lying above or below it.

CIE specification for one set of samples was reported by MacAdam (1977). The OSA uniform color scales have not yet been used in the study of color defects; however, since their design incorporates equivalent perceptual steps for normal trichromats on both purity and hue scales, the uniform color scale samples may see use in the future. Color samples should be viewed on a neutral gray background, matching the (0, 0, 0) sample under CIE standard illuminant D$_{65}$.

SPECIFICATION OF COLOR—COLORIMETRY

There are many ways to produce the same hue sensation. For example, a "yellow" can be produced by a monochromatic radiation of 590 nm or by the additive mixture of 545 nm (appearing yellowish-green) and 670 nm (appearing red with a slight tinge of yellow). A human observer looking at a yellow object has no way of knowing from its appearance the spectral composition of the physical stimulus. The aim of colorimetry is to provide an economical system of color measurement and specification based upon the concept of equivalent-appearing stimuli.

Principles and Procedures

ADDITIVE AND SUBTRACTIVE MIXTURES

There is an important physical difference between mixing lights and mixing pigments. When two or more colored lights are superimposed, an additive mixture results. For example, suppose the outputs of two projectors, each containing a spectral filter, are superimposed; if one filter transmits principally short wavelengths (blue) and the other a wavelength band near 580 nm (yellow), the resulting mixture will contain all the wavelength components of both filters, and the hue reported by an observer would probably be white or gray. When light is directed on a mixture of pigments or through the two filters in series (Chapter 1, Fig. 1.3), a subtractive mixture results. The resultant mixture contains only the wavelengths common to both filters and would give a correlated hue probably of dark green. While most painting involves subtractive mixtures, the painters of the pointillist school of art (e.g., Seurat) achieved the effect of additive mixture by using tiny adjacent dots of color that are unresolvable at the natural viewing distance of the painting. Light reflected from the dots is integrated by the visual system to form additive mixtures.

METAMERS

Figure 2.5 shows a typical example of a color-matching experiment using additive primaries. The two halves of the bipartite field contain dissimilar spectral radiations and yet are seen as the same by the observer. The two matching half-fields are called metameric lights. There are three important properties of metamers; these properties allow treatment of color mixture as a linear system, and they date back to notions and hypotheses postulated by Grassmann (1854):

1. The additive property. When a radiation is identically added to both sides of a color mixture field, the metamerism is unchanged.
2. The scalar property. When both sides of the color mixture field are changed in radiance by the same amount, the metamerism is unchanged.
3. The associative property. Suppose spectral radiation is known to be metameric to a mixture. The associative property states that in a color match, the mixture may be substituted for the metameric spectral field; the metameric property of the fields will be unchanged. Thus if a yellow is metameric to a mixture of spectral red and green, then the spectral mixture may be interchanged in any match that contains the yellow.

From these properties it is deduced that a color match is invariant under a variety of experimental conditions that may alter the appearance of the matching fields. If an observer looks at a metameric match to white after preexposure to a moderately bright green field, both halves of the field will appear reddish in hue (see below) but will still appear identical. Likewise, if a chromatic surround is placed around the matching fields, they both will change in appearance but the metamerism still holds.

TRICHROMACY

A fundamental property of normal human color vision is that it is possible to find a metamer for any spectral hue by variation of only three primary colors. For spectral colors, the primaries and the spectral hue will be arranged pairwise in the bipartite field, so that the spectral hue and one primary match the two other primaries. The terms trichromat (i.e., a three-color mixer) and trichromacy (the property of being a three-color mixer) come from this property of normal vision. The importance of the property relates not to the appearance of hue but to the equivalence of hue in the bipartite field.

There is wide freedom in the choice of primaries. A formal requirement is that one primary cannot be metameric to a mixture of the other two. In practice, it is desirable that the primaries be spectrally separated as much as possible. Apart from these considerations, the choice of primaries is dictated largely by experimental convenience. Primaries may or may not themselves be spectral.

THE COLOR-MATCHING EXPERIMENT

The basic color matching data are those of Wright (1929, 1946) and Guild (1931). Wright's experiment and analysis will be described below. Wright used a 2° foveal bipartite field and spectral primaries at 650 nm (R), 530 nm (G), and 460 nm (B). The spectral wavelengths were scanned in 10-nm steps between 410 and 700 nm. At each step, the test and primary lights were arranged pairwise and a color match was obtained. Table 2.3 shows the arrangement of the primaries for various wavelength regions. For

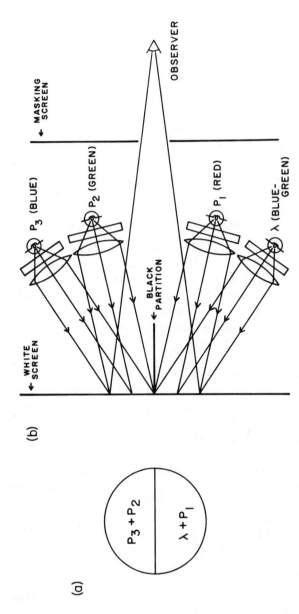

Fig. 2.5. Representation of a color mixture experiment. (a) Appearance of the field. The top half of the field is illuminated by an additive combination of blue and green primaries. The bottom half of the bipartite field is illuminated by the additive combination of light transmitted by blue–green test color and red primary. (b) Hypothetical arrangement of stimuli.

Table 2.3
Arrangement of Primaries in Wright's Color Mixture Experiment

Spectral Wavelength	Spectral Field	Mixture Field
400–450	$\lambda + P_{530}$	$P_{460} + P_{650}$
460	λ	P_{460}
470–520	$\lambda + P_{650}$	$P_{460} + P_{530}$
530	λ	P_{530}
540–640	$\lambda + P_{450}$	$P_{530} + P_{650}$
650	λ	P_{650}
650–680	$\lambda + P_{530}$	$P_{450} + P_{650}$

convenience of representation, the half-field containing the spectral radiation is shown in the left column as "test field," while the other half-field in the right column is called the "mixture field." For each spectral wavelength, the amounts of the primaries were measured at the color mixture match.

These mixtures are represented as a linear equation. Taking 490 nm as an example,

$$a_{490}\ 490 + a_R R \equiv a_G G + a_B B, \tag{2.4}$$

where $\equiv$ reads matches. This equation may be rewritten in terms only of the variable wavelength:

$$a_{490}\ 490 \equiv -a_R R + a_G G + a_B B; \tag{2.5}$$

a_R, a_G, and a_B represent the amounts of the primaries R, G, and B and are called the tristimulus values.

In a similar manner, every spectral wavelength can be specified in terms of the three primaries, with one of the three being negative or zero. The hue of all spectral lights can be matched by a mixture of two of the three primaries. Negative amounts for the third primary occur when the mixture color appears less saturated than the test wavelength alone. Addition of the third primary to the test field lowers its colorimetric purity and allows a metameric match to be made.

Representation of the Data

There are many ways to specify the unit of measurement for the primaries. For example, both radiometric units (Stiles, 1955; Stiles & Burch, 1959) and photometric units (Wright, 1946) have been used. There are two other important methods of specifying the primary unit.

NORMALIZATION TO WHITE

The units for the primaries may be normalized at the match to white. In this case, the amounts necessary for the three primaries (all together on one side of the colorimetric field) to match a specified white are taken as unit amounts of primary. This normalization may be thought of as reflecting the "coloring power" of each primary in rendering the match to white.

With this normalization the amounts of the primary units (tristimulus values) for each spectral wavelength may be plotted for an equal-energy spectrum. The tristimulus values define a set of functions called color-matching functions (or distribution coefficients). For a set of three primaries, identified as P_1, P_2, P_3, the color matching functions are identified as $\bar{p}_1(\lambda)$, $\bar{p}_2(\lambda)$, and $\bar{p}_3(\lambda)$. Figure 2.6 shows Wright's color matching functions normalized to his source S (a white of color temperature 4800 K) and plotted for the equal energy spectrum. P_1 is the red primary of 650 nm, P_2 is the green primary of 530 nm, and P_3 is the blue primary of 460 nm.

CHROMATICITY DIAGRAM

The results of color-matching experiments can be expressed on a color mixture diagram designed so that distances are proportional to the amounts of each color used (Fig. 2.7). The tristimulus values are converted into a form where the sum of the three always equals unity:

$$p_1(\lambda) = \frac{\bar{p}_1(\lambda)}{\bar{p}_1(\lambda) + \bar{p}_2(\lambda) + \bar{p}_3(\lambda)} , \qquad (2.6)$$

$$p_2(\lambda) = \frac{\bar{p}_2(\lambda)}{\bar{p}_1(\lambda) + \bar{p}_2(\lambda) + \bar{p}_3(\lambda)} , \qquad (2.7)$$

$$p_3(\lambda) = \frac{\bar{p}_3(\lambda)}{\bar{p}_1(\lambda) + \bar{p}_2(\lambda) + \bar{p}_3(\lambda)} . \qquad (2.8)$$

For the color-matching function, $\bar{p}_1(\lambda)$, $\bar{p}_2(\lambda)$, and $\bar{p}_3(\lambda)$, the coefficients p_1, p_2, and p_3 are called the chromaticity coordinates (or trichromatic coefficients). If p_1 is plotted against p_2 on cartesian axes, the values at the spectral wavelength fall on a horseshoe-shaped curve called the spectrum locus.

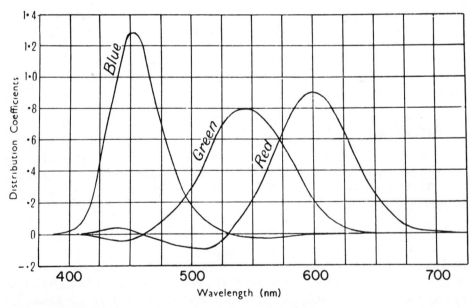

Fig. 2.6. Spectral distribution curves for the equal-energy spectrum, using primaries of 650, 530, and 460 nm normalized to Wright's source S. [From Wright, W. D. *Researches in normal and defective colour vision.* London: H. Kimpton, 1946 (reproduced by permission of H. Kimpton).]

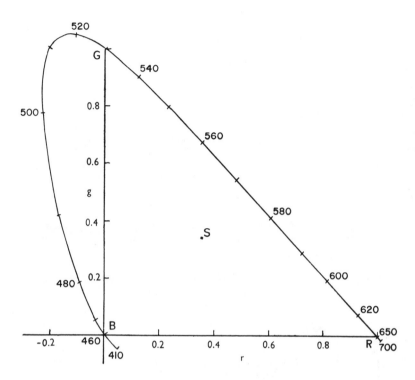

Fig. 2.7 The spectrum locus in the chromaticity diagram for primaries 650, 530, and 460 nm. [From Wright, W. D. *Researches in normal and defective colour vision*. London: H. Kimpton, 1946 (reproduced by permission of H. Kimpton).]

All colors can be specified in the space by their chromaticity coordinates. White occurs in the center. The bowing of the spectrum locus in Fig. 2.7 represents the negative values that the primaries take on in the specification of the spectral colors: $p_1(\lambda)$ is slightly negative for the spectral region ranging from blue to green, and $p_3(\lambda)$ is slightly negative for the spectral region including green, yellow, and red.

WDW NORMALIZATION

Another important method of normalization was devised by Wright and is called the WDW system. Two wavelengths, one in the yellow (Wright used 582.5 nm) and one in the blue-green (494 nm), are chosen as normalizing wavelengths. The amounts of P_2 primary and P_1 primary are set equal to each other at 582.5 nm and the amounts of P_2 primary and P_3 primary are set equal to each other at 494 nm. This normalization can be achieved either physically in the apparatus or algebraically by weighting the various P_1 primary amounts by the factor $P_{2582.5}/P_{1582.5}$ and the various P_3 primary amounts by the factor P_{2494}/P_{3494}. The trichromatic coefficients are computed. Fig. 2.8a shows the coefficients and chromaticity diagrams for Wright's ten observers. The ranges of the coefficients for the ten observers are constricted at the normalization wavelengths and at the primaries but spread out at other wavelengths. In the chromaticity diagram, the

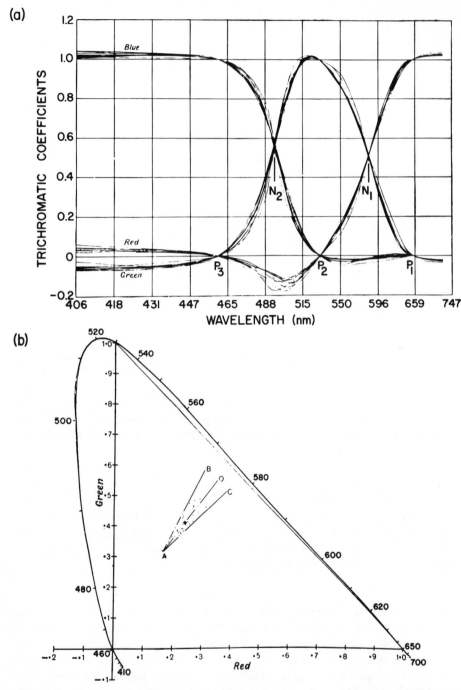

Fig. 2.8. (a) Superimposed spectral coefficient curves for ten observers. N_1 and N_2 are wavelengths 582.5 and 494 nm, respectively.   (b) Chromaticity diagram showing the spectral locus derived from the mean coefficient curves for 10 observers and the white points for 36 observers. The chromaticity diagram is plotted in terms of the matching primaries 650, 530, and 460 nm with units based on matches of 582.5 and 494 nm. The color temperature of the white stimulus was 4800 K. [From Wright, W. D. *Researches in normal and defective colour vision*. London: H. Kimpton, 1946 (reproduced by permission of H. Kimpton).]

coefficients for the 4800 K white are now spread out for the different observers. In comparison, the coefficients of Fig. 2.7 are all normalized to the white, and all occupy the same locus.

The importance of this normalization is that it separates interobserver variance caused by receptor variation from variance caused by inert pigment variation. It may be shown algebraically that in the WDW system interobserver variation greater than experimental error must be attributed to interobserver variation in the spectral absorption characteristics of the visual photoreceptors. Individual variation in the lens and macular pigment shows its effect in the distribution of the coefficients for white (Wright, 1946; Wyszecki & Stiles, 1967, pp. 419–425.) WDW normalization is important in distinguishing different causes of color matching abnormalities (see Chapters 4 and 6).

Experimental Variables

The Wright (1929) and Guild (1931) data were based on a 2° field viewed with foveal fixation. The variables of field size, retinal illuminance, and fixation are important in color-matching experiments.

EFFECT OF FIELD SIZE

Color matches depend on the field of view. A match for a 2° field will not hold for a larger or smaller field. There is a continuous change in the amounts of the primaries required for the color match as field size is changed (Pokorny & Smith, 1976.)

The 10° data.   Stiles (Stiles, 1955; Stiles & Burch, 1959) and Speranskaya (1959; 1961) measured the color-matching functions using a 10° field. Two experimental problems became evident in the measurement of 10° color-matching characteristics. First, for many fields a Maxwell spot appeared at the area of fixation. The Maxwell spot is a color inhomogeneity that appears as an ill-defined ellipse with major axis horizontal, extending 1° or 2°. The spot follows fixation and is best observed by switching rapidly from one half of the bipartite field to another. The Maxwell spot is usually, although perhaps not correctly, attributed to higher density of macular pigment in the central 1°–2° of the fovea. Speranskaya (1959; 1961) used a 10° annulus with the central part blocked. Stiles and Burch (1959) instructed their observers to ignore the Maxwell spot. A second problem is that of rod intrusion. The 10° field allowed stimulation of many rods. Since photopic color-matching functions were desired, Stiles and Burch (1959) made mathematical corrections to the data using a theoretical expectation of the nature of rod intrusion.

Small-field tritanopia.   When the color mixture field is reduced below 30′ of arc, there is a severe loss of discrimination. With stable fixation, if the field subtends 15′ or 20′ and is viewed either foveally or at 20′ or 40′ from the fovea, the normal trichromatic observer becomes dichromatic, requiring only two primaries for full spectrum color matching (Thomson & Wright, 1947). The color matches resemble those of a stationary congenital color defect—tritanopia (Chapter 7).

EFFECT OF RETINAL ILLUMINANCE

The scalar property states that metamers hold for all levels of retinal illumination; however, the range for which the small-field trichromatic metamers hold is limited to about 1–8000 td. Chromatic discrimination is optimal in a similar range of retinal illuminance.

With reduction in retinal illuminance there is discrimination loss, especially of the blueness-yellowness content of the stimuli. The effect is similar to that of small-field tritanopia; however, tritanopic color-matching characteristics have been reported only for fields of 15' and 20', not for larger fields under reduced illumination. With reduction in retinal illuminance, color matches continue to hold as long as the observer maintains foveal fixation.

When the retinal illuminance exceeds 8000 td, metamers no longer hold (Wyszecki, 1978). In the match of spectral yellow to a mixture of red and green primaries, more red is required. While the change in match is a failure of the scalar property, the matches remain trichromatic. The effect and its explanation are described further in Chapter 3.

PERIPHERAL COLOR MATCHING

Color matching may also be performed using the parafoveal or peripheral retina. With the dark-adapted eye and a scotopic illuminance, the normal observer is monochromatic, using the rod mechanism for color matching. At mesopic and photopic levels, parafoveal and peripheral color matching is trichromatic.

Color-matching data that allow the representation of peripheral color matches in terms of foveal color vision have been presented by Moreland and Cruz (1959). They presented a spectral test field of 40' × 80' to peripheral view and a 40' × 80' mixture field to the fovea. They used WDW normalization at the foveal match and presented proportions of foveal red and green primaries necessary to match various peripherally viewed stimuli. The chromaticity coefficients for peripherally viewed spectral stimuli all fall within the unit triangle for the 2° foveal data, indicating that a spectral radiation viewed in the peripheral retina is desaturated in appearance compared with its appearance at the fovea.

CIE Standard Colorimetric Observers

COLORIMETRY AND PHOTOMETRY

Provided the relative radiances of the spectral colors are known, a set of color matching functions, $\bar{p}_1(\lambda)$, $\bar{p}_2(\lambda)$, and $\bar{p}_3(\lambda)$, may be obtained directly; however, neither Wright (1929) nor Guild (1931) had such measurements. Wright (1929) therefore proposed to obtain color-matching functions by use of a luminosity function. The technique depends on the assumption that the luminance of the test field is equivalent to the sum (noting sign) of luminances of the primary amounts. Following Abney's law, at the color match the luminance of a spectral wavelength is equivalent to the sum of the luminances of the three primaries (in the amounts used for the color match). For wavelength λ,

$$S(\lambda) = S_{P_1}\bar{p}_1(\lambda) + S_{P_2}\bar{p}_2(\lambda) + S_{P_3}\bar{p}_3(\lambda), \qquad (2.9)$$

or in terms of the chromaticity coordinates $p(\lambda)$,

$$S(\lambda)/[\bar{p}_1(\lambda) + \bar{p}_2(\lambda) + \bar{p}_3(\lambda)] = S_{P_1}p_1(\lambda) + S_{P_2}p_2(\lambda) + S_{P_3}p_3(\lambda), \qquad (2.10)$$

where $S(\lambda)$ is the luminance of λ and S_{P_1}, S_{P_2}, and S_{P_3} are luminances of unit amounts of P_1, P_2, and P_3. Given a measured luminosity function $S(\lambda)$, the chromaticity coordinates

$p_1(\lambda)$, $p_2(\lambda)$, and $p_3(\lambda)$, and the luminance of unit amounts of the primaries, i.e., S_{P_1}, S_{P_2}, and S_{P_3}, the color matching functions may be calculated using the relation

$$\bar{p}_1 (\lambda) = p_1 (\lambda)[\bar{p}_1 (\lambda) + \bar{p}_2 (\lambda) + \bar{p}_3 (\lambda)] \tag{2.11}$$

$$= p_1 (\lambda) \frac{S (\lambda)}{S_{P_1}p_1 (\lambda) + S_{P_2}p_2 (\lambda) + S_{P_3}p_3 (\lambda)} . \tag{2.12}$$

This method of deriving color-matching functions incorporates the properties of photometry. The color-matching functions in Fig. 2.9 were derived in this manner. The technique was significant in the development of the colorimetric standard observer.

RGB AND XYZ SYSTEMS

Discussion of the Wright data is limited to the three chosen primaries. In fact, there are many sets of primaries that can be used. Furthermore, other chromaticity systems and diagrams can be algebraically derived from the original set of primaries using systems of linear equations.

The value of a standard observer for colorimetry was recognized as it had been for photometry, and a CIE standard observer for colorimetry was defined in 1931. The chromaticity coordinates of Wright and Guild were combined and transformed into a primary system based on primaries R, G, and B of 700, 546.1, and 435.8 nm. Normalization was to the equal-energy white. The $r(\lambda)$, $g(\lambda)$, and $b(\lambda)$ coefficients were then converted to color matching functions $\bar{r}(\lambda)$, $\bar{g}(\lambda)$, and $\bar{b}(\lambda)$ using the technique described by Wright. In this procedure the $V(\lambda)$ of the standard observer (see above) was

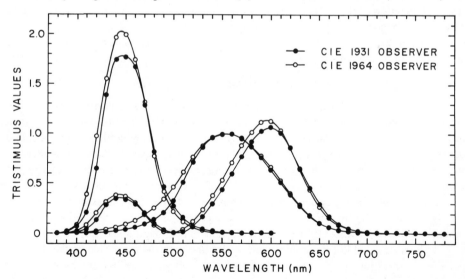

Fig. 2.9. Comparison of the color-matching functions of the CIE 1931 standard colorimetric observer with those of the CIE 1964 supplementary standard colorimetric observer. The differences are due to the different field sizes that apply to the two observers. The CIE 1931 observer data are based on color matches made in 2° fields; the CIE 1964 observer data are based on color matches made in 10° fields.

used as the luminosity function. This set of characteristics is known as the RGB system and is one of the standard observers adopted by the CIE. Color-matching functions and chromaticity coordinates were tabulated by Wyszecki and Stiles (1967).

It is possible by algebraic manipulation to devise a system in which all values of the three primaries are positive. The CIE developed an all-positive system of units by a linear transformation of the RGB system. The advantage of an all-positive system is that it allows more rapid, simpler computations. Figure 2.9 shows the color-matching functions of the system called the XYZ system, a system established to satisfy the criterion that there be no negative numbers. Normalization to the equal-energy white was maintained. A third and important new property was introduced: the transformation was defined so that the color-matching function $y(\lambda)$ for the spectrum might be equivalent to $V(\lambda)$ (the CIE photopic luminous efficiency function for the standard observer). Thus photometric quantities can be computed using $\overline{y}(\lambda)$.

The RGB and XYZ systems of units are two equivalent statements of the color-matching behavior of the 1931 CIE standard observer. The systems incorporate both colorimetric and photometric behavior. The XYZ system is more widely used and is tabulated at 1-nm intervals (Wyszecki & Stiles, 1967).

THE 10° OBSERVER

In 1964 the CIE defined a large-field standard observer based on color-matching data from the laboratories of Stiles and Burch (1959) and Speranskaya (1959; 1961). The color-matching functions are shown in Fig. 2.9.

The CIE transformed the corrected data into an all-positive system with properties similar to those of the 1931 XYZ system. The result is the 1964 large-field standard observer specified by a set of $\overline{x}_{10}(\lambda)$, $\overline{y}_{10}(\lambda)$, and $\overline{z}_{10}(\lambda)$ color-matching functions and an (x_{10}, y_{10}) chromaticity diagram. The $\overline{y}_{10}(\lambda)$ represents the relative spectral luminous efficiency function of the 10° standard observer. The color-matching functions of the CIE 1964 and chromaticity coordinates for the spectrum were tabulated at 10-nm intervals in Wyszecki and Stiles (1967). The characteristics of the large-field observer should be used for visual stimuli whose extent exceeds 4°.

PROPERTIES OF THE CHROMATICITY DIAGRAM

Figure 2.10 shows the x, y chromaticity chart for the CIE 1931 observer. In the XYZ system, the isosceles right triangle completely encloses the experimentally determined chromaticity diagram. The abscissa $(y = 0)$ has no luminance by definition and is called the *alychne* ("without light"). In the chromaticity diagram, spectral hues and whites are represented as loci on the perimeter and the center, respectively. The line connecting the coordinates for 380 and 700 nm is identified as the line of nonspectral purples.

Color mixtures of any two colors can be represented by joining the pair of colors with a straight line on the diagram. A mixture is a point on the line specified by relative amounts of the two colors. By drawing a straight line through a spectral color and the point designated as white, the intersection of the line with the other side of the diagram specifies the position of the complementary color. Many greens do not have spectral complementaries; their intersections occur at the line of mixtures of blues and reds (purples).

Assignment of hue names and saturations to loci is valid only for conditions of neutral adaptation and represents only an approximation of the hue an average normal observer might report. It is helpful in an intuitive understanding of the color space. The

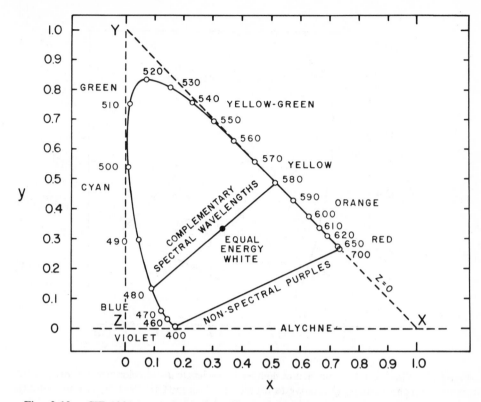

Fig. 2.10. CIE 1931 (x, y) chromaticity diagram. The three primaries, X, Y, and Z are not experimentally realizable. All computations utilizing this diagram involve positive numbers (the spectrum locus is entirely contained within the triangle XYZ).

primaries X, Y, and Z are sometimes called "imaginary primaries" and can be thought of as being more saturated than spectral colors.

A color Q whose chromaticity coordinates are known may be specified by its dominant wavelength λ_d excitation purity p_e (Fig. 2.11). The dominant wavelength of a sample of chromaticity Q for a source C is the wavelength occurring at the intersection of the spectrum locus and a line extending from C through Q. Both dominant wavelength and excitation purity may be estimated graphically. Precise computational methods for calculation of dominant wavelength are detailed by Wyszecki and Stiles (1967). If Q occurs in a region of the diagram for which the line extending from C to Q has no intersection on the spectrum locus, then the complementary wavelength may be used and should be noted by $-\lambda_d$ or λ_c. The hue of dominant wavelength λ_d or λ_c may be loosely considered as indicating the predominant hue quality of the color Q under neutral adaptation. The excitation purity is the ratio of the distance from C to Q and the distance from C to λ_d,

$$p_e = \frac{x_Q - x_c}{x_\lambda - x_c} \, . \tag{2.13}$$

In the case of a color whose dominant wavelength is $-\lambda_d$, the intersection with the purple line is used. Excitation purity is zero when C and Q coincide and unity when Q and λ_d

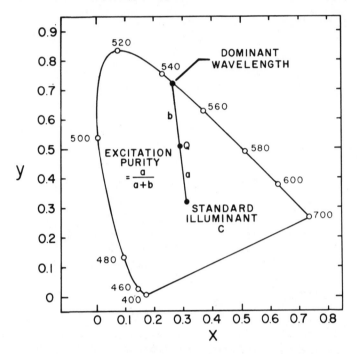

Fig. 2.11. Graphical determination of dominant wavelength d and colorimetric purity p_e of a stimulus with chromaticity Q relative to illuminant C on the CIE 1931 (x, y) chromaticity diagram.

coincide, and it gives an approximate idea of the apparent saturation of color Q on a scale from white to the dominant wavelength (or purple). Excitation purity is related to colorimetric purity by

$$p_c = \frac{y_\lambda}{y_Q}\, p_e. \tag{2.14}$$

Dominant wavelength and excitation purity are often calculated for color filters and provide a useful way of specifying color stimuli provided that the illuminant used in the calculation is identical to that used in the research application.

REPRESENTATION OF OBJECT COLORS
IN THE x, y CHROMATICITY DIAGRAM

All physically realizable colors are represented in the x, y diagram; chromaticity coordinates (x, y) may be calculated for any color surface whose reflectance $\rho(\lambda)$ is known. Suppose there is a pigment sample of spectral reflectance $\rho(\lambda)$ viewed under an illumination of spectral distribution $H(\lambda)\Delta\lambda$. The object color Q may be thought of as a continuous sum of varying amounts of spectral wavelengths. The tristimulus values of Q are given by

$$X = K \, \Sigma \, \rho\,(\lambda)\, H\,(\lambda)\, \bar{x}\,(\lambda)\, \Delta\lambda, \tag{2.15}$$

$$Y = K \, \Sigma \, \rho\,(\lambda)\, H\,(\lambda)\, \bar{y}\,(\lambda)\, \Delta\lambda, \tag{2.16}$$

$$Z = K \sum_i \rho (\lambda) H (\lambda) \bar{z} (\lambda) \Delta\lambda, \tag{2.17}$$

where K is a normalizing factor usually set at $100/\Sigma H(\lambda)y(\lambda)\Delta\lambda$. The chromaticity of Q is given by computing the proportions of x and y:

$$x = X/(X + Y + Z), \tag{2.18}$$

$$y = Y/(X + Y + Z). \tag{2.19}$$

These calculations may be made using the color-matching functions of the 1931 CIE standard observer or the 1964 CIE large-field standard observer. For a chromatic filter, the spectral transmission $\tau(\lambda)$ replaces the term $p(\lambda)$ for spectral reflectance. Figure 2.12 illustrates the necessary calculations for a Wratten gelatin filter (#78) and standard illuminant A.

With K set at $100/\sum H(\lambda)y\Delta\lambda$, Y has the value $100\sum [p(\lambda)H(\lambda)y(\lambda)\Delta\lambda]/\sum [H(\lambda)\bar{y}(\lambda)\Delta\lambda]$. If the object is a perfectly diffusing surface, with $\rho(\lambda) = 1.0$ for all wavelengths, or a perfectly transmitting object, with $\tau(\lambda) = 1.0$ for all wavelengths, Y has the value 100. Thus Y may be interpreted as the percentage luminous reflectance or percentage luminous transmittance. Calculation of the percentage luminous reflectance or transmittance is appropriate only for the 1931 CIE colorimetric standard observer (Wyszecki & Stiles, 1967), since the standard luminous efficiency function $V(\lambda)$ corresponds to the 1931 $\bar{y}(\lambda)$ function.

There are tables of products of $H(\lambda)\bar{x}(\lambda)$, $H(\lambda)\bar{y}(\lambda)$, and $H(\lambda)\bar{z}(\lambda)$ at 10-nm intervals for different illuminants (Wyszecki & Stiles, 1967) to assist computation. When the spectral reflectance or spectral transmittance is weighted by these products and summed, the technique is called the weighted ordinate method. Wyszecki and Stiles (1967) also describe a technique called the selected ordinate method that allows easier hand computation, although it may not be as accurate. Today, it is possible to link a dedicated computer to a spectrophotometer to give a rapid calculation of the spectral reflectance curve and x, y coordinates for any chosen illuminant. Some filter manufacturers give x, y coordinates for given illuminants for color filters. Use of x, y coordinates is another useful way for specifying a filter or paper, provided the identical illuminant and filter combination is used for the research application as for the calculation.

UNIFORM COLOR SPACE

The XYZ system represents the results of color matching and includes properties of the standard photometric observer. However, a fixed distance in the XYZ space does not represent a fixed perceptible color difference. During the past years, a major effort has been made by researchers in many countries working under the aegis of the CIE to develop a system that would incorporate the property of a uniform color space. In such a space, pairs of colors separated by equivalent distances would appear equally discriminable. It was recognized that such a space could not be a linear transformation of the XYZ space.

In 1964 the CIE adopted a color space called the u, v uniform color space. It was generally found unsatisfactory, and in 1976 the CIE recommended adoption of two separate uniform color spaces, the choice between them being governed by the user application. These spaces should be regarded as approximations, since color appearance and color discrimination are dependent on rather specific aspects of stimulus presentation.

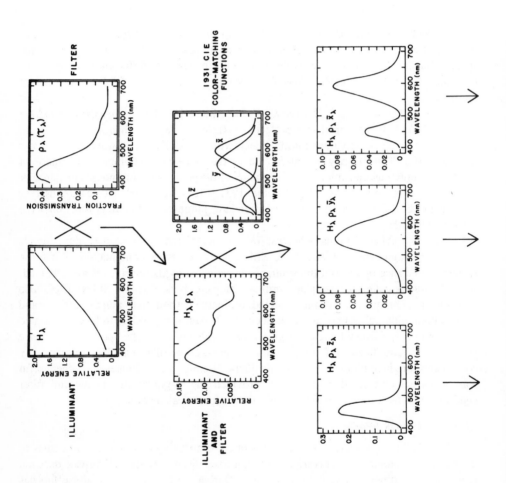

TRISTIMULUS
VALUES

$\sum H_\lambda \rho_\lambda \bar{z}_\lambda \, \Delta\lambda = Z$ 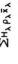 $\sum H_\lambda \rho_\lambda \bar{y}_\lambda \, \Delta\lambda = Y$ $\sum H_\lambda \rho_\lambda \bar{x}_\lambda \, \Delta\lambda = X$

CHROMATICITY COORDINATES $x = \dfrac{X}{X+Y+Z}$ $y = \dfrac{Y}{X+Y+Z}$

1931 CIE
CHROMATICITY
DIAGRAM

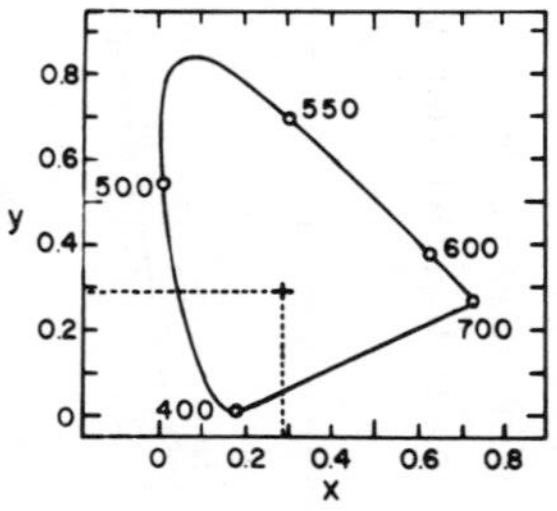

Fig. 2.12. Calculation of chromaticity coordinates (x, y) for an arbitrary sample of spectral transmittance $\tau(\lambda)$. The CIE tristimulus values X, Y, and Z of a color are obtained by multiplying together the relative energy of a CIE standard light source, the transmittance of the object, and the tristimulus values of the equal-energy spectrum colors, $\bar{x}(\lambda)$, $\bar{y}(\lambda)$, and $\bar{z}(\lambda)$. The products are summed for all the wavelenghts in the visible spectrum to give the tristimulus values as indicated in the diagram and by Eqs. (2.15)–(2.17). The chromaticity coordinates (x, y) are found using Eqs. (2.18 and (2.19).

53

One of the new uniform color spaces, the u', v' space (a revision of the 1964 u, v space), is related to the 1931 XYZ system by:

$$u' = 4x/(-2x + 12y + 3),$$

$$v' = 9y/(-2x + 12y + 3). \tag{2.20}$$

The diagram is shown in Fig. 2.13. Distances in the color space represent approximately proportional changes in perception.

PHENOMENA AFFECTING COLOR APPEARANCE

It must be emphasized that the assignment of color names to the Munsell or OSA colors, to spectral wavelengths, or to x, y coordinates in the CIE x, y diagram is valid only for a restricted set of conditions. The assignment of color names to Munsell colors (Munsell renotation) and use of the uniform color terms proposed by Kelly and Judd (1955) are valid for Munsell colors viewed under illuminant C. The OSA colors are to be viewed on a medium gray (sample 0, 0, 0, which has a uniform spectral reflectance) with

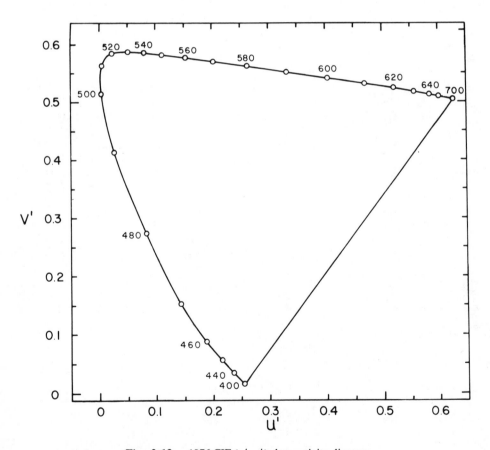

Fig. 2.13.   1976 CIE (u', v') chromaticity diagram.

luminous reflectance of 30 percent under CIE standard illuminant D_{65}. Many researchers think that assignment of color names to spectral wavelengths or to x, y coordinates of the CIE chromaticity diagram is entirely inappropriate; however, the practice is widespread and helps in intuitive understanding of color space or as an abbreviated way of describing a spectral region.

Assignment of color terms must be restricted to spectral colors, their mixtures, and surface colors viewed under conditions of neutral adaptation: either the eye is dark adapted or, if light adapted, the adaptation should be to an equal-energy white (Jameson & Hurvich, 1959). The reason for these restrictions is that color appearance is sensitive to the conditions of presentation. Color appearance of a sample viewed in a neutral equiluminant surround will change if the observer views it in a surround of differing spectral appearance or luminance. The phenomenona are called color and brightness contrast. Color appearance is also affected by interactions of saturation and brightness or saturation and lightness with hue. Two phenomena, named after the scientists who first described them, are the Bezold-Brücke and Abney effects (Le Grand, 1968), which result from interactions of hue with luminance and saturation, respectively.

Color and Brightness Contrast

Suppose a circle of 575 nm light is presented either within an equiluminant achromatic surround area or an equiluminant 650 nm surround area. The 575 nm will appear greenish when it occurs within the 650 nm surround and yellow when it occurs within the achromatic surround. A white area presented within a 575 nm surround will appear tinged with blue. These are examples of simultaneous color contrast (simultaneous color contrast refers to a change in the appearance of a field as a result of the presence of a second chromatic stimulus, for example, a surround field). Change in color appearance of a field produced by adapting with a chromatic stimulus is called "successive color contrast." The surround or adapting field is said to induce color in the test field. Color contrast is quite complicated. The relevant stimuli and their effects are reviewed in depth by Graham and Brown (1965); the theoretical basis of chromatic adaptation is discussed by Jameson and Hurvich (1972).

Colors may also be induced by luminance contrast. "Dark" colors occur when a test light is presented within a more radiant surround, which may be neutral or have the spectral characteristics of the test. Brown is an example of a dark color. Brown occurs when a 575–600 nm light is presented within a highly radiant neutral or 575–600 nm surround. The majority of dark colors are perceived as darker versions of the hue percept obtained without luminance contrast. Brown is an exception (Bartleson, 1976); few observers who have not seen the demonstration would consider brown to be dark yellow-red. In this sense, brown is a unique color but is not comparable to the spectral unique hues.

The Bezold-Brücke Effect

The Bezold-Brücke phenomenon refers to the change in hue of spectral lights with changes in radiance. Three hues called invariant hues associated with spectral wavelengths appear the same when energy is changed. They are a blue of about 478 nm, a green of about 503 nm, and a yellow of about 578 nm (Purdy, 1937). At low luminance, hues correlated with wavelengths 470–578 nm (blue-greens, greens, and yellow-greens) tend to appear greener, while hues correlated with wavelengths about 578 nm (oranges and reds) tend to appear redder than at an intermediate luminance. At a higher luminance, hues correlated with wavelengths below 500 nm (blues and blue-greens) appear bluer, and hues correlated with wavelengths above 500 nm (yellow-greens, yellows, and reds) appear yellower than at an intermediate luminance.

The Abney Effect

The Abney effect refers to the fact that when a hue associated with a spectral wavelength is desaturated by adding a small amount of equal-energy white, the apparent hue changes. There is one exception—a yellow of 570 nm appears invariant with change in saturation. With desaturation, hues correlated with wavelengths below 570 nm appear greener (blue-greens) or yellower (yellow-greens); hues asociated with wavelengths above 570 nm appear yellower. The apparent hue shift is variable for different wavelengths.

Bibliographic Note

Many textbooks contain tabulations of the photopic and scotopic relative spectral luminous efficiency functions. In addition, Wyszecki and Stiles (1967) describe a variety of useful tabulations of the CIE color-matching functions. Alternative developments of the concepts of colorimetry are given by Bouma (1971), Graham (1965), LeGrand (1968), and Wright (1946). Billmeyer and Saltzman (1966) have written a book introducing many concepts of color measurement and color technology to the nonspecialist.

Joel Pokorny, Ph.D.
Vivianne C. Smith, Ph.D.
Guy Verriest, M.D.

3
Physiological and Theoretical Bases of Normal Color Vision

Two major features characterize the observer with normal color vision: color-matching performance and chromatic discriminative ability. Since the early 19th century there has been a vigorous and continuous debate over theories to explain these features of normal color vision. It is the purpose of this chapter to provide a brief summary of some modern concepts of color theory that are relevant to studies of color defect. Although there are still many unsolved issues and debates, our intent is to provide a simple theoretical framework of normal color vision from which to view color vision deficiency.

In 1802, Thomas Young suggested that the eye required only three independent modes of excitation, with each of these being differentially sensitive in the visible spectrum and having peak sensitivities in different regions of the spectrum [Weale (1957) and Brindley (1960) summarize the earlier history of trichromatic theory]. There have been many attempts to derive or measure the relative spectral sensitivity of these fundamentals. Modern notions of trichromacy start with the fact that color-matching performance is trichromatic (as described in Chapter 2). Recent theoretical interpretations of trichromacy (e.g., Vos & Walraven, 1971; Smith & Pokorny, 1972; 1975) agree that the physiologic substrate mediating color-matching performance lies in the number and shapes of the absorption spectra of the cone visual photopigments.

Chromatic discriminative ability, as in judgments of hue differences, reflects two major and independent dimensions of perceptual color space—judgments of redness–greenness and judgments of blueness–yellowness. Such judgments are independent in two ways. A normal observer can abstract these qualities independently from a colored surface. With color-defective observers, chromatic discriminative loss occurs independently on the red–green axis or on the blue–yellow axis. Many theorists think that this organization of the hue space reflects the way in which the signals generated by the visual photopigments are processed by the nervous system. The biologic substrates of the perceptual phenomena are a set of independent neural processing channels.

Hering (English translation, 1964) in the late 19th century proposed an opponent-process theory to account for color perception. Based upon the complementary nature of blue and yellow and of red and green, Hering suggested that these four colors, together with black and white, form three pairs of unique sensory qualities. Further, since the members of each pair are never simultaneously perceived in a single hue percept, the two are considered mutually exclusive, or opponent sensory qualities. Jameson and Hurvich (1955) and Hurvich and Jameson (1955) revised Hering's notions with the publication of a modern quantitative opponent-process theory.

The majority of modern theories of the color mechanisms thus hypothesize three classes of photoreceptors with three visual photopigments exhibiting overlapping absorption spectra. The outputs of these receptors (directly or indirectly) may be either excitatory or inhibitory in their effects on higher-order neurons, thus allowing for mutually antagonistic responses. The postulated psychophysical equivalents of these neural substrates are the achromatic channel and two opponent chromatic channels (Hurvich & Jameson, 1957; Guth & Lodge, 1973).

SELECTIVE FILTERS IN THE EYE

Luminosity, color matching, chromatic discrimination, and color perception are affected by the selective transmission properties of the optic media that lie in front of the visual photopigments. The major sources of selective transmission in the human eye are absorption and dispersion in the lens and absorption by the macular pigment. The lens and macular pigments are called inert pigments because they do not participate in the generation of a visual response but act as selective filters modifying the spectral distribution of incident light.

The Lens

The lens does not transmit equally all wavelengths of light incident upon it (Fig. 3.1). The lens absorbs strongly at short wavelengths, having high optical density (about 1.2) at 400 nm. The optical density function decreases rapidly above 450 nm, and the lens transmits over 90 percent of incident light for wavelengths longer than 580 nm. Wyszecki and Stiles (1967) and van Norren and Vos (1974) have reviewed the many experimental studies of the lens transmission function. During life, physiologic changes in the lens are accompanied by increases in the optical density function of the lens (Ripps & Weale, 1976) (Fig. 3.2). The pupil narrows with age, so that the mean path length through the lens becomes longer (Weale, 1961). To a first approximation, the spectral density function of an old lens can be predicted as a linear (Said & Weale, 1959) or polynomial (Coren & Girgus, 1972) function of the spectral density function for a young lens; that is, the change in the lens absorption function represents normal maturational events occurring in the lens from youth. These calculations are only an approximation, since the possibility that pigments not present at birth can accumulate in the lens during life (e.g., Tan, 1971) is ignored.

Macular Pigment

The macular pigment is a substance that appears in the fundus as a yellowing or darkening at the posterior pole around the foveal area. Neither the extent nor the optical density of the macular pigment is precisely known, and both vary from individual to

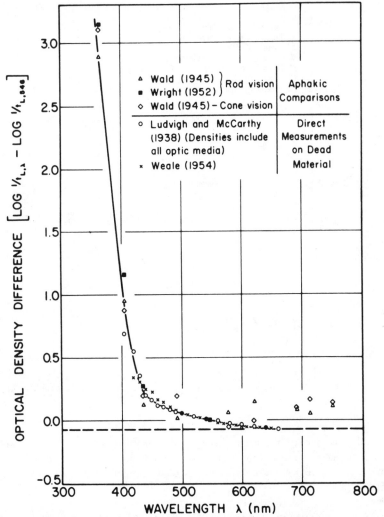

Fig. 3.1 Various determinations of the optical density of the human eye lens relative to that at 546 nm. Comparison of visual sensitivities of normals and aphakics (Wald, 1945; Wright, 1952). Direct measurements on excised material (Ludvigh & McCarthy, 1938; Weale, 1954). To each set of data a constant has been added to make the resultant density zero at λ = 546 nm. [From Wyszecki, G., & Stiles, W. S. *Color science*. New York: John Wiley & Sons, 1967 (reproduced by permission of John Wiley & Sons, Inc.).]

individual. The macular pigment appears to extend over a roughly elliptical area, with the long axis horizontal. The pigment may extend over 5°–10° on the horizontal meridian. Estimates of the optical density vary widely. A commonly accepted range is 0.35–0.5 log unit at 460 nm, the wavelength of maximal density (Wald, 1945; Stiles, 1953; Vos, 1972). 1972).

The density spectrum of the macular pigment has been measured by a variety of techniques, including psychophysical, reflection, photographic, and polarization. Vos (1972) reviewed these studies and showed that there is general agreement on the absorption spectrum (Fig. 3.3). Wald (1945) observed that the spectrum has the spectral

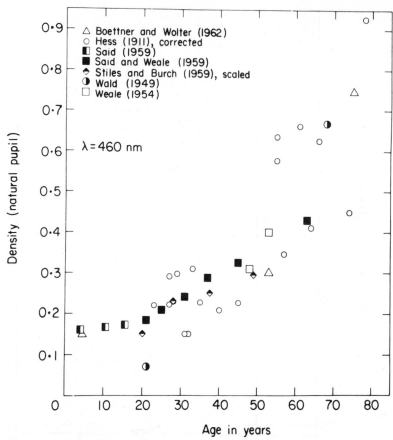

Fig. 3.2. The density of human crystalline lens measured with light of $\lambda = 460$ nm as a function of the age of the lens. [From Ripps, H., & Weale, R. A. *The visual stimulus in the eye* H. Davson (Ed.), (Vol. IIA). London: Academic Press, 1976 (reproduced by permission of Academic Press).]

characteristics of xanthophyll, a carotenoid pigment. Although there have been occasional reports of increases in macular pigment density with age, studies that separated lens effects from macular pigment effects show that macular pigment changes little (Stiles & Burch, 1959) or not at all (Ruddock, 1965b; Verriest, 1974b) with age.

VISUAL PHOTOPIGMENTS

Techniques of Measuring Visual Photopigments

The visual photopigments are situated in the outer segments of the photoreceptors. One method of studying a visual photopigment is to measure transmittance of a solution (as in Chapter 1) containing the outer segments of photoreceptor cells (Dartnall, 1957; 1972; Knowles & Dartnall, 1977); a density spectrum (also called extinction spectrum) is obtained. In this way early measurements were made of rhodopsin, the visual photopigment of the rods in many species (Knowles & Dartnall, 1977). It proved harder to

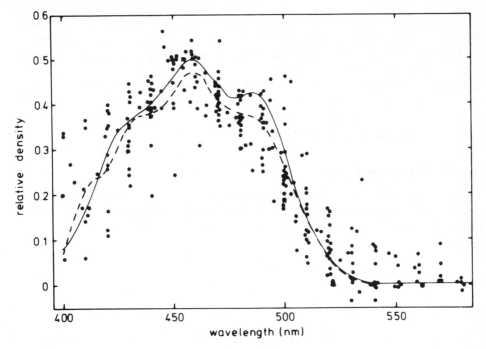

Fig. 3.3. Estimates of the average density spectrum of macular pigment based on a survey of experimental techniques. [From Vos, J. J. *Institute for Perception TNO Report* 1972-17, Soesterberg, 1972 (reproduced by permission of the Institute for Perception).]

measure a photopigment in cones, but a cone visual photopigment of the chicken retina, called iodopsin, has been isolated (Wald, 1937; Bliss, 1946; Wald, Brown, & Smith, 1955).

Modern technology allowed the development of microspectrophotometry [reviewed by Liebman (1972) and Knowles & Dartnall (1977)]. In this technique, light is transmitted through single cones or sections of retina containing cones. Using a light-sensitive photocell placed behind the cone, the experimenter compares the transmission at each wavelength of the beam passing through the cone with that of a reference beam. When a bleaching light is used, measurements may be made of the change in absorbance (pre- and postbleaching) at various wavelengths. The resulting function is called a difference spectrum. This is an extremely difficult undertaking, since the cone outer segments are small and the photopigments absorb only a small percentage of the incident light. In addition, the measuring light itself bleaches the pigment during the course of the experiment. Marks, Dobelle, and MacNichol (1964) were able to obtain recordings from ten primate cones and Brown and Wald (1964) from four human cones. The different spectra of these individual cones show a maximum change in absorbance of 0.02. The wavelengths of peak sensitivity are quite variable but appear to group in three classes, with peak sensitivities at 565, 536, and 445 nm. Both laboratories reported extreme difficulty in locating and measuring the 445 nm or short-wavelength–sensitive cones. Bowmaker, Dartnall, Lythgoe, and Mollon (1978) reported on a sample of 82 cones from the rhesus monkey and found 40 cones with a λmax of 565 ± 2.5 nm and 42 with a λmax of 536 ± 3.5 nm. They did not find a bleachable short-wavelength–sensitive cone.

Another technique of assessing visual photopigments is the in vivo technique of retinal densitometry [reviewed by Weale (1965a, b), Ripps & Weale (1970), and Rushton (1972)]. In retinal densitometry, a bright light is directed into the eye, and measurements are made of that portion of the light reflected back out of the eye. The reflected light has suffered attenuation and scatter in the ocular media, neural structures, and pigment epithelium as well as absorption by the visual photopigments. The rod photopigment and two cone photopigments can be detected in the normal human trichromat; one cone photopigment peaks near 560 nm, the other near 540 nm; a photopigment peaking in the short-wavelength region is not found with the technique.

The Absorption Spectrum

In vision, light must be absorbed to be seen. The absorbed light is that portion that was neither transmitted nor reflected. The measure of transmittance is discussed in Chapter 1. Assuming that the reflected light is negligible, the fraction of light absorbed, $F(\lambda)$, is

$$F(\lambda) = 1 - T(\lambda), \tag{3.1}$$

where $T(\lambda)$ is the transmittance. This may be expressed in terms of the absorbance $A(\lambda)$,

$$F(\lambda) = 1 - 10^{-A}(\lambda), \tag{3.1a}$$

where $A(\lambda)$ is a term describing the product of the concentration c of the pigment, the path length l of the light beam, and the decadic molar absorptivity spectrum $\epsilon(\lambda)$, a characteristic of the pigment. Absorption spectra are sometimes called fractional or partial absorption spectra.

An important property of the relative fractional absorption spectrum $F(\lambda)/F(\lambda_{max})$, given by

$$\frac{F(\lambda)}{F(\lambda_{max})} = \frac{1 - 10^{-A}(\lambda)}{1 - 10^{-A}(\lambda_{max})}, \tag{3.2}$$

is that its shape depends on the optical density $A(\lambda)$ of the pigment. The greater the optical density, the broader the shape of the spectrum. In comparison, the relative density spectrum $A(\lambda)/A(\lambda_{max})$ reduces to $\epsilon(\lambda)/\epsilon(\lambda_{max})$ and is independent of optical density (Dartnall, 1957). As optical density decreases to a minimal value, the relative absorption spectrum $F(\lambda)/F(\lambda_{max})$ will approach the relative density spectrum $A(\lambda)/A(\lambda_{max})$, as shown in Fig. 3.4. When a psychophysical experiment is designed to derive an estimate of the spectral response of a photoreceptor or to calculate the effect of a bleaching light, the psychophysical functions must be referred to fractional absorption spectra of appropriate optical density (see below).

Psychophysical Correlates

Brindley (1960; 1970) summarized evidence that in normal human color vision there are three classes of visual photopigment contained in separate cone types. There have been two basic approaches to deriving the spectral sensitivities of the three cone types. One approach is analytical and involves calculating a linear transformation of color-matching

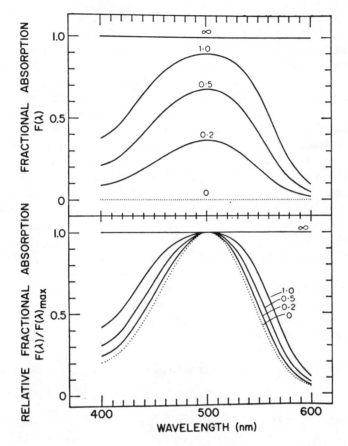

Fig. 3.4 Upper diagram shows in a schematic manner fractional absorption spectra for different concentrations of the same visual pigment. The lower diagram shows these curves plotted as a function of their maximum values. Note the broadening of these curves as the pigment concentration increases. [After Dartnall, H. J. A. *The visual pigments.* London: Methuen & Co., 1957 (reproduced by permission of Methuen & Co., Ltd.).]

data; the second is psychophysical and involves the measurement of spectral sensitivity when the eye is adapted to chromatic stimuli.

COLOR MIXTURE

Early trichromatic theory stated that a linear transform of the color mixture data should yield the spectral sensitivities of the color mechanisms *(Grundempfindungen)* or the fundamental response curves. There are infinitely many transformations of color mixture data; each requires solving sets of equations for nine unknowns. A major analytical advance was the König and Dieterici (1886, 1893) suggestion of incorporating data from certain types of color-defective observers to restrict the number of arbitrary choices (spectral sensitivity curves that are derived using data of color-defective observers are discussed in Chapter 7).

A modern interpretation states that color mixture data are linearly related to the absorption spectra of the cone visual photopigments (Smith & Pokorny, 1972). This interpretation reflects the following reasoning: A perceptual difference across an isomeric bipartite field can occur only if the quantal flux is made different between the two halves (i.e., two fields of identical spectral distribution but differing flux). For each active visual photopigment, the quantal catch is similarly different. The signals generated by the photoreceptors reflect these differences, giving rise to the perception of a brightness or lightness difference. When the quantal flux and hence the quantal catch rate is equivalent for each visual photopigment, a uniform circular field is seen. In the metameric field, the same principle holds—when the quantal catch is equivalent on both halves for each visual photopigment, the two halves will appear identical. Achieving this identity is, however, a more complicated process, since the different spectral radiations on the two halves cause different quantal catch rates in the three photopigments. An adjustment in the total quantal flux of one half-field can equalize the quantal catch only for one of the photopigments. The requirement that three primaries are needed for color matching reflects the fact that three adjustments will be necessary to balance the quantal catch rates for each of three photopigments and achieve the perception of uniform hue in the bipartite field. This requirement of simultaneous balance of each active photopigment can be expressed by means of three simultaneous equations, one for each photopigment.

Expressing the quantal catch as the absorption sensitivity S weighted by the radiance at tristimulus values a, b, c, and d for test wavelength 490 nm and primaries 650, 530, and 460 nm, respectively, we find

Photopigment 1: $aS_1 (490) + bS_1 (650) = cS_1 (530) + dS_1 (460)$,   (3.3)

Photopigment 2: $aS_2 (490) + bS_2 (650) = cS_2 (530) + dS_2 (460)$,   (3.4)

Photopigment 3: $aS_3 (490) + bS_3 (650) = cS_3 (530) + dS_3 (460)$.   (3.5)

Neither a spectrally shape-invariant change in sensitivity of one or more photopigments nor a change in radiance will change the color match, since multiplying any one of the equations by a constant factor will not alter the relative values of a, b, c, or d. Similarly, color matches do not depend on the relative cone populations; color matches depend only on the shapes of the absorption spectra.

According to this interpretation, a linear transformation of color-matching data can yield the spectral sensitivities of the cone visual photopigments. Figure 3.5 shows a set of relative sensitivities for human foveal cone visual photopigments proposed by Smith, Pokorny, and Starr (1976). These sensitivities were principally derived from color-matching data and satisfy a variety of theoretical and experimental considerations. In particular, the proposed curves can fit color-matching data of normal and color-defective observers and are consistent with recent theoretical accounts explaining the shape and λmax of visual photopigments in the animal kingdom (Honig & Ebrey, 1974; Ebrey & Honig, 1977). Following the suggestion of De Valois (1971), these absorption spectra are termed short-wavelength sensitive (SWS) for the function peaking near 435 nm, middle (or medium)-wavelength sensitive (MWS) for the function peaking near 534 nm, and long-wavelength sensitive (LWS) for the function peaking near 555 nm. The estimated relative spectral sensitivity is shown in Fig. 3.5 plotted in two different ways—as the relative quantal sensitivity as a function of wave number at the outer segment and as the relative sensitivity as a function of wavelength at the corneal surface.

Measurements of energy flux form the basis of radiometry and photometry.

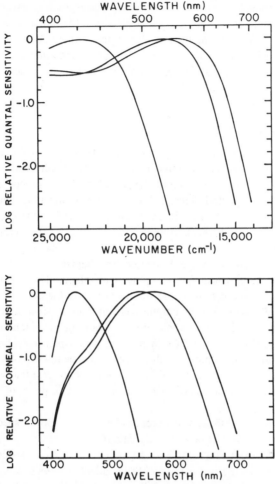

Fig. 3.5. Proposed relative spectral sensitivity of the cone visual photopigments. Upper panel shows log relative quantal sensitivity at the outer segment. Lower panel shows log relative sensitivity (radiant energy) at the cornea. All curves are normalized to their own maxima.

Consequently, visual sensitivity functions are usually referred to an equal-energy spectrum in which an equal amount of radiant energy is presented at each wavelength. In vision, however, each quantum absorbed bleaches a single unit of visual photopigment; this event may then initiate a visual response in a manner only partially understood. Provided an absorption occurs, the actual energy of the quantum, whether of short wavelength (high energy) or long wavelength (low energy), is irrelevant. It is the quantal flux rather than the energy flux that is important in the study of visual photopigment. The relation between energy flux and quantal flux was described in Chapter 1. The functions of Fig. 3.5 have other differences. In the intact eye, inert ocular pigments occur between the cornea and the outer segment. The upper panel of Fig. 3.5 shows estimates of relative quantal sensitivities at the receptors. This form of presentation is required for comparison with absorption spectra of visual photopigments (Dartnall & Goodeve, 1937; Dartnall,

1953). The lower panel of Fig. 3.5 shows the corresponding estimates of sensitivity curves for equal radiant energy at the corneal surface of the human eye, thus including the filtering properties of the lens and the macular pigment; these curves are sometimes called relative corneal sensitivities and are in the form of presentation used in the majority of psychophysical studies. The various corrections cause changes in the λ_{max}. The λ_{max} of the corneal sensitivity curves are displaced to longer wavelengths than the corresponding quantal sensitivity curves.

PARTIAL BLEACHING STUDIES

Spectral sensitivity curves of the receptors are derived in psychophysical procedures that isolate one or another cone photoreceptor class. Psychophysical methods to isolate a receptor in a normal trichromat depend on the partial bleaching procedure—the observer is adapted to an intense spectral light, following which matching equations or relative spectral sensitivity thresholds are obtained (Brindley, 1953). Alternatively, thresholds may be measured on steady backgrounds (Stiles, 1939; 1959; Wald, 1964; see also Chapter 6). If, for example, a 650 nm light is used for a bleaching or adapting field, it is hypothesized that the long-wavelength receptor mechanism is bleached or adapted more than the middle- or short-wavelength receptor mechanisms. Thus the observer's matches or thresholds after red adaptation should reflect primarily the activities of the middle- or short-wavelength receptors. The technique has limitations, since as Fig. 3.5 shows the receptor sensitivities overlap and the majority of adapting lights tend to adapt more than one class of receptor (Walraven, 1976). Wald's (1964) adaptation technique in the normal trichromat yields three overlapping functions with peaks near 442, 546, and 571 nm (these were termed "blue," "green," and "red" receptor mechanisms) that were assumed to be the corneal sensitivities associated with the absorption sepctra of three cone visual photopigments.

There are small but consistent differences between proposed spectral sensitivites of cone photopigments derived from sensitivity data of color-defective observers (or, for that matter, from color mixture data using König's assumptions, as the spectra of Fig. 3.5) and the spectral sensitivities derived using the Stiles adaptation techniques (Boynton, 1963; see Chapter 6). These discrepancies have been a source of research activity and are still unresolved (e.g., Piantanida, Bruch, Latch, & Varner, 1976; Estévez & Cavonius, 1977; Pugh & Sigel, 1978). It is not clear whether the differences represent experimental variation, methodologic or analytical artifact, or interobserver differences. In any event, we emphasize the general agreement rather than the small differences between the derivations.

Factors Affecting Color Matches—The Role of Optical Density

Color matches do depend on the effective optical density of the underlying visual photopigments. The optical density of a single photoreceptor for incident light parallel to its long axis is calculated as the peak absorptivity per unit length multiplied by the length of the outer segment. The highest optical densities are calculated for the long cylindrical photoreceptors of the foveola. Parafoveal and peripheral photoreceptors have lower optical densities. In a psychophysical experiment many cones are stimulated, and the stimulus field will be characterized by an effective optical density representing some average function of the individual photoreceptors. Differences in color matches made in a

2° or 10° field may be partly attributed to differences in the effective optical densities characterizing these fields (Pokorny, Smith, & Starr, 1976).

Foveal color matches are *not* affected by changes in radiance as long as there is no substantial bleaching of the cone visual photopigments. At very high levels of radiance (called bleaching levels) a large proportion of visual photopigment is bleached. The effective optical density is reduced, and as in Fig. 3.4 the effective absorption spectra are narrower. The color matches change; in a match of red plus green to yellow, more red is required (Brindley, 1953; 1955a; 1970). This effect, sometimes called "self-screening," was measured quantitatively by Brindley (1953; 1955a), who correctly deduced that the cause was reduction in effective optical density. The complete explanation is complicated and involves understanding of the waveguide nature of light propagation in the inner and outer segments of the photoreceptors (Starr, 1977). The effect, however, is simple: when effective optical density is reduced, the absorption spectra are narrower and red–green matches shift to red.

There is another way to reduce the effective optical density of the visual photoreceptors in the human eye: when the entering light is primarily diagonal to the long axis of the photoreceptors, effective optical density is reduced. Again, the full explanation is complicated (Starr, 1977), but the effects are simple: optical density is reduced and red–green matches shift to red. Physically, this condition occurs in the normal eye when the light in a narrow beam is directed through the edge of the maximally dilated pupillary aperture. Alternatively, the plane of the photoreceptors may tilt relative to normally incident light. This condition can occur in eye disorders [for example, in central serous choroidopathy, when serious fluid elevates the retina and tilts the cones out of their normal alignment (Smith, Pokorny, & Diddie, 1978)].

NEURAL PROCESSING—THE BASIS OF COLOR PERCEPTION

The signals generated by the three classes of cone photoreceptors are subject to a complex interaction in the retinal neural layers. The concept that retinal processing may show opponency dates from the studies of Svaetichin [reviewed by Svaetichin, Negichi, & Fatehchand (1965)]. Studies demonstrating opponency in retinal ganglion and lateral geniculate cells of macaque monkeys are reviewed by DeValois (1971), DeValois and DeValois (1975), and Rodieck (1973).

Techniques of Studying Neural Processing Channels

The electrophysiologic approach involves recording changes in nerve impulse activity of single units in the optic nerve or lateral geniculate body due to light stimulation of the eye. DeValois, Abramov, and Jacobs (1966), recording in the lateral geniculate of the macaque monkey, found that in the absence of a visual stimulus cells were spontaneously active, exhibiting a temporally random pattern of nerve impulse firing. When a spectral stimulus was flashed, there were two possible response patterns: the cell may respond with an increased or decreased firing rate to all wavelengths (spectrally nonopponent) or with increased firing rate to some wavelengths and decreased firing rate to others (spectrally opponent). Of the cells sampled, about one-third were spectrally nonopponent and the remaining two-thirds were spectrally opponent. The spectrally opponent cells were classified into four categories: the $+B-Y$ cells increase in firing rate when short-wavelength light is flashed and decrease in rate when long-wavelength light is flashed; the $+Y-B$, observed with about equal frequency, were considered mirror images of the $+B-Y$ cells, showing increased firing for yellow and decreased firing for blue. The two other types of cells $+R-G$ and $+G-R$, showed spectrally opponent behavior over a different portion of the spectrum.

Spectral response studies were expanded by Wiesel and Hubel (1966) to include spatial properties and by Gouras (1968; 1969) to include both spatial and temporal properties of macaque retinal ganglion cells. Gouras (1968; 1969) found a basic two-part distinction; he classified cells as either phasic or tonic. Some properties of phasic and tonic cells were summarized by Ingling (1978). Currently, the electrophysiology seems more complicated than the original phasic–tonic distinction (reviewed by MacLeod, 1978), but the general two-part classification seems a valid generalization. Phasic cells, whose spectral response is similar to the DeValois, Abramov, and Jacobs (1966) nonopponent cells, respond to rapid temporal stimulation but do not have good spatial resolution. Their occurrence is infrequent near the fovea and increases rapidly outside the fovea. The tonic cells have a spectral opponent response similar to that of DeValois, Abramov, and Jacobs (1966) $R-G$ opponents. These cells respond continuously to steady light and have poorer temporal resolution but good spatial resolution. These cells appear to be most numerous at the fovea, their numbers decreasing outside the fovea. This dual processing of visual information has analogues in other vertebrates [the $X-Y$ dichotomy first described by Enroth-Cugell and Robson (1966) for the cat]. In the primate, from the ganglion cell level to the visual cortex, there are parallel systems—one system (tonic system) that one might speculate is specialized for form and color vision with maximal representation at the fovea and the other (phasic system) specialized for detecting temporal changes.

Psychophysical Correlates

In 1955, Jameson and Hurvich (1955; also, Hurvich & Jameson, 1955) first published their modern version of the opponent process theory. This theory was designed to explain the "quality" coding of visual information—how the perceptual quality of color occurs. It was based on experimental studies of hue cancellation. In hue cancellation, a light, for example, a long-wavelength red, is added to a spectral blue-green; the mixture then appears as a desaturated bluish color tinged with either redness or greenness. A measure is taken of the amount of red necessary to cancel exactly the "greenness" of the blue-green light. This measure gives the strength of the greenness component of the blue-green light. The data are plotted as valences of redness–greenness and blueness–yellowness. It was noted that the experimental data could be approximately fitted by a linear transformation of CIE data previously described by Judd (1951b). Larimer, Krantz, and Cicerone (1974) have shown that the redness–greenness valence fulfills the requirements for being a linear transform of color-matching functions; the blueness–yellowness valence, however, exhibits minor nonlinearities (Larimer, Krantz, & Cicerone, 1975).

According to a recent statement of the theory (Jameson, 1972), signals generated by absorptions in the three cone visual photopigments are recorded in the nervous system to give three new and different quality coding channels, V_1, V_2, and V_3 (Fig. 3.6)—V_1, representing a summation of cone inputs, signals whiteness or brightness; V_2, representing a summing and differencing of cone inputs, signals redness for positive values and

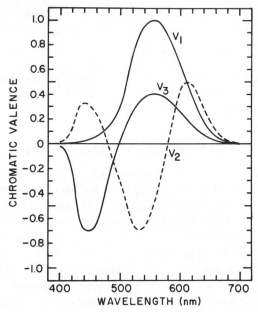

Fig. 3.6. Theoretical curves for three quality coding channels of normal 2° foveal color vision. V_1, V_2, and V_3 are linear combinations for the 1931 CIE standard observer (Judd, 1951b): $V_1 = 1.0[\bar{y}(\lambda)]$; $V_2 = 0.4[\bar{y}(\lambda) - \bar{z}(\lambda)]$; $V_3 = 1.0[\bar{x}(\lambda) - \bar{y}(\lambda)]$.

greenness for negative values; V_3, also representing a summing and differencing of cone inputs, signals blueness for negative values and yellowness for positive values. V_2 and V_3 are usually called chromatic (or color) opponent channels.

Experimental evidence for opponent chromatic channels was obtained by Guth and co-workers (Guth & Lodge, 1973, and earlier papers referenced therein). They measured the threshold of visibility of lights of many wavelengths and then evaluated the visibility of additive pairs of wavelengths. Suppose one of the wavelengths in the pair is attenuated to half of its threshold value and the radiance of the other, variable member of the pair is adjusted by the subject until the combination just reaches visibility. Whenever dissimilar wavelengths are added, more radiance is required than is predicted by additivity. For colors adjacent in the spectrum (e.g., red and yellow), the deviation is small. The greatest effect is observed for complementary pairs of colors. For red and green pairs, a green light of sufficient radiance to be just above threshold by itself is rendered invisible by the addition of a small amount of red light. As much as 20 percent more green light must be added to restore the red–green mixture to visibility.

It is possible (although speculative) to view the Hurvich and Jameson three quality coding channels, the achromatic V_1 and the two chromatic V_2 and V_3, as the psychophysical correlates of a phasic and two tonic neural channels similar to those described by Gouras (1968). This type of approach was made specific by Ingling and Drum (1973). Ingling and his co-workers further attempted to derive the sensory coding channels directly from absorption spectra of visual photopigments similar to those of Fig. 3.5 (Ingling, 1977; Ingling & Tsou, 1977). Since the intial reports of DeValois and colleagues in the 1960s, many investigators have looked at color opponent neurons in the retina and at geniculate nuclei of primates. It is becoming clear that classification of the color opponent neurons by suspected cone input is not simple, nor is there a simple correlation between psychophysical opponent color channels and the measured opponent neurons. The physiologic data have given a basis for the theoretical concept of a phasic achromatic channel and two tonic opponent color channels, but the exact relation between the psychophysical and the physiologic data has not yet been made explicit. The concepts, however, provide a framework within which to view certain aspects of defective color vision (see Chapters 4 and 6).

Interpretation of Luminosity and Sensitivity Curves

Relative spectral sensitivity curves obtained for different visual criteria have different shapes (see Chapter 2). The differences may be interpreted as reflecting differing sensitivities of and interactions between the achromatic and chromatic channels.

A recent advance in color theory has concerned the treatment of brightness. The work of Guth, Donley, and Marrocco (1969), Kaiser (1971), and Boynton and his co-workers (reviewed by Boynton, 1973) demonstrated that the differences in the shapes of the heterochromatic flicker photometry (HFP) or minimally distinct border (MDB) functions compared with the brightness-matching function were reproducible and reflected different underlying physiologic mechanisms. Guth and Lodge (1973) postulate that the HFP and MDB functions represent activity in the achromatic channel formed by a summed output of LWS and MWS cone types. The brightness-matching function represents combined activity of the achromatic and two chromatic opponent channels. Kaiser, Herzberg, and Boynton (1971), Guth and Lodge (1973), and Ingling and Tsou (1977) suggested that achromatic and chromatic channels combine with a vector law of combination. The achromatic channel that is isolated by HFP and MDB techniques is to a first approximation linear, at least under the usual conditions of measurement (comparison to a midspectral or white standard retinal illuminance of about 100 td and a $1°-2°$ viewing field). The obtained functions obey Abney's law (Wagner & Boynton, 1972), and thus HFP and MDB are techniques of choice for photometry. Nonlinearities can, however, be detected and become evident when the HFP and MDB data are collected for spectrally disparate stimuli over a wide range of radiances (de Vries, 1948a; Ingling, Tsou, Gast, Burns, Emerick & Reisenberg, 1978).

Sensitivity to chromatic stimuli presented on white background appear to be determined by the achromatic channel (King-Smith, 1975; King-Smith & Carden, 1976), by chromatic channels (Sperling & Harwerth, 1971), or by a combination of achromatic and chromatic channels (King-Smith, 1975; King-Smith & Carden, 1976). King-Smith, Kranda, and Wood (1976) showed that flicker detection of chromatic stimuli on white backgrounds followed the unimodal shape postulated to be the spectral sensitivity of the achromatic channel when a high flicker rate was used (30 Hz). In comparison, for detection of a 250-msec pulse the sensitivity function showed three maxima, which King-Smith, Kranda, and Wood (1976) ascribed to the joint activity of achromatic and chromatic opponent channels. With high-radiance white adapting fields, Sperling and Harwerth (1971) suggested that increment detection is dominated by chromatic differencing channels.

A. J. L. G. Pinckers, M.D.
Joel Pokorny, Ph.D.
Vivianne C. Smith, Ph.D.
Guy Verriest, M.D.

4

Classification of Abnormal Color Vision

CLASSIFICATION SYSTEMS FOR COLOR DEFECTS

The existence of individuals with abnormalities of color vision has been known for a long time, perhaps even by the ancient Greeks (Bell, 1926; Trevor-Roper, 1970). The first published reports of color vision abnormalities stem from the late 18th century (Huddart, 1777; Lort, 1778). Halbertsma (1949) has summarized much of the historical information. Dalton (1798) is often credited with establishing the condition by identifying his difficulties of recognizing chemicals by color. Terms such as Daltonism, color blindness, and dyschromatopsia have been used to describe abnormalities of chromatic discrimination and color-matching performance as well as anomalies or distortions of color perception. The term dyschromatopsia (meaning "seeing color amiss") is commonly used in Europe in relation to acquired color vision defects but applies equally to congenital abnormalities. Typically, persons with congenital color vision defects show no deterioration of their remaining color vision with time other than the usual effects due to aging, whereas color vision defects accompanying disease or injury to the eye, optic nerve, optic tract, or visual cortex can lead to deterioration and subsequent loss of vision. The toxic effects of drugs can also lead to a loss of color vision.

There have been several attempts to classify color defects. These include classification according to the presumed origin of the disorder, according to performance on color vision tests, and according to the presumed mechanism.

Classification by Origin

In classification by origin an attempt is made to distinguish those color vision defects characterized by a primary abnormality of color vision without evidence of organic disease from those color defects associated with other abnormalities of the visual system for which color vision once may have been normal. Color vision abnormalities that occur without other symptoms are usually called "congenital," stationary, or hereditary defects (because they are for the most part congenital, stationary, and hereditary). Color vision abnormalities that accompany another disorder are usually called "acquired" defects (i.e., acquired during the course of an eye disease). As with any classification system, this system is arbitrary and has some contradictions. For example, many eye diseases are present at birth, stationary, and hereditary, and we may ask why the concomitant color defect is termed "acquired." An alternative approach might be to call congenital defects "primary" ones and the acquired defects "secondary" ones; however, the terminology of the division of color vision defects into congenital and acquired types is now well accepted.

There are a number of differences between congenital and acquired color vision defects (Jaeger, 1956; Jaeger & Grützner, 1963; Verriest, 1964; Krill, 1972; Pinckers, 1976b), that are summarized in Table 4.1. In the congenital color vision defects the color defect is nearly always easy to classify, constant, and identical in the two eyes; there is usually no other complaint; and the observer may not even know he has a color defect. A characteristic and consistent result occurs on clinical color vision testing. The color defect does not show any gross change with age, although discrimination loss typical of normal aging occurs (Lakowski, 1974). Observers with congenital color defects make characteristic color confusions; a common confusion is of colors that to the normal trichromat appear green and tan. Such characteristic color confusions are easily evident in clinical color testing. However, observers with congenital color defects do name many object colors correctly, since in childhood they were constrained to use the normal terminology with the greatest accuracy possible. An occasional observer with congenital color vision defect even may show remarkable accuracy in correct color identification of everyday objects.

In contrast, the acquired defect is less clearcut and shows variation depending on the format of the clinical color test used. The two eyes are often affected to different degrees.

Table 4.1
Differences Between Congenital and Acquired Color Defects

Congenital	Acquired
Usually color discrimination loss in specific areas	Often no clearcut area of discrimination loss
Less marked dependence of color vision on target size and illuminance	Marked dependence of color vision on target size and illuminance
Characteristic results obtained on various clinical color vision tests	Conflicting or variable results may be obtained on various clinical color vision tests
Many object colors are named correctly or predictable errors are made	Some object colors are named incorrectly
Both eyes usually affected to same degree	Two eyes sometimes affected to different degrees
Usually no other visual complaint	Sometimes a visual complaint, e.g., reduced visual acuity or field loss
Defect does not change	Defect may show obvious progression or regression.

There is usually a concomitant complaint of blurring, reduced vision, or visual field abnormality. The defect may show an obvious progression (or regression) with time, and the observer may remember having had normal color vision. The observer with an acquired color vision defect will often name object colors incorrectly, using terminology learned when color vision was normal. In a disorder that affects primarily one eye the observer may notice a remarkable difference between the color perceptions of the two eyes. In a disorder with rapid onset observers may suddenly discover themselves in unusual disagreement with family and friends on such events as setting the hue balance of a color television or choosing clothes.

Classification by Performance

Classification by performance in given experimental procedures is empiric. Observers may be classified by their color-matching performance or by two aspects of chromatic discriminative ability, one qualitative and the other quantitative.

COLOR-MATCHING PERFORMANCE

The nomenclature is derived from the color-matching performance of the observer. An observer who needs three primaries for full-spectrum color matching is defined as a trichromat (Chapter 2). An observer who needs only two primaries for full-spectrum color matching is defined as a dichromat. An observer who needs only one primary for full-spectrum color matching is defined as a monochromat.

CHROMATIC DISCRIMINATION*

Both a qualitative and a quantitative aspect of chromatic discriminative ability may also be classified. A qualitative assessment of the axis (red–green or blue–yellow) of major chromatic discriminative loss may be made. In addition, the extent of the defect may be assessed on an ordinal scale using terms such as mild, moderate, and severe.

Classification by Mechanism

The first attempt to classify a color defect by its presumed mechanism was that of von Kries (1897).

VON KRIES MECHANISMS—ABSORPTION, ALTERATION, AND
REDUCTION SYSTEMS

von Kries (1897) showed that defective color vision can be subdivided according to features of color matches that allow prediction of the mechanism of the defect. It is possible to recognize absorption systems, alteration systems, and reduction systems.

In the absorption system, some color matches differ from those of normal color vision; however, color matches reported with WDW normalization (Chapter 2) will agree with those of normal trichromats. An absorption system is caused by an abnormal prereceptoral filter; the retinal mechanisms are normal. Most absorption systems can be mimicked in a normal eye by placing before it an appropriate color filter or even by placing this color filter before the illuminant. Examples of "absorption systems" in the normal eye are the lens and the macular pigment. Pigments in the lens and the macular pigment cause considerable variation between color matches and spectral sensitivities of normal observers.

*We use the conventional nomenclature of "blue-yellow defect" in this book, but thoroughly agree with Professor Wright's comment in the foreword (J. P. and V. S.).

In the alteration system, color matches also differ from those of normal color vision; in addition, color matches reported with WDW normalization will still differ from those of normal trichromats. An alteration system occurs when one (or more) of the visual photopigments differs from those of normal trichromats. An alteration system is primary evidence of an abnormality or change in the photopigment absorption spectra. Specialized psychophysical techniques to distinguish the absorption and alteration system are described in Chapter 6.

The reduction system is characterized by the fact that normal color matches are accepted by the color-defective observer. Of course, allowance must be made for normal variation in prereceptoral absorption and normal receptoral variations. Chromaticity discrimination is usually much worse than in the normal trichromat. A reduction system occurs either by the loss of one of the normal receptor mechanisms [called a König mechanism (Chapter 7)] or by the collapse (or fusion) of two normal receptor mechanisms [called a Leber-Fick or Aitken-Leber-Fick mechanism (Chapter 7)]. A reduction system caused by loss (König mechanism) is usually attributed to loss of function of one class of photoreceptors; a reduction system caused by fusion or collapse (Leber-Fick mechanism) is often considered postreceptoral.

OTHER MECHANISMS

The ideas developed by von Kries (1897) may also be applied to acquired color vision defects. In addition, Verriest (1964) and others introduced three interrelated concepts to describe conditions frequently found in acquired color vision defects— *mesopization, scotopization,* and *eccentration.* Verriest (1964), in using the term mesopization [introduced by Ourgaud & Etienne (1961)], specifically refers to acquired color defects that occur when the thresholds for the photopic mechanism are increased. Mesopization results in a condition such that qualitatively the effective level of retinal illuminance is reduced for the affected observer. In this condition the acquired blue–yellow defect shown by the affected observer is like color discrimination losses occurring in a normal subject in mesopic (or low light level) vision (Chapter 6).

By scotopization Verriest (1964) refers to the intrusion of rod activity in color vision when assessed using photopic observation conditions and the preferred fixation of the observer. The photopic luminous efficiency function does not describe the sensitivity of the observer. The actual function is intermediate between the photopic and scotopic functions and in extreme cases will follow the form of the scotopic function. The exact relation between normal parafoveal color vision and scotopization is unknown. The majority of disorders showing scotopization involve cone degeneration, and parafoveal cone vision is probably also abnormal. Related to the concept of scotopization is eccentric fixation (eccentration). In strabismic amblyopia, some observers with reduced visual acuity do not use foveal fixation in the amblyopic eye. They fixate photopic stimuli on the parafoveal retina, therefore showing poorer chromatic discrimination (Chapter 8).

CLASSIFICATION OF CONGENITAL COLOR VISION DEFECTS

The modern study of color vision defects began in the early 19th century. An attempt at qualitative classification involved the terms red-blind, green-blind, or blue-blind according to the hypothetically absent color sensation. An atheoretical nomenclature was introduced by von Kries (1897) using Greek words, protan (first, applied to the red-blind), deutan (second, applied to the green-blind), tritan (third, applied to the blue-blind), and tetartan (fourth). Today these terms refer to characteristic color confusions that may be displayed on the CIE chromaticity diagram (as in Chapter 7). Observers were also classified by their color-matching performance as trichromats, dichromats, or monochromats and according to the von Kries (1897) concepts of alteration and reduction systems. In addition to characteristic behavior on color matching, the majority of observers with congenital color defect have a deficit in color discrimination that allows another classification according to the major axis and severity of chromatic discrimination loss.

The congenital color defects include the red–green defects, the blue–yellow defects, and the achromatopsias. The names and classification by mechanism and performance for these defects are summarized in Table 4.2. These defects are presumed to be congenital, hereditary, stationary defects of color perception. It is difficult to establish the congenital nature of a red–green or blue–yellow color vision defect. Recent studies of infant color perception do suggest that red–green abnormalities may be identified in infants who are at risk for a red–green defect (Teller, D.Y.: Personal communication). Although inheritance patterns are established for the majority of congenital color defects, the hereditary natures of tritanomaly and achromatopsia with normal visual acuity are largely unknown. Any of the congenital defects may be affected by normal aging (Verriest, 1963) and thus may appear to show a progressive loss of chromatic discrimination (Lakowski, 1974). Progression in achromatopsia is variable; in some cases rod function is affected (Pinckers, 1972a). Classically, the achromatopsias are considered to be functional disorders within the classification of congenital color defects; however, from the ophthalmologist's point of view achromatopsia with reduced visual acuity may be better included among the cone dysfunction syndromes (Goodman, Ripps, & Siegel, 1963), a group of stationary and progressive dystrophies and degenerations of the cone photoreceptors.

The Red–Green Defects

The red–green defects are the most common defects of color vision. Visual acuity is normal, but there is a disorder in color matching and there is chromatic discrimination loss on the red–green axis. Two qualitatively different forms exist—the protan defects and the deutan defects. Each has a reduction form, protanopia and deuteranopia, in which the observers are dichromatic and for whom the discrimination loss on the red–green axis appears on clinical tests to be moderate or severe. Each has an alteration form, protanomaly and deuteranomaly, in which observers are trichromatic and for whom the chromatic discrimination loss on the red–green axis is mild or moderate. Some anomalous trichromats show no or minimal chromatic discrimination loss. The rod mechanism is normal.

The Blue–Yellow Defects

The blue–yellow defects are more rare. Again, visual acuity is normal, but there is a disorder of color vision. The autosomal dominant tritan defect is a variable form of reduction disorder that may be dichromatic (tritanopia) or trichromatic (incomplete tritanopia, sometimes inappropriately called tritanomaly). The severity of chromatic discrimination loss ranges from mild to severe. Further, an alteration form of tritan defect, tritanomaly, that is trichromatic is classically recognized. This defect is of unknown inheritance and extremely rare. The rod mechanism is normal.

Table 4.2
Classification of Congenital Color Vision Defects

Name	Classification by Performance			Classification by Mechanism (von Kries)
	Color Matching	*Discrimination Deficit*		
		Axis	Severity	
Red–green defects				
Protanopia	Dichromatic	Red–green (protan)	Moderate	Reduction
Deuteranopia	Dichromatic	Red–green (deutan)	Moderate	Reduction
Protanomaly	Trichromatic	Red–green (protan)	Mild to moderate	Alteration
Deuteranomaly	Trichromatic	Red–green (deutan)	Mild to moderate	Alteration
Blue–yellow defects				
Tritan defect (tritanopia and incomplete tritanopia)	Dichromatic, trichromatic	Blue–yellow (tritan)	Mild to moderate	Reduction
Tritanomaly	Trichromatic	Blue–yellow (tritan)	Mild	Alteration
Achromatopsias				
Complete with reduced visual acuity	Monochromatic	Red–green and blue–yellow	Severe	Alteration
Incomplete with reduced visual acuity	Dichromatic, trichromatic	Various	Severe	Alteration
Complete with normal visual acuity	Monochromatic	Red–green and blue–yellow	Severe	Reduction

Finally, the tetartan defect is a hypothetical blue–yellow defect based on some early theoretical ideas. Tetartanopia was postulated by Müller (1924) to allow for two forms of blue–yellow defect parallel to the two forms of red–green defect. The theoretical notion in its development considered protanopia as a "red" (receptoral) color defect, deuteranopia as a "red–green" (postreceptoral) color defect, and tritanopia as a receptoral "blue" color defect, and therefore tetartanopia as a "blue–yellow" (postreceptoral) color defect (Judd, 1943). To date there has been no documented case of congenital tetartanopia. Nevertheless, there are color tests designed on theoretical grounds to screen for tetartan defect.

The Achromatopsias

The achromatopsias comprise a varied group of disorders characterized by a very severe abnormality of color vision.

In complete and incomplete achromatopsia with reduced visual acuity, there are visual defects evident from infancy, and the individual is usually referred to an eye clinic. These disorders involve a severe abnormality of cone photoreceptors. Normal color matches are not accepted, and therefore the defects cannot be considered as a reduction form of normal color vision. Vision may be dominated by the rod system under all illuminations; thus these congenital defects may be viewed as examples of scotopization. In addition, there is evidence for the existence of cone photoreceptors containing a visual photopigment whose spectral absorption characteristics are similar to those of rhodopsin, the rod visual photopigment. These cone photoreceptors form the basis for a true alteration system. The rod mechanism is presumed to be normal, although Pinckers (1972a) has questioned this assumption. In complete achromatopsia with reduced visual acuity, there is no basis for chromatic perception. These observers may be considered "color-blind" in the sense that they cannot distinguish any pair of colors on the basis of a pure chromatic difference. In other types of color defects, the term color-blind is inappropriate.

There is also a form of complete achromatopsia with normal visual acuity (a very rare disorder) in which cones mediate normal visual acuity but there is no discrimination of color. As with red–green and blue–yellow defects, rods are presumed to be normal.

CLASSIFICATION OF ACQUIRED COLOR VISION DEFECTS

Acquired defects of color vision were recognized as early as the 19th century. The research on these defects developed in Germany at the beginning of the 20th century. In 1912 Köllner concluded that lesions in the outer retinal layers gave rise to blue–yellow defects while damage to the inner retinal layers and the optic nerve caused progressive but initially mainly red–green defects. Today it is known that red–green defects also occur in diseases of the outer retinal layers, such as central cone degeneration.

Classification of acquired color vision defects may be based on color-matching performance. As with the congenital defects, cases resembling trichromatism, dichromatism, and monochromatism are found; however, the distinction is not meaningful in this context and should not be confused with specific malfunction or nonfunction of one of the three cone receptor mechanisms.

Classification by absorption, alteration, and reduction mechanisms may also be applied to the acquired color vision defects. Typically a selective absorption system affecting the short-wavelength section of the spectrum occurs with aging, yellow cataracts, and jaundice. This color defect manifests itself as a loss of discrimination in the blue–yellow and as a shift of the Rayleigh match toward green. An alteration defect occurs in diseases that show the Rayleigh match shifting to red. A reduction defect occurs in diseases of the optic nerve. The Verriest mechanisms of mesopization and scotopization can also be observed. Mesopization occurs primarily in retinal disorders. Scotopization is usually evident when there is a severe loss of both chromatic discrimination and visual acuity, as in cone degenerations.

Classification of acquired color vision defects by the major axes of discrimination loss was proposed by Verriest (1963). There are three basic patterns: a nonspecific loss, a loss whose axis corresponds to the red–green axis of discrimination, and a loss whose axis corresponds to the blue–yellow axis of discrimination. The discrimination loss may range from mild to severe.

The relation of the acquired color defect to visual acuity is complex. In some diseases an acquired color vision defect is observed when visual acuity is normal or slightly affected. In retrobulbar neuritis, for example, a color vision defect is still present when visual acuity has returned to normal. On the other hand, visual acuity may have dropped to 0.2 in strabismic amblyopia (squint) without a concomitant acquired color defect. In degenerative disease, the severity of the color vision defect may parallel the decreasing visual acuity.

When the visual acuity is reduced to 0.2–0.25 there may be increased variability in making a color match with an anomaloscope or in making any psychophysical judgment that requires stable fixation of a foveal test field subtending 1° or less. If the visual acuity is reduced below 0.1, the question of where preferred fixation occurs must be raised—the patient may be using eccentric fixation. In this event the patient's preferred fixation may be documented by use of the visuscope or by fundus photography with a fixation target. A word of caution is in order here. Most methods for establishing the retinal locus for fixation use bright lights. For a patient with a relative central scotoma, fixation may be foveal at high light levels but parafoveal for dimmer fixation targets. A fundus photographic device, such as the one described by Siegel and Bruno (1964), is necessary to document foveal fixation for dim light conditions. On the other hand, if fixation is parafoveal under bright light conditions, we can assume that it will also be parafoveal for dim illumination.

Table 4.3 shows the Verriest classification, which is primarily based on the axis of major chromatic discrimination loss. Color vision findings are more variable in acquired than in congenital color vision defects, since acquired color vision defects involve variable losses in visual acuity and patients are tested at various·stages of the causal disease. The acquired color vision defects shown in Table 4.3 include types I and II acquired red–green defects and type III acquired blue–yellow defect.

Type I Acquired Red–Green Defect

In the type I acquired red–green defect the chromatic discrimination on the red–green axis progressively deteriorates, showing a moderate or severe loss accompanying a parallel defect in visual acuity. At the same time, the photopic luminosity curve also changes, and finally only a scotopic curve similar to that of a complete achromat is observed. In an advanced stage, there is total color blindness in the affected visual field, resembling congenital achromatopsia. The type I acquired defect is observed

Table 4.3
Classification of Acquired Color Vision Defects

Name	Classification by Performance			Classification by Mechanism	Usual Visual Acuity	Usual Outcome
	Color Matching	Discrimination Deficit				
		Major Axis	Severity			
Type I, acquired red–green	Trichromatic → Monochromatic	Red–green	Mild → Severe	Alteration or scotopization	Moderate to severe reduction	Achromatopsia (scotopic)
Type II, acquired red–green	Trichromatic → Monochromatic	Red–green; Concomitant blue–yellow	Mild → Severe, mild	Reduction	Moderate to severe reduction	May recover or progress to severe
Type III, acquired blue–yellow	Trichromatic → Dichromatic (monochromatic rarely)	Blue–yellow	Mild → Moderate	Reduction or absorption or alteration	Mild to severe reduction	Various

79

in retinal disease primarily involving the photoreceptors of the posterior pole. It is associated with a major loss of visual acuity and eccentric fixation. The type I defect is assumed to reflect a destruction of the macular cones and is thus primarily a reduction system accompanied by scotopization.

Type II Acquired Red–Green Defect

In the type II acquired red–green defect hue discrimination for the red–green axis deteriorates progressively, showing moderate or severe loss; there is a concomitant milder blue–yellow loss. The relative luminous efficiency function remains approximately normal. The chromatic discrimination in early stages is characterized by reduction in apparent saturation of most chromatic stimuli. In advanced stages there is a neutral zone in which colors appear gray at about 500 nm. With severe loss in visual acuity, the neutral zone widens to include the whole midspectral region. The Rayleigh match is often not only widened but may be displaced toward the green primary. In advanced stages anomaloscopic investigation indicates acceptance of all red–green mixtures but with normal relative luminous efficiency function. In extreme cases patients may have eccentric fixation, and the color vision can approach achromatopsia, showing scotopization. The type II defect is observed in optic nerve involvement—namely, optic neuritis, retrobulbar neuritis, optic atrophies—and in optic nerve intoxications, in malformations of the optic disc, and in tumors of the optic nerve or chiasm. The defect is primarily a reduction system. The report of green-shifted Rayleigh matches implies an absorption or alteration system in addition to reduction (Verriest, 1963).

Type III Acquired Blue–Yellow Defect

The type III acquired blue–yellow defect is the most frequent acquired color vision defect. The type III defect is characterized by mild or moderate loss of discrimination on the blue–yellow axis, and the visual acuity deficit is similarly mild or moderate. The early stage is characterized by confusions in the "blue" region of the chromaticity diagram. These occur for some chromaticities that to the normal trichromat appear purple, violet, blue, and blue-green; the discrimination is normal elsewhere, and there is no neutral point in the spectrum. In an advanced stage the vision is dichromatic and there is a neutral zone at about 550 nm. The spectral luminous efficiency curve may be normal or abnormal.

The type III acquired blue–yellow defect occurs in many choroidal, pigment epithelial, retinal, and neural disorders; these include nuclear cataract, most chorioretinal inflammations and degenerations, vascular disorders, senile macular degeneration, papilledema, glaucoma, autosomal dominant optic atrophy, and even prechiasmal optic nerve disorders (Ohta, 1970; Pinckers, 1975a). This blue–yellow defect therefore cannot be ascribed to a specific lesion of the visual system or to a specific mechanism. The type III defect may be the result of a selective absorption system, e.g., in brown nuclear cataract, and it also occurs as an alteration system in central serous choroidopathy with pseudoprotanomaly (Smith, Pokorny, & Diddie, 1978). As a reduction system with mesopization, the type III defect occurs in retinal vascular disease and in retinitis pigmentosa. The type III defect is also observed in glaucoma and autosomal dominant optic atrophy.

Aging gives rise to blue–yellow defect (Verriest, 1963) caused primarily by (senile) discoloration of the lens but perhaps also by age-related changes of the retina and pigment epithelium (Lakowski, 1962). Notwithstanding the fact that statistical evaluation of different age groups is of great help for the diagnosis of type III defect, the decision as to whether a blue–yellow defect is a physiologic or a pathologic one in an individual case sometimes remains difficult.

Other Abnormalities of Color Vision

CHROMATOPSIA

Chromatopsia, or perversion of color vision, may be defined as a condition in which white stimuli appear colored. The condition is called *ianthinopsia* if white is perceived as violet, *cyanopsia* if white is perceived as blue, *chloropsia* if white is perceived as green, *xanthopsia* if white is perceived as yellow, and *erythropsia* if white is perceived as red. Chromatopsias have been described as occurring in intoxications; they can be due to either quickly formed absorption systems (as, for example, in fluorescein angiography) or an imbalance in the retinal physiologic mechanisms. Chromatopsia is a temporary condition, since color perception adapts to the new equilibrium and white surfaces are again perceived as white. In cases such as jaundice, chromatopsia may not be accompanied by an impairment in chromatic discrimination. In the majority of cases, however, chromatopsia does accompany an acquired color vision defect. Chromatopsia may also occur in cortical defects, and it has been termed coloropsia. Coloropsia may show recurrent episodes over a period of years.

CORTICAL DEFECTS

Color vision abnormalities caused by cortical defects are rare. The abnormalities do not fit within usual classification schema and must be treated as unique entities. Color agnosia is the total or partial inability to recognize or appreciate colors. Color agnosia can occur as an isolated phenomenon but is often a symptom of visual agnosia. The defects accompanying color agnosia have been termed cerebral achromatopsia (Meadows, 1974). Aphasia and alexia for color names may also occur. In these cases colorimetric performance and chromatic discrimination are normal; however, the affected observer may be unable to name colors correctly or unable to associate color names with their usual meanings. Cortical defects are discussed in Chapter 8.

New Approaches to the Study of Acquired Color Vision Defects

Acquired color vision defects are usually classified in the clinic according to the Verriest classification. Sophisticated psychophysical testing has also been used to analyze acquired color vision defects. Marré developed the chromatic adaptation technique for the study of acquired color vision defects, the Wald-Marré technique (reviewed by Marré, 1973). The Wald-Marré technique is described in Chapter 6.

Smith and Pokorny and their colleagues (Smith, Pokorny, Ernest, & Starr, 1978; Smith, Pokorny, & Diddie, 1978; Pokorny, Smith, & Johnston, 1979) have analyzed pseudoprotanomaly, an alteration condition in which there is an abnormal Rayleigh match by psychophysical testing that includes an extended Rayleigh series (see Chapter 6) and measurements of the Stiles-Crawford effect (see Chapter 6). The data showed that pseudoprotanomaly occurs because the photoreceptor layer is disoriented (Smith,

Pokorny, Ernest & Starr, 1978; Smith, Pokorny, & Diddie, 1978; Pokorny, Smith, & Johnston, 1979). The causes are many (Pokorny, Smith, & Ernest, in press) and include serous elevation as in central serous choroidopathy, deposits in the pigment epithelium as in vitelliform macular degeneration, degeneration or atrophy of pigment epithelium/choroid as in choroideremia, fibrous scars occuring as sequelae of chorioretinal inflammation or vitelliform macular degeneration, and in neovascular membranes in advanced senile macular degeneration, familiar drusen, and various forms of choroiditis. In some disorders further degeneration occurs at the photoreceptor layer at the fovea, and the color vision defect may progress to a type I defect with scotopization. In some disorders, e.g., central serous choroidopathy or acute posterior multifocal placoid pigment epitheliopathy, there may be recovery of vision and color discrimination.

Another new approach to the study of acquired color vision defects is analysis of the defect according to whether or not neural processing of chromatic information reveals specfic losses in chromatic opponent channels. The psychophysical procedures (see Chapter 6) are increment detection (Sperling & Harwerth, 1971; Sperling, Piantanida, & Garrett, 1976) or flicker detection (King-Smith, Kranda, & Wood, 1976; Zisman, Bhargava, & King-Smith, 1978) of chromatic stimuli on white backgrounds. These techniques are particularly well suited to the study of disorders of the optic disc and optic nerve. Verriest and Uvijls (1977a,b) adapted a Tübinger perimeter to allow clinical evaluation of increment thresholds on white backgrounds.

Jennifer Birch, M. Phil.

I. A. Chisholm, M.D.

Paul Kinnear, Ph.D.

A. J. L. G. Pinckers, M.D.

Joel Pokorny, Ph.D.

Vivianne C. Smith, Ph.D.

Guy Verriest, M.D.

5

Clinical Testing Methods

Clinical tests are designed for easy and rapid evaluation of color vision. The majority of clinical tests are designed to screen from the normal population those individuals who have a congenital red–green color vision defect. Although laboratory measurements allow sophisticated analysis of color vision characteristics, such measurements take a good deal of time to perform and require a high degree of cooperation from the patient. Clinical tests evolved separately; they provide abridged versions of colorimetric measurements in the context of rapid and simple judgments. The purpose of the chapter is to review some of the tests used for clinical examination of color vision.

PLATE TESTS*

In a plate test the observer is usually required to read or identify a figure, usually a numeral, embedded in a background. Plate tests, the most popular color vision tests, are quick and easy to use. There are many different tests available, but all tend to reproduce similar aims and formats. The variety represents lack of international cooperation rather than significant innovation (Sloan & Habel, 1956; Belcher, Greenshields & Wright, 1958; Frey, 1963). The main purpose of plate tests is to screen congenital protan and deutan color-defective observers from normals; however, some plate tests attempt a more specific diagnosis of both the type and the degree of the defect, and some contain plates designed to detect tritan defects.

The majority of plate tests are based on the pseudoisochromatic principle in which the elements are placed in such a way that the figure appears in shades of a chromatic quality on a background of a different chromatic quality. The individual elements of the

*Contributed by Jennifer Birch, M. Phil.

designs are dots or spots of color in various sizes and contrasts. Hardy, Rand, and Rittler (1945) characterized the four types of pseudoisochromatic design as follows: The vanishing design contains a figure (numeral, etc.) that is correctly read by the normal but is not seen by the defective observer, since the colors in the figure are confused with the background colors (i.e., the vanishing figure is pseudoisochromatic to the color defective). The qualitatively diagnostic plate is a more sophisticated version of the vanishing plate that allows differentiation of a protan from a deutan observer. In the transformation plate two figures are embedded in the background: one figure has the appropriate color and lightness contrast to be read by the normal observer, and the other has the appropriate chromatic and lightness contrast to be read by the defective observer. In the hidden digit design the figure is not seen by the normal observer but is seen by color defectives (i.e., the plate is a vanishing plate for normal trichromats). Lakowski (1965b; 1966; 1969b; 1976) has analyzed the colorimetric properties of several existing pseudoisochromatic plate tests.

The Design of Plate Tests

Pseudoisochromatic tests capitalize on the color confusions characteristic of different types of deficiency. The efficiency of each plate depends on the accurate choice of color, size, and positioning of the dots, the dimensions of the figure, and the luminous contrast between the elements contained in the symbol and those in the background (Hansen, 1963; Birch, 1975). It is important that the color differences employed are kept small so that slight defects can be detected; however, if the color difference is too small, then some normal subjects (such as those with poor visual acuity or the elderly) will also fail to distinguish the figure. Conversely, if the color difference is too large, then some color defectives will be able to interpret the plate correctly. It is this necessity for the discrimination to be difficult but not too difficult that introduces the need for statistical analysis of each plate in a given test so that the best plates (and tests) can be identified. Such analysis makes use of results obtained for previously diagnosed color defectives of various types together with a group of normal subjects. Different age populations may also be studied and the responses of disadvantaged groups obtained.

Careful control of the color difference is not the only factor governing the accuracy of the design; the luminance contrast between the elements of the symbol and the background has to be kept within about 5 percent or the symbol will be distinguished by achromatic contrast alone. Most pseudoisochromatic designs use colors in a variety of tones specifically to reduce luminance contrast and to allow for interobserver differences in relative luminous efficiency. However, some pseudoisochromatic plates are designed specifically to exploit interobserver differences in relative luminous efficiency. For example, the long-wavelength luminosity loss of protanopes can be used to construct diagnostic plates for protan observers.

Most pseudoisochromatic tests do not employ a full range of colors but exploit the loss of chromatic discrimination characteristic of red–green–defective observers. Such tests have only limited application to the study of acquired color defects, where it is desirable that a full range of colors be used. For example, in acquired color vision defects, failure to read the red–green screening plates does not indicate a congenital color defect but only that reduction in chromatic discriminative ability has occurred. Conversely, the prescription of tinted lenses, although enabling congenital color defectives to pass a pseudoisochromatic screening test, does not result in correction of their defect.

Congenital blue–yellow defects are rare, but acquired defects are predominantly of this type. The design of pseudoisochromatic screening plates for blue–yellow defects is particularly difficult due to wide variations among normal observers in the luminous efficiency for the short-wavelength portion of the visible spectrum (Chapters 3 and 8). Congenital blue–yellow defects do not often give rise to serious occupational difficulties, and many pseudoisochromatic tests do not include blue–yellow plates. The plates that are available suffer from the difficulty of setting an appropriate color difference that will both screen for slight defects and pass normal trichromats with dense ocular pigmentation. Further, most tests were designed before detailed information became available concerning the typical color confusions of blue–yellow defectives and differences between congenital and acquired blue–yellow defects.

The colors for diagnostic pseudoisochromatic plates are chosen so as to lie upon appropriate isochromatic lines for each type of defect (see Chapter 7). The colors for diagnostic plates to distinguish between protan and deutan defects have to be carefully chosen, since the isochromatic lines are close together (Chapter 7). Pairs of colors whose chromaticity coordinates are represented along isochromatic lines will be confused only if the relative luminance (that is, the contrast) is appropriate. Most diagnostic protan and deutan plates make use of the confusions of blue–greens and purples with neutral grays. The tritanopic isochromatic lines converge to a point just outside the blue corner of the chromaticity diagram (Chapter 7); therefore most appropriate colors for diagnostic plates are blues, grays, and yellows. This choice introduces difficulties for the printer because yellows are normally much lighter colors than blues and it is therefore more difficult to get appropriate contrast.

Ishihara Plates

The Ishihara test is the most popular screening test for congenital protan and deutan defects, and it is generally accepted as the best pseudoisochromatic test for this purpose. It has appeared in many different editions, including an abridged version. Different editions of the Ishihara plates have slight variations in the color printing. It is usual to allow normal trichromats to make two partial errors of interpretation, but the frequency of partial errors may vary slightly with the edition. An introductory plate is provided for both the standard section of the test (24 plates) and for the illiterate section (12 plates). No scoresheet is provided, and the instructions to the examiner are minimal. The test has worldwide distribution.

The different formats employed in the Ishihara include vanishing, transformation, hidden digit, and diagnostic plates (Hardy, Rand, & Rittler, 1945; Lakowski, 1965b). The employment of a range of designs makes the Ishihara test unique. However, the hidden digit is usually possible. When neither of these digits is seen, it is more difficult to work well. For example, anomalous trichromats may be able to see both digits on the diagnostic plates, but a tentative diagnosis of either protan or deutan can be obtained by asking if one of the digits looks clearer. A consistent choice of either the left- or right-hand digit is usually possible. When neither of these digits is seen, it is more difficult to interpret the result. Protanopes and occasionally deuteranopes make this response; in this case it is the effect of either dense macular pigmentation or increased lens density that "spreads" the color confusions to encompass both digits. Patients with either poor visual acuity or poor hue discrimination may fail both the vanishing and transformation designs without seeing the hidden digit; this result should not be interpreted as a red–green defect.

The Ishihara test is excellent for screening patients with both slight and severe defects from the normal population (Belcher, Greenshields, & Wright, 1958; Frey, 1958; Sloan & Habel, 1956). The severity of the defect can be estimated according to the number of errors made. If some of the confusion and vanishing plates are interpreted correctly, then the defect is probably slight. It is not possible to distinguish dichromats from severe anomalous trichromats with this test.

American Optical Company Plates (Hardy, Rand, & Rittler or AO HRR Plates)

The AO HRR (Hardy, Rand, & Rittler, 1954) plate test, now out of print, is still widely used and is one of the most popular pseudoisochromatic tests because it provides screening and diagnostic plates for tritan defects in addition to diagnostic and grading plates for protan and deutan defects (Belcher, Greenshields, & Wright, 1958; Frey, 1958; Walls, 1959a). The test is less good for distinguishing between normals and red–green color defectives, since normal trichromats are allowed two partial errors and only four screening plates are provided. The AO HRR plates are therefore usually used together with a more efficient screening test such as the Ishihara plates. The results obtained from these two tests provide perhaps the most complete information about the nature of the color defect that can be expected from pseudoisochromatic designs. However, it is still not possible to distinguish consistently between dichromats and severe anomalous trichromats. A slight disadvantage is the inclusion in the test of plates designed to detect "tetartanopia." Tetartanopia defects have been very much disputed (see Chapter 4), and no known congenital case has been fully established. Nevertheless, occasional patients with acquired blue–yellow color defects show this pattern (3 of 77—Pinckers, 1975a). The blue–yellow plates appear to work well for both congenital and acquired color defectives, although it is sometimes necessary to ask the patient which of the symbols on the diagnostic plates appears clearer.

There are four introductory plates, four protan/deutan screening plates, and two tritan screening plates. These are followed by the diagnostic and grading plates (classifying defects as either "mild," "medium," or "strong") for protan/deutan defects and four tritan diagnostic plates. The instruction manual is specific, and a scoresheet is provided.

The use of symbols rather than numerals and the concept of increasing the saturation of the colors in steps to provide a grading series was a unique innovation for pseudoisochromatic designs. Although two editions were made available, the test was printed only once and the plates are identical.

The HRR classification of severity of red–green color defects has been interpreted as being not fully representative of the degree of defect, and an improved scoresheet was developed by Vos, Verkaik, and Boogaard (1971; 1972). The new classification system is designated HRR-R (HRR-reevaluated).

Velhagen Plates

The first pseudoisochromatic tests to be constructed were the Stilling plates, which first appeared in 1877. The original test was subsequently modified firstly by Stilling himself, then by Hertel, and more recently by Velhagen. Therefore unlike the Ishihara plates this pseudoisochromatic test has changed in format over the years. While some designs have been retained and are common to the various editions, other designs have been introduced and subsequently discarded. The number of plates varies slightly, and when referring to tests in this series it is essential to indicate which edition is being used. The Velhagen test is as of this writing in the 26th edition, but older tests are still in use (Frey, 1975c; Neubauer & Harrer, 1976).

The tests contain one or two introductory plates. There are a large number of protan/deutan screening plates, which are mainly of the vanishing design. Diagnostic plates to distinguish between protan and deutan defects are usually included, but no attempt is made to provide systematic grading of the severity of the defect other than according to the number of errors made. Screening plates for tritan defects are usually included, as are specific designs for examining simultaneous color contrast. Some editions in this series contain plates for illiterates, and some do not. Since the design parameters used in the screening plates show quite large variations (e.g., in the dot size and in the overall size and stroke width of the symbols), there are also large variations in the relative efficiency of the plates. Normal trichromats are allowed up to four partial errors.

The 26th edition of the Velhagen plates (printed in 1977) is slightly different from the 25th edition (1974). Both use a combination of numerals and upper case letters and have 30 plates in all. There are two introductory plates, and emphasis is placed on protan/deutan screening and broad classification of the type of defect. Tritan screening plates are also included. Neither test contains plates for illiterates, but both have simultaneous contrast designs. The diagnostic plates are somewhat scattered through the test, which makes interpretation of the results rather difficult until the examiner becomes familiar with the test. The protan diagnostic plates make use of the poor relative luminous efficiency suffered by protan observers for red wavelengths. The test instructions are in German, and no scoring sheet is provided.

Okuma Plates

The Okuma (Okuma, Masuda, Kawada, & Shinjo, 1973) charts introduce the novel idea of using a Landolt ring for the symbol in pseudoisochromatic designs. In the transformation designs, the gap in the ring is seen at different orientations by normal trichromats and by color defectives. The colors used in the screening plates are similar to those employed in the Ishihara test. There is a single introductory plate, and a sample Landolt ring card is provided that can be given to the patient to orient according to the design seen. There are seven screening plates, four of the transformation type, two vanishing plates, and one hidden digit plate. A further six plates, designed for diagnosis and grading of protan and deutan defects, are of the vanishing design. There are three protan grading plates and three deutan grading plates in which both the size of the Landolt ring is altered and the saturation of the colors is increased. Each three-plate series is therefore similar to the system employed in the AO HRR plates but using red-purples and blue-greens for the diagnostic colors throughout.

Some patients see both breaks in the ring on the transformation plates and some see neither. No scoresheet is provided, and the test instructions are in Japanese only. It is easy for the examiner to lose his place since the test is composed of individual cards. The recommended test distance is 0.75 m.

F$_2$ Plate

Farnsworth designed a tritan plate that was reproduced by Wright (1952) to obtain patients for his survey of the characteristics of tritanopia. Farnsworth subsequently improved the design in the F$_2$ plate, which consists of two overlapping squares, one yellow-green and the other blue, embedded in a purple background. Normal trichromats see both squares, but the yellow-green square is much clearer (or brighter). Tritanopes should fail to see the yellow-green square, and incomplete tritanopes, while seeing both squares, should indicate that the blue square is clearer. Congenital protans and deutans fail to see the blue square, and this fact seems to be an unexpected bonus (Lakowski, 1965; Verriest, 1968; Taylor, 1970; Pinckers, 1972c). The plate may therefore seem to be an ideal screening plate for congenital and acquired color defects. However, the plate does not work well for acquired blue–yellow defects (Legras & Coscas, 1972; Pinckers, 1972c; 1975a; Ohtani, Ohta, Kogure, & Seki, 1975). Although congenital tritanopes fail to see the yellow-green square, observers with type III acquired blue–yellow defects tend to see only the yellow-green square and not the blue square, leading to confusion of interpretation. Care has to be taken in interpreting the patient's responses. It is necessary for the patient to say how many squares there are and to indicate the position of the square seen more clearly so that the examiner can confirm which one it is without having to rely on the patient's color naming.

The F_2 plate has been available gratis from the New London Submarine Base, Groton, Connecticut. It is not available commercially, but it is possible to construct the plate from Munsell papers (Taylor, 1975).

Boström-Kugelberg Pseudoisochromatic Plates (B-K)

A new edition of the Boström-Kugelberg plates has been introduced (Hedin, 1974) with 21 plates. The aim is protan/deutan screening, and there are 15 plates of the vanishing type, 3 plates with no digit to detect malingering, and 2 plates for illiterates. There is no introductory plate. The colors are desaturated, and a small dot size is employed. Hedin (1974) observed that there is an age effect for the red–green plates (older color normals are more frequently misclassified as red–green defective than younger color normals). These plates replace the previous editions of Boström-Kugelberg and Boström plates. The latter test contained 16 plates screening for color defect and 4 plates for detection of malingerers. A period of fifteen seconds is allowed for viewing each plate. The instructions are in Swedish.

Dvorine Pseudoisochromatic Plates

In the Dvorine test an introductory plate is provided for the standard part of the test, which consists of 14 plates of the vanishing type designed for screening red–green defect. There are 7 plates for illiterates, and an introductory plate for this section (Peters, 1956).

Screening efficiency for protan and deutan defects is very good, and an estimation of the severity of the defect can be made according to the number of errors recorded (Dvorine, 1946; Frey, 1962). The instruction manual is good, and a scoresheet is provided. The recommended viewing time is given as 5 sec per plate and the test distance as 30 inches. Two partial errors are allowed by color normals. Although two of the plates are designed to be diagnostic for protan and deutan defects, this is not explained in the manual. The Dvorine (Dvorine, 1946) test is unique in providing a color-naming test in addition to pseudoisochromatic designs.

Tokyo Medical College Plates (TMC)

The Tokyo Medical College plates (Umazume, Seki, & Obi, 1954; 1955; 1956) are constructed differently from other printed pseudoisochromatic tests. In this case, the dot format is achieved by superimposing a white matrix upon painted colors. The use of painted colors is intended to avoid fading. The dot size used is one of the smallest employed in pseudoisochromatic tests, and the interstitial spaces are relatively large; the stroke width of the numeral is also narrower than in most other tests. These factors require that the test be used only with patients who have good visual acuity. Reduction to about 0.5 can be sufficient to produce failure on the protan/deutan screening plates. There is no introductory plate. Screening plates are of the vanishing type. Five screening plates for protan/deutan defects are provided along with two screening plates for tritan defects. Two sets of grading plates, and diagnostic plates for protan and deutan defects each containing three designs, are also included. The test provides very good screening of congenital protan and deutan defects, but the tritan plates do not work well for either congenital or acquired defects. Diagnosis of the type of the defect is not very reliable. Again, it may be necessary to ask the patient which of the numerals is clearer (but the more likely response is that the severe defectives will see neither digit). Grading of the severity of the defect agrees well with that found with other tests (Sloan, 1961; Umazume, 1958; Vos, Verkaik, & Boogaard, 1971; 1972). No scoresheet is provided.

American Optical Company Plates (1965, AOC Plates)

The 14-plate American Optical Company Plates test aims to reproduce the best plates found in other tests and is only partially successful in doing so. The introductory plate and 6 confusion designs are taken from the Ishihara test, but color quality is only moderate and the plates do not have quite the same efficiency. The remaining 7 plates, which are vanishing designs, appear to be taken from the Velhagen and Polack tests. A scoresheet is provided, and normal trichromats are allowed up to four partial errors. Only 2 sec are allowed for viewing each design.

The City University Color Vision Test (TCU Test)

The City University test (Fletcher, 1972) consists of a series of ten charts. On each is displayed a central color subtending 1° and four peripheral colors of equal subtense mounted on a matte black ground. The patient is asked to select which of the four outer colors is most simlar to the central color. This test criterion is therefore different from that used in other plate tests. The colors employed are all selected from the Munsell series and are identical with those used in the Farnsworth Panel D-15 test (below) with the addition of a neutral and a yellow-green. An adjacent color taken from the Farnsworth Panel D-15 is designated as the normal choice on each for the diagnostic colors typical of either protan, deutan, or tritan defects. The diagnostic colors are selected from the opposite side of the hue circle used in the Farnsworth Panel D-15 sequence and represent isochromatic confusions for each type of defect.

The rationale of the design is that manipulation of the colors is not required, which prevents soiling. The format is considered to be more appropriate for the elderly or for the very young, who may find either the manipulation of the colors in the Farnsworth Panel

D-15 test to be difficult or the concept of constructing a color sequence beyond their comprehension. On the other hand, use of the TCU test in clinical practice indicates that some patients, regardless of age, find the selection criterion difficult; some complain that none of the colors is in any way similar to the test color, while others select more than one color that appears to be identical.

Since it is based on the Farnsworth Panel D-15, the TCU test is not designed for screening; approximately 20 percent of color defectives pass the test. Although the protan/deutan diagnosis is not always clear (e.g., plates 1 and 7 appear to give protan results for deuteranopes), most moderate and severe defects are diagnosed correctly, and the degree of the defect is indicated by the number of errors made. Instructions on test procedure are included with the test, and a scoresheet is provided. Desaturation of the displays is recommended, presumably to obtain more efficient screening, but how this can be achieved is not explained.

The TCU test is similar in performance to the Farnsworth Panel D-15 test; they can be used to confirm each other or substituted according to which format is preferred for a particular patient. Recent evaluations of the TCU test are given by Hill, Connolly, and Dundas (1978), Ohta, Kogure, Izutsu, Miyamoto, and Nagai (1978), and Verriest and Caluwaerts (1978).

Standard Pseudoisochromatic Plates (Ichikawa, Hukami, Tanabe, and Kawakami)

This new set of pseudoisochromatic plates is designed to screen for red–green color defects and to separate and classify protan and deutan color defectives. The plates are constructed from uniform-sized dots that form digits (embedded in a background) designed to resemble those found on electronically generated numeric displays (e.g., pocket calculators). There are four demonstration plates to familiarize the testee with the form of the test. The authors suggest that two of the demonstration plates may be useful in diagnosing tritan defects. The ten screening plates are designed so that one numeral on each plate is visible to normal observers and the other visible to color-defective observers. The plates use reasonably highly saturated colors. An observer is considered normal if eight or more of the numerals for normals are read correctly. Finally, there are five classification plates in which color-defective observers may be distinguished as either protan or deutan on the basis of which of two digits on each plate can be read (or which of the two is more distinct). Three of these plates have colored digits on colored backgrounds; the other two have colored digits on gray backgrounds.

The test is designed to be administered under natural daylight from a north window (northern hemisphere) or under artificial light of similar spectral composition. The plates are placed 0.75 m from the observer, and a maximum viewing time of 3 sec is permitted. A limited number of scoring sheets of clear design are provided.

The plates are attractive in design and are easy to administer. It is necessary to postpone evaluation of the test until independent verification of the screening and classification efficiencies of the plates is reported.

Tests for Achromatopsia

The Sloan achromatopsia test consists of seven plates; each plate contains a series of 17 gray rectangles whose reflectance increases gradually in small steps across the card from almost white to almost black. The rectangles are numbered from 1 to 9 in 0.5 steps.

In the center of each rectangle appears a colored circle of fixed hue and reflectance. The seven cards each have a differently colored circle—gray, red, yellow-red, yellow, green, purple-blue, and red-purple. Complete achromats can find an exact match of the color circle and one of the rectangles on each card. Others can make only a brightness match of a color circle to a rectangle, except for the gray card, for which an exact match exists for all observers.

The observer must indicate for which gray rectangle the center circle is a match either in color or in brightness. The test starts with the gray card (for which there is an exact match of rectangle and center circle). The other cards are then presented. The cards are presented at 0.5 m at right angles to the line of sight under daylight illumination. Test time is 2–3 min per eye. The examiner notes the number of the rectangle chosen. The instructions include the numerals of rectangles chosen as complete matches by achromats and those chosen as brightness matches by normal observers in photopic and scotopic (rod vision) illumination. The test results are compared with these sequences.

The FVS (François, Verriest, & Seki) test plates are designed for evaluation of achromatopsia. A pilot model of the test was described by Verriest and Seki (1965). The test is available through the Murakami Color Research Company in Tokyo. The plates look like pseudoisochromatic plates, the symbol being a cross. There is one introductory plate and two diagnostic plates on which the cross is invisible only in achromatopsia with a scotopic spectral luminosity curve (normal scotopic vision, typical achromatopsia, scotopic stage of cone degenerations).

Tests Designed for Use With Children

The Guy's Hospital test (Gardiner, 1973) attempts to reproduce the colors and format of the Ishihara test but uses upper case letters. Plastic letters are included with the test so that children can select the letter they see. The page surface is glossy; while this allows the pages to be wiped clean, it may also introduce specular reflection if the illuminant is not carefully placed. There are two introductory plates, four screening plates of the confusion type, and two diagnostic plates. A scoring sheet is provided, but the significance of the diagnostic plates is not explained in the manual. It is suggested that a viewing distance of 2 feet be used but that satisfactory results can be obtained at 4 feet. No comparative data on the efficiency of the test are available, but the indications are that the test is poorly designed, since both the correct and confusion letters appear equally visible to normal trichromats (Alexander, 1975).

The Matsubara Color Vision Test Plates for the Infants (Koyima & Matsubara, 1957) is a pseudoisochromatic design with pictographs, symbols of items familiar in Japanese culture. There are ten plates, six for screening and four for diagnostic purposes. The test is available from the publisher (Handaya Co., Ltd.) but has not received full validation in a European population.

Miscellaneous Plate Tests

The Freeman Illuminant Stable color vision test (Freeman, 1948; Freeman & Zaccaria, 1948) was designed so that the colors chosen for the screening plates should retain their appearance under different types of illumination. The test was not successful (Farnsworth, Paulson, & Connolly, undated) and is no longer available.

The Polack pseudoisochromatic plate test contained approximately 50 plates in a variety of designs. Vanishing, confusion, and hidden digit principles were employed. Some designs contained numerals and some pictograms. Plates for illiterates were included, and protan/deutan diagnosis was possible. The Polack plates are no longer available, and the test has been superseded by others.

A number of visual screening devices, e.g., the Titmus vision tester, the Bausch and Lomb Orthorater, and the Keystone Ophthalmic Telebinocular, contain color slides or photographic reproductions of one or more pseudoisochromatic plates. Since neither the reproduction nor the illuminant has correct color relations, these plates are unsuitable for color vision screening.

ARRANGEMENT TESTS*

In an arrangement test the observer is required to organize a set of color samples according to a specified order—for example, a hue or saturation order. Arrangement tests allow evaluation of chromatic discriminative ability of normal and color-defective observers. Their origin dates to tests developed by Pierce (1934) at the National Institute of Industrial Psychology. The arrangement tests that have proved important in evaluation of congenital and acquired color vision defects have been the two tests designed by Dean Farnsworth and recent modifications. Some industries have their own versions of arrangement tests; however, such tests are not standardized for general use.

Farnsworth (1943) originally designed two arrangement tests, the Farnsworth-Munsell 100-hue test (FM 100-hue test) and the Farnsworth Dichotomous Test for Color Blindness. Both tests were subsequently modified: the test known as the FM 100-hue test now contains 85 hues (Farnsworth, 1957), and the dichotomous test, the Farnsworth Panel D-15, contains 15 hues (Farnsworth, 1947). Both tests used Munsell papers (see Chapter 2) of fixed value and chroma, and the samples are selected from the entire hue circle. In the FM 100-hue test the color differences between adjacent color samples are small. Correct arrangement of the color samples requires not only normal color vision but also good chromatic discriminative ability. Since the samples are divided into four separate boxes completing the hue circle, errors can occur in adjacent color regions (yellow-greens, greens, blue-greens) but not across the color circle. In the Farnsworth Panel D-15, the color differences between adjacent samples are large and all 15 samples are presented in one box. Thus errors across the hue circle (e.g., placing green next to purple) are possible, and the test evaluates color confusions of the color-defective observer. New versions of both tests have been derived including for the FM 100-hue test a 40-hue version using approximately every second sample (Ohta 40-hue test: Ohta, 1966) and a 28-hue version (the Roth 28-hue test) using every third sample. Farnsworth designed a high-chroma version of the Farnsworth Panel D-15 (the H-16 test) that used slightly larger, high-chroma samples, and Lanthony (1974b) devised a low-chroma version, the desaturated Panel D-15, in which the samples have lower chroma but higher value than the standard Panel D-15. The City University test was derived from the Farnsworth Panel D-15 test. Of these modified versions, the Roth 28-hue and the Lanthony desaturated Panel D-15 are commercially avilable. A completely new arrangement test using Munsell colors is the Lanthony New Color Test (Lanthony, 1975a), which incorporates both a hue series and multiple chroma levels.

---

*Contributed by I. A. Chisholm, M.D., A. J. L. G. Pinckers, M.D., and Vivianne C. Smith, Ph.D.

Farnsworth-Munsell 100-hue Test (FM 100-hue Test)

The FM 100-hue test (Farnsworth, 1943) was designed to test hue discrimination among persons with normal color vision and to evaluate chromatic discrimination loss in observers with congenital color vision defects. François and Verriest (1956) applied the FM 100-hue test to acquired color vision defects. Today the FM 100-hue test is recognized to provide a sensitive evaluation of chromatic discriminative ability (Lakowski, 1968a).

The test consists of 85 movable color samples arranged in four boxes of 21 or 22 colors each. The 85 samples were chosen to represent perceptually equal steps of hue and to form a natural hue circle. The caps are of approximately equal lightness for a color-normal observer. The colors are set in plastic caps and subtend 1.5° at 0.50 m. They are numbered on the back according to the ideal color order of the hue circle. Two pilot colors are fixed at either end of each box.

EXAMINATION PROCEDURE

One box is presented at a time (box I, Nos. 1–22; box II, Nos. 23–43; box III, Nos. 44–64; box IV, Nos. 65–85). The colored caps are arranged in random order on the upper lid.The subject is required "to arrange the caps in order according to color" on the lower panel between the fixed end caps. The test is performed under standard illuminant C providing at least 250 lux. Under usual testing circumstances, the subject is allowed as long as necessary to complete the task (contrary to the suggestion of a time limit of 2 min/box given in the manual).

The subject's arrangement of the cap sequence is recorded using the numbers on the reverse side. The score for each cap is calculated as the sum of the absolute differences between adjacent caps. The error score is the cap score minus 2 (in a perfect arrangement each cap has a cap score of 2). The cap scores are also presented on a circular graph (Fig. 5.1), where the score for each cap is plotted as a distance on a radial line (Farnsworth, 1957). Alternatively, the cap scores can simply be plotted serially according to Kinnear (1970), who states that the merit of this method is to make the defect easier to identify and categorize (Table 5.1, Fig. 5.2).

The recording of the results and production of the circular graph can be tedious and time consuming and is open to simple arithmetical errors. The ultimate refinement has been the design of a dedicated minicomputer (Donaldson, 1977) that has been linked to the caps (without altering them in anyway) so that not only is the computation of the error score performed automatically, but the 100-hue chart can be printed simultaneously in either the Farnsworth or Kinnear mode. This technological advance can reduce the workload per test to less than 2 min (Taylor & Donaldson, 1976).

INTERPRETATION OF RESULTS

Characteristic FM 100-hue plots for subjects with congenital color vision defects show concentrations of errors in two well-defined areas (confusion zones); these zones are termed poles. For subjects with congenital color deficiency the poles occur in characteristic positions according to the type of defect. When poles are diametrically opposite, their combined effect is that of an axis (Fig. 5.2).

The locus of the center cap of the pole is also characteristic of the congenital deficiency. The center cap can be determined accurately only on the average of several tests. Representative center caps found by Farnsworth (1943), confirmed by François and

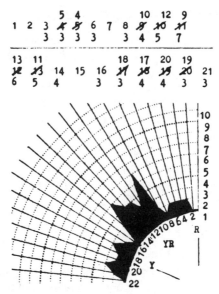

Fig. 5.1. Specimen test result and plot according to Farnsworth. [From Chisholm, I. A., Bronte-Stewart, J., & Awduche, E. D. *Acta Ophthalmologica,* 1970, *48,* 1146–1156 (reproduced with permission of Acta Ophthalmologica).]

Verriest (1957a) and Perdriel (1962), are shown in Table 5.2. For observers with abnormal spectral luminous efficiency function (protans, achromats, and those with type I red–green defects) a lightness cue is present; this cue forms the basis for the axis shown by complete achromats (Verriest, Buyssens & Vanderdonck, 1963).

The fact that confusion zones may overlap two boxes is sometimes inconvenient. To overcome this, Taylor (1974) suggested rearrangement of the caps: box I, nos. 7–27; box II, nos. 28–48; box III, nos. 49–69; box IV, nos. 70–85 and 1–6. Taylor (1974) further suggested that starting with box II (green range) would enable naive subjects with congenital protan or deutan defects to grasp the idea behind the test more readily than if they were to start the test with box I (red-yellow), where their chromatic discrimination would be poor.

Aspinall (1974a) calculated the upper limit of error scores based upon a random series of cap arrangements to be 200 for any one box or 984 for all four boxes and suggested that only error scores below this theoretical upper limit could be assumed to arise from specific color confusions. High error scores of 1000 or so do occur in achromatopsia. The Aspinall (1974a) calculation may be helpful in evaluating malingering.

EFFECT OF AGE

Colors are perceived and discriminated most accurately between the ages of 16 and 35 years (Lakowski, 1958). After age 55 years there is a deterioration in the ability for fine color discrimination, which affects mainly blue–yellow or violet/blue-green discrimination (acquired type III defect), red–green discrimination remaining stable (see Chapter 8). Verriest (1963) demonstrated that for normal healthy subjects the FM 100-hue test score increased in a positive manner with age after 35 years. Verriest (1963)

Table 5.1

Comparison of Scoring Methods Recommended by
Farnsworth and by Kinnear

Normal Cap Order:	9 10 11 12 13 14 15 16 17 . . .
Subject's Cap Order:	9 10 11 21 13 18 14 15 16 . . .
Cap Score:	2 11 18 13 9 5 2 . . .

Graphic Representation			
Farnsworth Mode		*Kinnear Mode*	
Cap Number	Error Plot of Cap Score	Cap Number	Error Plot of Cap Score
10	2	10	2
11	11	11	11
12	—	12	18
13	13	13	13
14	5	14	9
15	2	15	5
16	—	16	2
17	—		
18	9		
19	—		
20	—		
21	18		

provided a guideline for the assessment of an acquired type III defect in which color defect is indicated by an error score in excess of the 95th percentile for the age-matched normal (Table 5.3).

REPEATABILITY

The FM 100-hue test may be used both as a diagnostic aid and in followup examinations for observing the evolution of pathologic changes in treated and untreated subjects. A statistical evaluation of the significance of the retest score (Chisholm, 1969a) showed that it was not influenced by subject age or directly by the initial error score. A guideline was provided whereby the significance of a change in error score on retest could be identified (Fig. 5.3). Provided that the increment of change lay outside the 95th percentile limits, the alteration in error score would be significant. In their reviews of analytical methods useful for intereye comparisons both Kinnear (1970) and Aspinall (1974b) concluded that the square root of the Farnsworth-Munsell 100-hue error score is statistically more informative than either the total error score or its logarithm.

Table 5.2

Center Caps Characterizing the Axes in Congenital Color Vision Defects

	Farnsworth (1943)	Verriest (1963)	Perdriel (1962)
Protan	19 and 65	63–67	22 and 66
Deutan	15 and 59	57–61	14 and 58
Tritan	84/2 and 46/47	46–48	84/5 and 52/64
Scotopic		50–57	

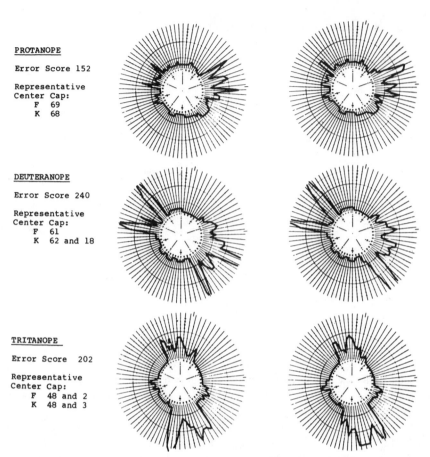

PROTANOPE

Error Score 152

Representative
Center Cap:
F 69
K 68

DEUTERANOPE

Error Score 240

Representative
Center Cap:
F 61
K 62 and 18

TRITANOPE

Error Score 202

Representative
Center Cap:
F 48 and 2
K 48 and 3

Fig. 5.2. Comparison of plot according to Farnsworth and Kinnear for observers with congenital color deficiencies. Total error score and representative center caps are indicated. [From Kinnear, P. R. *Vision Research,* 1970, *10*, 423–433 (reproduced with permission of Pergamon Press).]

Table 5.3*
Upper Limit of Error Scores (95th Percentile) Made by
Normal Trichromats of Different Ages

Age Range (Years)	95th Percentile
16–20	100
21–25	74
26–30	92
31–35	106
36–40	120
41–45	134
46–50	144
51–55	154
56–60	164
61–65	174

*Based on data of Verriest, G. *Journal of the Optical Society of America,* 1963, *53*, 185–195.

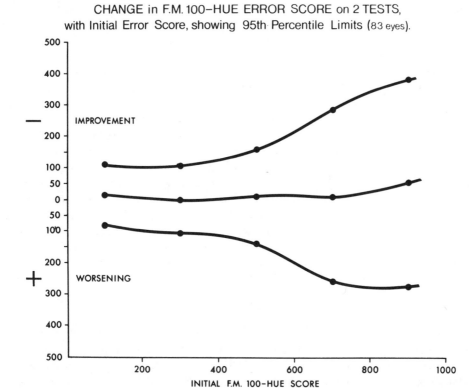

Fig. 5.3. Change in FM 100-hue error score on two successive tests (83 eyes). [From Chisholm, I. A., Foulds, W. E., & McClure, E. *Transactions of the Ophthalmological Society of the United Kingdom,* 1975, *95,* 167–172 (reproduced with permission of the Ophthalmological Society of the United Kingdom).]

Dichotomous Test for Color Blindness (Panel D-15)

The Farnsworth dichotomous test for color blindness (Panel D-15) (Farnsworth, 1947) is designed to select those observers with moderate and severe chromatic discrimination loss. Among congenital red–green defects, such observers comprise 5 percent of the males, or one-half of the color defective population. In addition, the test indicates blue–yellow discrimination loss, detects achromatopsia, and is useful in evaluation of acquired color vision defects (François & Verriest, 1956; Verriest, 1963; Linksz, 1966). The test consists of 15 movable color samples placed in a box with one fixed color sample. The samples are chosen to represent approximately equal hue steps for the natural color circle. The colors are similar in chroma to those of the FM 100-hue test. They are set in plastic caps and subtend 1.5° at 0.50 m. The movable caps are numbered on the back according to the ideal color circle. An instruction manual and scoring sheets are provided.

EXAMINATION PROCEDURE

The caps are prearranged in random order on the upper lid of the open box. The subject is instructed to "arrange the caps in order according to color" in the lower panel, starting with the cap closest to the fixed reference cap. The box is presented at a comfortable distance under daylight illumination providing at least 250 lux. The majority of individuals with normal color vision can complete a box in 1 min. The observer is allowed as long as is necessary to complete the task.

The order of the caps is plotted directly on the scoresheet on a diagram that shows correct cap positions extending in a circle from the reference cap. An error occurs when caps are misplaced from the ideal order. The scorer draws a line connecting the caps in the order arranged by the patients. In correct order the line retraces the hue circle. A minor error—say, caps 4 and 3 misplaced—leads to a reversal in the plot at caps 4 and 3, since cap 4 is connected to cap 2 and cap 3 is connected to cap 5. A major error occurs when distant caps—e.g., 3 and 12—are placed next to each other; the line connecting these caps crosses the hue circle. Subjects with normal color vision will sometimes make one or two minor errors or occasionally a single major error, as, for example, when the observer reverses part of the series. These are common errors in young children (Adams, Balliet, & McAdams, 1975; Cohen, 1976). The single major error that may be considered normal is the placement of cap 15 next to cap 7. This error occurs because the color difference step from cap 7 to cap 8 is unduly large. Occasionally an observer will make a few minor errors and a few major errors. In this case, a retest is required.

INTERPRETATION

The major errors give rise to lines crossing the color circle. In congenital color defects these major errors fall on consistent axes corresponding to protan, deutan, and tritan defects. These axes are indicated on the scoresheet. A fourth axis, that of achromats, indicating a scotopic pattern, lies between the deutan and tritan axes (Sloan, 1954; Verriest, 1963). Two or more major errors constitute failure. Among observers with congenital color defects, the Panel D-15 was designed to fail those with severe chromatic discrimination loss (Farnsworth, 1947). Such observers include dichromats, extreme anomalous trichromats, and occasional simple anomalous trichromats (Majima, 1969; Paulson, 1974). The concept of "pass–fail" is relevant only when the test is used as part of the SMRL test battery (see below—Using Color Vision Tests) for which it was designed.

PINCKERS FM 100-HUE VERSION OF THE FARNSWORTH
PANEL D-15 TEST

Pinckers (1971c) suggested that 16 of the FM 100-hue test caps are sufficiently similar to the Panel D-15 caps to be used in place of them. Higgins and Knoblauch (1977) confirm that for red–green color-defective observers equivalent results are obtained with the Panel D-15 and the version derived from the FM 100-hue test. Pinckers (1971c) further specifies a method for combining Panel D-15 and FM 100-hue test results on a single 100-hue scoresheet.

Lanthony Desaturated Panel D-15 Test

The Lanthony Desaturated Panel D-15 (Lanthony & Dubois-Poulsen, 1973; Lanthony, 1974a, b, 1978b) test was designed specifically for acquired color vision defects. The test is used in conjunction with the standard panel (Farnsworth Panel D-15 test) and has identical format. The color samples are paler and lighter (lower chroma, higher value) than those of the Panel D-15 test. If an observer makes many major errors on the standard Farnsworth Panel D-15, it is unnecessary to give the desaturated panel.

EXAMINATION PROCEDURE

The Desaturated Panel D-15 is performed following the Farnsworth Panel D-15. The results are plotted side by side on the specially designed scoresheet. Administration of the test is identical to that of the standard Farnsworth Panel D-15. The majority of individuals with normal color vision can complete a box in 1 min. The observer is allowed as long as is necessary to complete the task.

The order of the caps is plotted directly on the scoresheet on a diagram that shows correct cap positions extending in a circle from the reference cap. An error occurs when caps are misplaced from the ideal order. The scorer draws a line connecting the caps in their actual order. In correct order, the line retraces the hue circle. Scoring of minor and major errors is as for the standard Farnsworth Panel D-15. Subjects with normal color vision may make one or two minor errors, and a single crossline may occur when the observer reverses part of the series.

INTERPRETATION

Observers with congenital defects make major errors on the Desaturated Panel with axis identical to that of the corresponding dichromat on the standard Panel. Simple anomalous trichromats fail the Desaturated Panel because of the lower chroma. The test may be used to classify severity of discrimination loss in congenital red–green color defects. In acquired color vision defects the test may be used to follow the progression of a defect (recovery or deterioration) (Perdriel, Lanthony, & Chevaleraud, 1975b; Pinckers, Nabbe, & Bogaard, 1976; Lagerlöf, 1978; Pinckers & Baron, 1978; Verriest & Caluwaerts, 1978).

Lanthony New Color Test (NCT)

The New Color Test (NCT) (Lanthony, 1975a, b, 1978c) was designed specifically for use in acquired color vision defects. The test allows determination of neutral zones (colors confused with gray) and evaluation of chromatic discriminative ability at each of four chroma levels.

The NCT includes four boxes each with 15 colored caps. The caps subtend 1.5° at 0.5 m. The 15 hues are the same in each of the four boxes; they are designated by their initials (in French). All the caps have equal lightness. The boxes differ in saturation; the first (high saturation) box has Munsell chroma 8 (box 8/6), the second (medium saturation) has Munsell chroma 6 (box 6/6), the third (medium saturation) has Munsell chroma 4 (box 4/6), and the fourth (low saturation) has Munsell chroma 2 (box 2/6). The hues represent approximately equal steps in the color circle. In addition to these 60 colored caps, the test includes 10 gray caps at values increasing from 4 to 8 (steps: 0.5, with two caps at value 6); they are designated by Munsell nomenclature, N4 to N8. An instruction manual and scoring sheets are provided. The test is presented at a comfortable distance using standard illuminant C providing 250 lux.

EXAMINATION PROCEDURE

The NCT is performed in two phases, a separation phase followed by a classification phase. The separation phase is one in which the 15 colored caps of box 8/6 and the 10 gray caps are mixed together and presented to the observer who must separate the caps into two groups: a group of caps that appear gray and a group of caps that appear colored. The classification phase has two parts. First, the observer arranges the caps appearing as gray in a row ranging from dark to bright. All observers can achieve a perfect arrangement of this set of gray caps. This part of the test allows determination of the position in the gray scale of the colored caps. Second, the observer arranges the remaining caps according to their natural color order. This procedure differs from that used in the Farnsworth Panel D-15 in that the observer chooses the starting cap, since no one cap is fixed. Further, since the classification phase follows the separation phase, there may not always be 15 colored caps remaining, although there may be some gray caps.

There are two score sheets, one for each phase of the test. For the separation phase, the errors are plotted on a circular diagram where hue is represented on the circumference and chroma as a radial distance from the center. The diagram includes four concentric rings (four chroma), each ring containing 15 compartments (for each of the 15 hues). The results of the test are expressed by penciling in the hue compartments corresponding to these colored caps wrongly placed among the grays. For the classification phase, the positions of those colored caps grouped among the grays are indicated on a diagram with hue on the abscissa and value on the ordinate. For each colored cap wrongly placed among the grays a circle is drawn at its position on the gray scale. Finally, the order of the colored caps is recorded on a diagram analogous to that of the Farnsworth Panel D-15, but with four concentric rings. At a given chroma level a line is drawn connecting colored caps placed adjacent to one another. The total procedure is then repeated for the other boxes.

INTERPRETATION

In the separation phase the colored caps grouped with gray give an indication of the neutral zone, namely, its position, its width, and its range of chroma levels. In congenital color defects (Lanthony, 1975a; 1976) the results are characteristic: the neutral zone includes hues RP (red-purple) and VB (green-blue) for protan defects, hues PR (purple-red) and V(green) for deutan defects, and hues PB (purple-blue) and J (yellow) for tritan defects. Observers with mild or moderate chromatic discrimination loss (anomalous trichromats) have neutral zones only for the low-chroma box (chroma 2). Dichromats and anomalous trichromats with moderate and severe chromatic discrimination loss show neutral zones for higher-chroma boxes. In acquired color vision defects the results are more variable (Lanthony, 1975b; 1978a).

In the classification phase, the ordering of the colored caps grouped among the grays on the gray scale may indicate relative luminosity change from the normal function. The ordering of the remaining colored caps into a natural color order is somewhat analogous to the Farnsworth Panel D-15, and the confusion axes will be similar to those of the Farnsworth Panel D-15. However, the classification is performed typically in two parts, one for each set of hues lying on either side of the observer's neutral zone. The connection between the two sides is somewhat arbitrary. If the examiner provides some gray caps among the colored caps (or if the subject has wrongly included some gray caps among them during the separation phase), the subject readily places these gray caps in the gap.

In summary, this is a new color vision test designed specifically for acquired color vision defects. The separation phase allows determination of neutral zones, according to the colored caps confused with the grays, at four saturation levels. The classification phase allows determination of relative luminosity by the position of colored caps in the gray scale and of chromatic discrimination according to the arrangement of the colored caps. A number of authors (Lanthony, 1978a; Pinckers & Baron, 1978; Pinckers, Nabbe,

& Bogaard, 1978; Pinckers, 1978a, b) are evaluating the NCT in acquired color vision disorders.

ILLUMINANTS*

The majority of the pigment tests described above were designed and standardized either for natural daylight or for CIE standard illuminant C with a correlated color temperature of 6774 K. By "natural daylight" is meant northern sky light in the northern hemisphere. The spectral distribution of natural daylight approximates that of standard illuminant C. However, the level of illuminance and the color temperature of natural daylight are not as constant as can be obtained with an artificial illuminant (Hardy, 1945). In the United States and continental Europe, standard illuminant C is typically used. An alternative source is standard illuminant D_{65}, a source with color temperature of 6504 K. This illuminant has been adopted by the British Standards Institution (1967) and is widely used in Great Britain and continental Europe.

Importance of the Illuminant

Theoretically, the importance of the illuminant is that the pigment colors will occupy different positions in the CIE chromaticity diagram (see Chapter 2) under different illuminants, i.e., their apparent color will change with the illuminant. If the figure and background colors of a given pseudoisochromatic plate fall on or near the protan or deutan isochromatic lines (see Chapter 7) under standard illuminant C, they may not fall on such isochromatic lines under other illuminants. The theoretical expectation is that the plates are most effective when test and background colors do fall on or near the isochromatic lines (Lakowski, 1966; 1969a, b). Ordinary window light is too variable in both illuminance level and spectral composition (Schmidt, 1952) to be an adequate source for color vision testing.

As a practical example of the importance of using the correct illuminant, a number of investigators (Reed, 1944; Hardy, Rand, & Rittler, 1946; Volk & Fry, 1947; Farnsworth, Reed & Shilling, 1948; Katavisto, 1961; Higgins, Moskowitz-Cook, & Knoblauch, 1978) have shown that unfiltered tungsten illuminants or illuminants with color temperatures lower than that of source C result in deutan subjects making fewer errors on pseudoisochromatic plate tests including the Ishihara, Stilling, American Optical, and AO Hardy-Rand-Rittler tests. Therefore many simple deuteranomalous observers may pass a screening test. Schmidt (1952) showed that the error percentage for normal and deutan observers continues to rise when color temperature is increased above that of standard illuminant C. As an exception, the Boström II plates are rather insensitive to illuminant (Katavisto, 1961).

For an arrangement test such as the FM 100-hue test or the Farnsworth Panel D-15, deutans may make fewer errors under incandescent illumination. In addition, protans may show axis rotation. Extreme protanomalous trichromats and protanopes show a deutan profile when tested with unfiltered tungsten illumination of color temperature 2850 K (Higgins, Moskowitz-Cook, & Knoblauch, 1978). The use of lamps simulating standard illuminant B or ordinary tungsten lamps (as illuminant A) will not give adequate results and should be discouraged.

Fluorescent tubes have also been investigated but with conflicting results. Katavisto

---

*Contributed by Joel Pokorny, Ph.D., and Vivianne C. Smith, Ph.D.

(1961) said that the Boström II and Ishihara plates (but not Stilling plates) are valid when viewed with an Airam "natural" fluorescent light. Sloan (1945) reported no difference in test results for the "Army" and "Navy" plates (selected AO plates) when viewed with a Macbeth daylight or a "daylight" fluorescent tube. Schmidt (1952) similarly suggested that the AO plates are valid when viewed under a "daylight" fluorescent. However, different fluorescent lamps vary greatly in their relative spectral energies and especially in the emissions of the line spectra (Chapter 1). Therefore test results with one fluorescent tube cannot be generalized to other or all fluorescent tubes. Ordinary commercially available fluorescent tubes are not generally appropriate for color vision testing (Farnsworth, Reed, & Shilling, 1948).

In recent years a number of high-quality fluorescent lamps have been developed especially for use in color comparison work. Richards, Tack, and Thome (1971) evaluated two U.S.-manufactured lamps, the GE Chroma 70 and the Verd-A-Ray Criticolor Fluorescent; they suggest that these lamps are comparable to the filtered tungsten of the Macbeth Easel Lamp for screening purposes.

The Freeman illuminant stable color vision test was designed as a rapid screening test that would be valid under all illuminants (Freeman, 1948; Freeman & Zaccaria, 1948). Although this concept is excellent, the test did not prove to be a successful screening test (Farnsworth, Paulsen, & Connolly, undated); it is no longer in production.

How to Obtain Illuminant C or Illuminant D_{65}

Illuminant C can be realized physically by an incandescent tungsten lamp operated at a correlated color temperature of 2854 K (source A) in conjunction with a specified liquid filter that raises its correlated color temperature to 6774 K. There are several glass filters that closely approximate the liquid filter. Some fluorescent lamps are available that have the required color temperature and good color rendition. D_{65} is obtained by filtered tungsten or fluorescent sources with correlated color temperatures of 6504 K. Table 5.4 summarizes some illuminants commercially avilable in the U.S. and Europe. Table 5.4 includes three illuminants that use a tungsten source with filters, ten fluorescent sources, and one xenon source and shows supplier and description; the correlated color temperature, the color rendering index, and the level of illumination are included for various illuminants. The color rendering index is a number that expresses how closely a test source (i.e., the particular fluorescent lamp) can reproduce color in comparison with a standard source. The standard source is either a blackbody radiator or a specified natural daylight source at the correlated color temperature of the test. The difference in reciprocal color temperature (see Chapter 1) between test and standard should not exceed 5 R. The x, y chromaticities of eight chosen Munsell chips are calculated for both the test and standard source. A statistical procedure then evaluates the distances between the two sets of CIE coordinates (Wyszecki & Stiles, 1967).

TUNGSTEN SOURCE WITH FILTERS

The spectral output of a tungsten lamp may be modified by filters to approximate standard illuminants. The filter may be placed between the source and the test material or between the test material and the observer.

The Macbeth Easel Lamp was designed for use with screening plate tests. It is a widely used illuminant in the U.S. The lamp and filter are mounted in a stand that allows source, plate test, and subject to be in correct spatial relationship. The daylight filters vary: on each is marked the correlated color temperature. These are usually close to that of standard illuminant C. The level of illumination varies with the daylight filter; a typical value is 100 lux. The daylight filter, for use with a 100-W tungsten lamp, is available separately and can be used with or without the easel stand. The Macbeth Daylight Executive, used in Europe and the U.S., consists of a metal light box providing diffuse illumination of 1850 lux. The various color tests placed in the box are viewed in correct spatial relationship to the observer.

The "color-test glasses" (Pokorny, Smith, & Trimble, 1977; Pokorny, Smith, & Lund, 1978) are a pair of color-correcting glasses designed to be used with a 200-W tungsten source. This combination provides 385 lux at a correlated color temperature of 6800 K. Crone (1961) and Higgins, Moskowitz-Cook, and Knoblauch (1978) have also described methods of using filters between observer and test material.

FLUORESCENT SOURCES

Fluorescent lamps with acceptable colorimetric properties are available from a variety of manufacturers in the U.S., Europe, and Japan. The color rendering indices (for those reported) are almost as good as those for the filtered tungsten sources or for the one filtered xenon source.

Fluorescent tubes Color 54 and Color 57 are available in Holland. Vos, Verkaik, and Boogaard (1971) evaluated and recommended the Color 57. One Color 57 tube at 1.5–1 m above table height provides 250–500 lux of 7400 K illumination; a bank of six provides 1750 lux. The Color 54 and Color 57 tubes may be used in combination. A bank of tubes using three Color 57 and one Color 55 gives a color temperature of 6460 K and color rendering index of 93. The Verivide Industrial Cabinet provides a fluorescent source giving 6500 K. This lamp is manufactured to meet the recommendation (1967) of the British Standards Institution. A number of U.S. companies manufacture fluorescents with good color rendering capabilities.

It should be noted that conventional commercially available fluorescent lamps do not have color rendering properties equivalent to those of the special lamps listed in Table 5.4. For example, a conventional commercially available daylight fluorescent lamp has a correlated color temperature of 6673 K but a color rendering index of only 76.

Level of Illumination

Very few tests specify the necessary level of illumination. The AO HRR should be viewed under 100–650 lux (Hardy, Rand, & Rittler, 1954); the FM 100-hue test and the Farnsworth Panel D-15 test should be viewed under 270 lux. The City University test is specified for 600 lux. The majority of researchers would consider 100 lux to be a minimal level for screening purposes, although Judd (quoted by Schmidt, 1952) recommended a minimal level of 215 lux. Screening test results are not affected by changes in level of illumination between 215 and 600 lux (Sloan, 1943), 108 and 650 lux (Hardy, 1945), 270 and 1076 lux (Schmidt, 1952) or 100 and 600 lux (Frey, 1964).

If the aim of the research is evaluation of color discrimination, an illuminant providing 2000 lux is preferable. Error scores on the FM 100-hue test vary with the level of illumination (Verriest, 1963). In Verriest's study the mean error score was slightly lower when the test was given under 1850 lux illumination than under 100 lux illumination; the standard deviation and highest score were similarly reduced. Thus the effect of increased illumination was improvement of error scores for those observers

Table 5.4*

Some Commercially Available Illuminants

Name and/or Description	Supplier	Correlated Color Temperature (K)	Color Rendering Index	Illumination (lux)
Tungsten sources with filters				
Macbeth Easel Lamp (with 100-W tungsten lamp and daylight filter)	Macbeth, U.S.	Various: marked on daylight filter		~ 100
Macbeth Daylight Executive	House of			1850
"Color-test glasses" (used with 200-W tungsten source)	Vision, U.S.	6800	96	385
Xenon sources				
150-W xenon arc, XBOF 6500 with one filter	Macbeth, U.S.	6580	97	
Fluorescent sources				
Fluorescent tube, Color 57, TL 57	Philips, Netherlands	7400	96	250–500
Fluorescent tube, Color 55, TL 55	Philips, Netherlands	5000	96	
Fluorescent combination, three Color 55 and one Color 77	Philips, Netherlands	6460	93	

Table 5.4 (Continued)

Name and/or Description	Supplier	Correlated Color Temperature (K)	Color Rendering Index	Illumination (lux)
Fluorescent Fl-20S	Shibaura Electric, Japan	6720	91	
Verivide Industrial	Leslie Hubble Ltd., Leicestershire, U.K.	6500	—	
Fluorescent tube, type 1416	Ch. Gamain, Paris	6500	—	1200
440 Luminaire (fluorescent), NL 6500	Macbeth, U.S.	6720	91	
Fluorescent Macbeth, NL 6500 — $F_{40}T_{12}$	Macbeth, U.S.	6710	90	
Chroma 75, $F_{15}T8$ C75	General Electric, U.S.	7500	94	
Criticolor fluorescent, $F_{15}T8$/CC	Verd-A-Ray, U.S.	5700	91	
Verilux daylight, $F_{15}T8$ VLX	Verilux, U.S.	6200	94	

*Data on which this table was based were in part suplied by Professor J. D. Moreland, University of Waterloo, Ontario, Canada.

whose chromatic discrimination was below average at the lower level of illumination specified. The Verriest age norms (Table 5.3) are for 100 lux. Lower norms would be expected with 1850 lux illumination. With reduction in illumination below 100 lux, Verriest, Buyssens, and Vanderdonck (1963) noted increasing error scores that showed first a blue–yellow axis at an illumination of 15 lux and then a scotopic axis as illumination was further reduced in the range of 0.04–0.2 lux.

Arrangement of Observer, Test, and Illuminant

The observer, test material, and illuminant should be arranged to allow a comfortable position during test performance. The observer is seated at a desk or table. The illuminant should be mounted above the test material and adjusted to provide even and direct illumination. The distance of the illuminant from the material determines the level of illuminance and the area of illumination (Chapter 1). The test material should be angled to be approximately perpendicular to the observer's line of regard to avoid glare or gloss (Chapter 1). Plate tests should be presented at a distance of about 0.75 m. Arrangement tests are presented at a distance comfortable for manipulation (about 0.5 m).

ANOMALOSCOPES*

An anomaloscope is an instrument designed to evaluate specialized color matches and diagnose color defect in a large population. As described in Chapter 2, normal observers can match all hues by appropriate adjustment of three primary lights. Usually, the test color and one primary are matched to the mixture of the remaining two primaries. Hence normal observers are known as trichromats. Different normal trichromats will use slightly different amounts of the primaries to match various hues, but it is the general similarities rather than the comparatively small differences among normal observers that allow us to classify an observer whose color vision we are evaluating as either normal or abnormal. In order to define normal trichromacy and diagnose color defect, there are special color matches (typically called equations) that make use of only two primaries. These matches are relatively quick and easy to perform compared with full-spectrum color matching (which requires three primaries). Full-spectrum color matching has not been performed in the general population, but there are many studies of large population samples using the anomaloscope.

Equations Measured by the Anomaloscope

The use of color matching to establish an abnormality of color vision dates to Lord Rayleigh's (1881) discovery that the color match of a yellow test light to a mixture of green and red primary lights distinguishes variations of color vision and allows diagnosis of congenital red–green color defects. Subsequently, a match or equation for evaluation of congenital blue–yellow defects was derived. This was the Engelking equation, the match of a blue-green test to a mixture of blue and green primary lights (Engelking, 1925), also called the Trendelenburg equation (Trendelenburg, 1941a). Moreland and Kerr (1978) recently optimized the match for tritanomalous vision with a modification of the Engelking-Trendelenburg equation. Pickford and Lakowski (1960) suggested the match of a white test to a mixture of blue and yellow primary lights. This Pickford-Lakowski equation has had special application in acquired color vision defects.

---

*Contributed by Joel Pokorny, Ph.D., and Vivianne C. Smith, Ph.D.

RAYLEIGH EQUATION

The Rayleigh equation involves matching a spectral (or nearly spectral) yellow light to a mixture of spectral (or nearly spectral) red and green lights. Although only two primaries are used, a perfect match occurs. The primaries and test light occur at wavelengths to which the SWS photopigment (Chapter 3) is not sensitive. Since only two photopigments (MWS and LWS) are active, only two primaries are required. The Rayleigh equation differentiates normal trichromats from observers with all types of congenital red–green color defect and allows classification of congenital red–green color defects.

The original test and primary lights used by Lord Rayleigh (1881) were spectral lights obtained by a spectroscope. The test light was at the sodium line (589 nm); the primary lights were at the thallium (535 nm) and lithium (670 nm) lines. In practice, however, the range of choices for primary wavelengths and the spectral purity of the lights has been wide. Although most anomaloscopes use relatively narrow-band radiations, the Rayleigh equation has been evaluated with colored papers on rotating wheels (Collins, 1929; Pickford, 1951).

It is desirable that the red and green primaries should be well separated. Willis and Farnsworth (1952) evaluated five anomaloscopes (including the Nagel model II, the Hecht-Shlaer, the Bausch and Lomb, double wedge, double dichroic Polaroid, and Dimmick single wedge) in which the dominant wavelength of the yellow test light varied from 577 to 589 nm and the dominant wavelengths of the primary lights ranged from 530 to 574 nm for the green primary light and from 605 to 670 nm for the red primary light, giving wavelength separations of 31–134 nm. Willis and Farnsworth (1952) noted that these anomaloscopes differed in their efficiencies of diagnosis, the best results occurring for the instruments in which the wavelength separation of green and red primaries was greatest (for example, the Nagel model II).

In practice, the choice of the red primary should be as far as possible to the deep red, provided the energy is sufficient to give a photopic field luminance (at least 3 cd m^{-2}). When spectral lights are used, the wavelength of the green primary should be chosen so that its x, y coordinates in the CIE diagram will lie on the linear portion of the spectrum locus, i.e., dominant wavelength above 540 nm (see Chapter 2). This is necessary so that the mixture field will not appear paler or desaturated compared with the spectral test field. If broadband stimuli are used—for example, gelatin filters—the green primary will typically have lower purity than the red primary and the mixture will have lower purity than the test field. In this case it may be necessary to desaturate the yellow test field (by adding white light) so that the x, y coordinates of the test light fall on the line joining the x, y coordinates of the primary lights (i.e., the test and primary lights are collinear; see Chapter 2). Pickford and Lakowski (1960) used such a desaturation in setting up the Rayleigh equation on the Pickford-Nicolson anomaloscope.

In summary, a wavelength near 545–555 nm is a good choice for the green primary and a wavelength above 640 nm will be adequate for the red primary. The main consideration in the choice of a wavelength for the yellow test field is to optimize wavelength discrimination so that matching ranges for normal trichromats will be narrow, giving a range of 585–600 nm for the yellow test field. In practice, the wavelength is usually near the sodium line at 589 nm.

The field luminance must be in the photopic range, i.e., above several cd m^{-2}. For diagnosis of congenital red–green defect, the size of the field of view should be between

1° and 2°. If the field of view exceeds 2°, the majority of dichromats will not accept a full range of matches (Smith & Pokorny, 1977), but with test fields below 1°, anomalous trichromats have broadened matching ranges and may appear to be dichromats. There is an advantage of having large fields of view (5°– 10°) available when the Rayleigh equation is evaluated in acquired color vision defects, as in pseudoprotanomaly (Smith, Pokorny, & Diddie, 1978).

The x, y, coordinates (Chapter 2) of the Rayleigh equation primary lights may be calculated for the two anomaloscopes in commercial production, the Nagel model I and the Pickford-Nicolson (Fig. 5.4). The Nagel primary lights lie on the linear portion of the spectrum locus and will therefore lie on the confusion lines of red–green dichromats, protanopes, and deuteranopes (Chapter 7). The meaning of the confusion line is that the dichromat can exactly match any colors on the line provided radiance adjustment of the yellow test field is allowed. Dichromats can match the yellow test field to either primary or to any mixture. The diagnosis of dichromacy hinges on this behavior. In the Pickford-Nicolson anomaloscope the primaries are desaturated but are collinear with the test field, allowing normal trichromats to make perfect matches. The x, y coordinates of

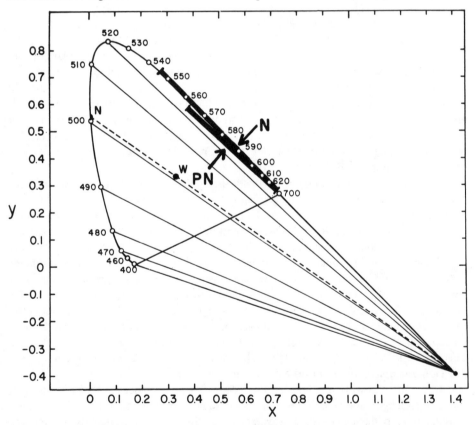

Fig. 5.4. Location of the x, y coordinates in the 1931 CIE diagram for primaries and test lights for the Rayleigh match on the Nagel model I (N) and the Pickford-Nicolson (PN) anomaloscopes. Deuteranopic confusion lines are shown for comparison. The primaries for the Nagel lie on the spectrum locus and will fall on confusion lines of protanopes and deuteranopes. The green primary of the Pickford-Nicolson is desaturated, and the primary mixtures do not coincide with the theoretical deuteranope confusion lines.

primaries and test field coincide with a protanopic confusion line but do not coincide precisely with a deuteranopic confusion line. Theoretically, some deuteranopes may not be diagnosed on the Pickford-Nicolson (i.e., they might be classified as extreme deuteranomalous trichromats), although no comparative data are available.

ENGELKING-TRENDELENBURG EQUATION

The Engelking-Trendelenburg equation is the match of a blue-green (or blue) test field to a mixture of blue (or blue-violet) and green primary lights. Engelking (1925) originally proposed this match for the investigation of congenital blue–yellow defects. The match is not as successful as the Rayleigh match. In the Engelking match, all three visual photopigments are stimulated by test and primary lights. The x, y coordinates of test and primary lights are not collinear, and the test field appears more saturated (higher in purity) than the mixture field. A perfect match is not obtained unless the instrument allows the addition of white light to the test field. Further, if the luminance of the short-wavelength (blue or violet) primary is low relative to that of the green primary, both normal and anomalous matches are forced toward the blue primary. Finally, the large variability in lens and macular pigment density among normal trichromats results in a large range of matches in this spectral region. An abnormal match, indicative of tritanomalous vision (anomalous blue–yellow vision), is not therefore easily defined.

The original wavelengths for the Engelking equation included a test wavelength of 490 nm and primaries of 470 nm and 517 nm (Engelking, 1925). Trendelenburg developed the Engelking equation in a "tritoscope" (1941a), which included the desaturation of the blue-green test field. The match is also known as the Trendelenburg equation. Other workers have used differing test and primaries. Crone (1955; 1956) used a desaturated 480 nm test matched to a mixture of 455 nm and 513 nm primary lights. Pickford and Lakowski (1960) used a broadband filter in the Pickford-Nicolson anomaloscope giving a green test light (496 nm with excitation purity of 0.43) matched to a yellow-green (555 nm, 0.717 excitation purity) plus a blue (470 nm, 0.937 excitation purity). The x, y coordinates of these various matches are shown in Fig. 5.5 compared with tritan confusion lines (see Chapter 7). The various equations do not lie on tritan confusion lines. Therefore the equation may not distinguish tritanopes who have a dichromatic form of blue–yellow defect from incomplete tritanopes who have a trichromatic form of blue–yellow defect. Tritanopic observers will probably not accept a full range of matches. The Engelking-Trendelenburg equation was available in the Nagel model II anomaloscope but not in the Nagel model I anomaloscope, the model currently in commercial production. Pickford's adaptation of the Engleking-Trendelenburg equation is available in the Pickford-Nicolson anomaloscope. Norms were published by Pickford and Lakowski (1960) and Lakowski (1971), but the match is not widely used.

MORELAND EQUATION

Moreland (1972; Moreland & Young, 1976; Moreland & Kerr, 1978; Moreland, 1978) has developed a three-primary color-match equation for tritan defect that allows a perfect match and minimizes the effect of macular pigment. Lens changes due to age, however, need to be taken into account (Moreland, 1978). This equation is

$$a\,579\ \text{nm} + b\,480\ \text{nm} \equiv c\,439\ \text{nm} + d\,499\ \text{nm}. \qquad (5.1)$$

The equation may prove useful in defining tritanomalous observers. However, the primary_

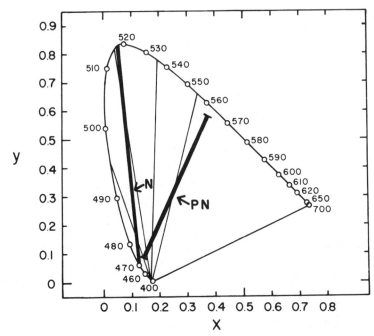

Fig. 5.5. Location of *x, y* coordinates in the 1931 CIE diagram for the primary and test lights for the Engelking-Trendelenburg equation on the Nagel model II (N) and the Pickford-Nicolson (PN) anomaloscopes. Tritanopic confusion lines are shown for comparison. The primary mixtures do not fall on the tritan confusion lines.

wavelengths, 499 and 439 nm, do not lie on a confusion line for tritanopes, and this equation may not be helpful in diagnosis of tritanopia.

The use of a three-primary color match is a genuine disadvantage. However, Moreland and Kerr (1978) suggest that it is possible to use a fixed ratio of 480 and 579 nm (i.e., fixed desaturation of the 480 nm test field), making the anomaloscope a two-variable instrument, as is true for the Trendelenburg (1941a) and Pickford-Lakowski (1960) equations.

PICKFORD-LAKOWSKI EQUATION

A match available in some anomaloscopes, e.g., the Pickford-Nicolson anomaloscope, is the match of a white test light to a mixture of blue and yellow primary lights. This match was originally used to evaluate the yellowing of the eye lens with age but has also proved useful in evaluating acquired color vision defects resulting from eye disease.

The match was suggested by Lakowski (Pickford, 1968), and Pickford and Lakowski (1960) and Lakowski (1971a) presented normal data for the match. The primaries are obtained from colored filters. For the blue primary the dominant wavelength is 470 nm with excitation purity of 0.937 (see Chapter 1); for the yellow primary the dominant wavelength is 585 nm with excitation purity of 0.955 (Fig. 5.6). The white test field is similar to standard illuminant A.

For evaluation of acquired color vision defects, the relevant statistic for the Pickford-Lakowski equation is the matching range. The matching range increases with age of the observer. For age-matched comparisons, ranges are larger for observers with

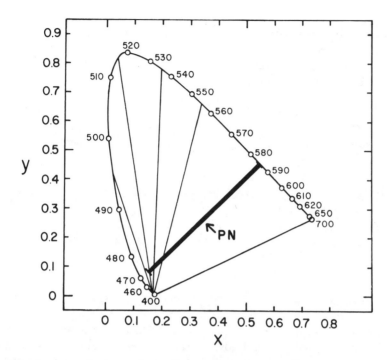

Fig. 5.6. Location of x, y coordinates in the 1931 CIE diagram for primary and test lights for the Pickford-Lakowski equation on the Pickford-Nicolson anomaloscope. Tritanopic confusion lines are shown for comparison. The primary mixtures do not coincide with the theoretical tritan confusion lines.

acquired color vision defects—for example, patients with macular degenerations or retinitis pigmentosa—than for normal observers (Lakowski, 1972). The equation does not lie on a tritan confusion line (Fig. 5.6) and may not be helpful in diagnosis of tritanopia, since a tritanope will not accept a full range of matches.

Treatment of the Data

Modern anomaloscopes are designed so that the manipulations required to obtain a metameric match are as simple as possible. Rather than having independent control of the radiances of the primaries as in most colorimeters, a single knob is used to vary the ratio of the primaries; as the radiant flux of one primary is increased, the flux of the second primary is decreased proportionally. As a result of this arrangement, the choice of the radiances for the primaries is important in the design of the anomaloscope. The second knob on an anomaloscope controls the radiant flux of the test field.

In full-spectrum color matching the primary energies are independently varied, and the primary energies are expressed in units of radiometric energy, photometric energy, coloring power, or as proportions of the various primaries (see Chapter 2)—units requiring precise calibration procedures. In anomaloscope matches, the primary ratio data are typically expressed relative to a normal observer's match (or mean normal match), obviating the need for precise calibration of the exact ratios or flux of the primary and test lights.

SCALE UNITS

The anomaloscope contains two scales from which may be read a number proportional to the primary ratio in the mixture field and a number proportional to the radiance of the test color. The scales that appear on the instrument are quite arbitrary, reflecting the whim of the manufacturer. For example, in the Nagel model I anomaloscope the red–green mixture scale (arbitrary divisions) goes from 0 at green to 73 at red and the yellow scale goes from 0 (dark) to 80. On the Pickford-Nicolson anomaloscope (Pickford & Lakowski, 1960) the red–green mixture scale is 0 at red and 80 at green. In testing an observer the examiner notes the scale values; these are then available for further transformation or comparison.

There are two statistics for the primary ratio: the range and the midpoint of the matches. In the case of the Rayleigh equation, the matching range comprises all the scale values on the red–green mixture scale that a given observer says match the yellow. A third statistic is also noted, the scale value indicating the value of the yellow scale. This scale value is used to evaluate relative luminosity losses of color-defective observers.

THE ANOMALOUS QUOTIENT

The anomalous quotient is a common method of presenting the midpoint of the red–green equation. The quotient was introduced by Trendelenburg (1929) as a technique for compensating for minor changes in line voltage and bulb aging. It involves calculation of the individual observer's match relative to that of another observer (or to the mean of many observers). The anomalous quotient for observer X relative to a group of normal observers is defined as

$$\frac{\text{Amount green}}{\text{Amount red}} \text{ for observer } X \div \frac{\text{Amount green}}{\text{Amount red}} \text{ for the group.} \qquad (5.2)$$

In the Nagel model I anomaloscope, for example, the mixture knob tells us how much red is in the match. At 0 the field is pure green and at 73 the field is pure red. Suppose for a group of 50 normal trichromats the average match midpoint is 45 on the mixture scale. This means that 45 is the amount of red. To obtain the amount of green, subtract 45 from 73 and find 28 as the amount of green. The ratio 28/45 is the green red ratio for the normal sample. A new observer with a match midpoint at 43 then has a green–red ratio of 30/43. To find this observer's anomalous quotient, divide the green–red ratio by the green–red ratio for the normal sample, obtaining (30/43) ÷ (28/45), or 1.12. Anomalous quotients for normal trichromats fall between about 0.74 and 1.33. Anomalous quotients may be used to compare data from different laboratories provided that the identical set of primaries is used in both laboratories. Calculation of the anomalous quotient is meaningless when matching range is large, as occurs in many color-defective observers.

A slide rule for rapid calculation of anomalous quotients (AQ) (Anomalquotientrechenschieber) is manufactured by Schmidt and Haensch. Hallden (1959) published a nomogram for easy calculation of the AQ.

COMPARATIVE SCALE UNITS (CSU)

An alternative to calculation of the anomalous quotient is to convert the anomaloscope raw scale units to comparative scale units (Willis & Farnsworth, 1952).

Comparative scale units range from 0 at the green primary to 100 at the red primary, with the normal match at 50. The equation to convert to comparative scale units is

$$\frac{\text{Raw score} \times \text{correction factor}}{(\text{Raw score} \times \text{correction factor}) + (\text{maximum score} - \text{raw score})} \qquad (5.3)$$

provided that the scale is adjusted to go from zero at green primary to maximum at the red primary. The correction factor is the ratio of raw score units of green to raw score units of red at the normal match. Thus in the Nagel model I anomaloscope with range of 0–73 and normal match at 45, we take 45 as the amount red and 73–45 or 28 as the amount green, giving a correction factor of 28/45 or 0.62. A raw score of 45 converts to 50 CSU. This conversion does allow comparison of matching ranges of observers with wide ranges. The CSU preserves the anomalous quotient (i.e., anomalous quotients will be identical when calculated from CSUs as from raw scores). Data from different instruments should be compared only provided that primary and test wavelengths are identical. The CSU conversion has not been widely used.

STATISTICAL UNITS

An alternative method of expressing the equation of a given observer relative to that of a population of normal observers is to use the statistical properties of the distribution of match midpoints made by normal observers (Pickford, 1957). For the Pickford-Nicolson anomaloscope, midmatching points (expressed as R/G ratios) of a population of normal observers show a normal (symmetrical peaked) distribution (Fig. 5.7). Such a distribution is characterized by its mean and standard deviation. A way of expressing deviation from the mean value is to define what is termed the normal deviate or z score,

$$z = \frac{x - \mu}{\sigma}, \qquad (5.4)$$

where x is the scale value of a given observer, μ is the mean scale value of the population, and σ is the standard deviation of the normal population. Using tables available in standard statistics textbooks, it is possible to estimate with what frequency any match (or a more deviant match) would be expected to occur as a variant of the originally sampled normal population.

The matching width data for the Pickford-Nicolson anomaloscope have a skewed distribution. Pickford (1957) suggested that these be characterized by their modal (most frequently occurring) value and data expressed in terms of the mode. Lakowski (1971) suggested that percentiles (observed frequency/total $\times$ 100) could be used.

JND UNITS

Finally, the midpoint and matching range may be plotted on the 1931 x, y chromaticity diagram and the data further transformed into one of the CIE's uniform color spaces to give data expressed as just noticeable differences (jnd units) in the uniform color space (Lakowski, 1965a). Lakowski (1965a; 1971) performed this transformation using the CIE 1960 uniform color space (Chapter 2). The idea is a good one, since observers may be directly compared no matter what primaries and test lights were used; however, the calculation requires calibration of the anomaloscope onto the jnd scale. Results should

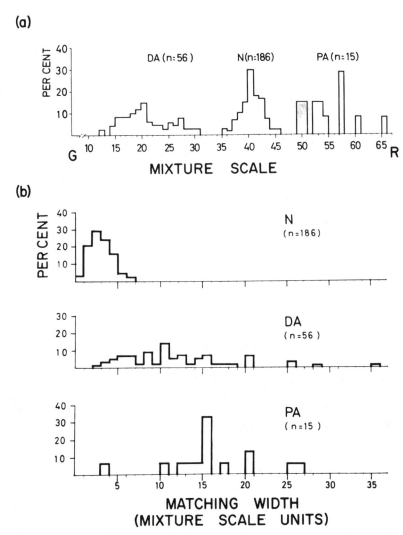

Fig. 5.7. Norms for the Nagel model I anomaloscope. (a) Histogram showing the percentage distributions of the midmatching points among the deuteranomalous (DA), normal (N), and protanomalous (PA) subjects (years of age). (b) Histograms showing the percentage distribution of the matching ranges among the normal (N), deuteranomalous (DA), and protanomalous (PA) subjects. The results refer to measurements made with the eye conditioned to white light. [From Helve, J., *Acta Ophthalmologica (Suppl.),* 1972, *114:*1–50 (reproduced with permission of Acta Ophthalmologica).]

be considered approximate, since there is a lack of agreement among colorimetrists as to the best color space to use.

Testing Procedures

Evaluation of an anomaloscope equation is a complex procedure requiring a skilled examiner who is trained in psychophysical techniques. It is easiest if the examiner understands the principles of colorimetry (Chapter 2). An untrained person can be given a set of steps to follow, but the examination will be time consuming and an occasional observer may prove too difficult to test. It is very helpful to perform a screening test beforehand to ascertain whether or not a congenital red–green defect exists.

The customary psychophysical procedure in colorimetry is the method of adjustment. The observer has control of the radiances of the primaries and adjusts them for an exact color match across the colorimetric field. Matches may be repeated to obtain a good estimate of the average match and its variance. In anomaloscope testing, the examiner usually makes all primary ratio adjustments, asking the observer for a verbal judgment; the self-adjustment method is rarely used. There are a number of reasons for this difference of procedures. First, anomaloscopes are primarily used with naive observers when a rapid evaluation of a specific equation is required. Many naive observers and especially color-defective observers do not at first understand how the color fields are changing as the knobs change; such observers are slow at setting a color match. In comparison, in the colorimetry laboratory the majority of observers are skilled, have normal color vision, and understand the principle of the equipment. For such an observer the method of adjustment is both economical and precise. Second, the anomaloscope has only two control features, the primary mixture ratio and the test radiance. It is therefore quite simple for the examiner to set the primary mixture control, to vary (or to allow the observer to vary) the test luminance, and to simply ask the observer, "Is this a color match?" This technique allows the investigator to establish the full range of primary mixtures that are acceptable (the matching range).

There are a variety of clinical procedures used for anomaloscope evaluation. Linksz (1964) has detailed a procedure for use with the Nagel anomaloscope. The Linksz (1964) procedure was primarily developed from Trendelenburg's (1929) methods of anomaloscope evaluation. Pickford (1951; 1957) and Pickford and Lakowski (1960) have detailed a procedure for use with the Pickford-Nicolson anomaloscope. The complete range of matching scale values is evaluated. It is inappropriate to characterize an observer by a single match; all experienced examiners agree that the full matching range must be evaluated.

LINKSZ PROCEDURE FOR THE NAGEL ANOMALOSCOPE

In the Linksz procedure the examination starts with a 3-min preadaptation to the lighted Trendelenburg screen on the front panel of the Nagel model I. The screen is extinguished and the observer is presented with a normal match prepared by the examiner in advance. If asked to comment on the color appearance, the normal or dichromat will say they look the same or are shades of the same color. The anomalous trichromat will say that the mixture field appears red (deuteranomalous trichromat) or green (protanomalous trichromat). At this point, some examiners allow the observer to use both red–green and yellow controls to adjust the two fields to equality.

If the normal match is accepted, or one close to it, the next step is to evaluate the range of acceptable values. For a normal observer this will be small (0–5 scale units). The examiner turns the red–green mixture ±5 scale units from the match and, alternating from +5 to −5 in 1-unit steps centers in toward the match, asking, "Is this a match?" on each trial. The observer (or examiner) will make minor adjustments of the yellow test knob if necessary. In the Nagel model I anomaloscope, the luminance of the primary lights is approximately equal for normal and deutan observers. The red–green knob changes only the hue of the mixture field for a normal trichromat. The 3 or 4 scale units that constitute the usual normal range are quickly established. For a dichromat a full range of red–green mixtures is acceptable; for an extreme anomalous trichromat a very wide range is acceptable. For these observers the examiner turns the red–green mixture knob to 0 and then to 73, and then alternates in 10-unit steps. The observer (or examiner) adjusts the yellow radiance knob. Deuteranopes and extreme deuteranomalous trichromats usually make minimal adjustments with the yellow knob on the Nagel anomaloscope, leaving it near the setting made by a normal observer (i.e., around 15). Protanopes and extreme protanomalous trichromats set the yellow control to high numbers (35–40) at the green end (0) on the mixture scale and low numbers (0–5) at the red end (near 73) of the mixture scale (see Chapter 7). When testing large ranges it is necessary to ask the observer to readapt to the Trendelenburg screen after each setting and to remind the observer not to stare at the match for more than a few seconds.

If the normal range was not accepted, the observer is an anomalous trichromat. Based on the color report at the normal match, the observer or examiner moves the red–green mixture into the appropriate range. The red–green matching range is then examined in a systematic way as described above. It is important to remind the observer not to stare at a match for more than 2–3 sec and to readapt after every setting. The obtained range of settings is the match range under neutral adaptation *(Neutralstimmung)*.

Following this procedure, Linksz recommends the so-called tuning procedure, in which the observer stares at his or her own color match for 15 sec *(Umstimmung)*. The examiner then again examines the matching range, asking, "Is this a match?" to establish a new tuned matching range (range under *Umstimmung)*. Normal trichromats do not usually show a widened range; those that do have been termed Farbenasthenopie in the German literature (Chapter 7). Some simple anomalous trichromats show a minor amount of tuning. Extreme anomalous trichromats, as defined by Trendelenburg and Schmidt (1935) (see Chapter 7), do show a widened tuning range that may enlarge to include one or even both primaries.

The midmatching points of the range are calculated, and these may be converted to anomalous quotients. Many laboratories simply report the scale units, including the usual normal range.

PICKFORD-LAKOWSKI PROCEDURE

The observer sits about 1 meter from the screen, which should be at eye level. A preliminary screening with a plate test is recommended so that the examiner knows if the observer does have a color defect. One eye is tested at a time. All manipulations of the anomaloscope are performed by the examiner. The test starts with presentation of a normal match, and the test luminance is adjusted if necessary. The observer reports on the field appearance. As with the Linksz procedure the responses indicate the examiner's next steps. In the Rayleigh equation a response of "equal" or "close" suggests a normal trichromat or dichromat; a response of mixture field "green" suggests a protanomalous trichromat; a response of mixture field "red" suggests a deuteranomalous trichromat. If the normal match was accepted or close, the matching range is examined using the method of limits. For the normal trichromat, the examiner moves in 1-unit steps. Starting with a mixture that is definitely not a match (e.g., mixture too "orange"), the examiner moves toward the match in 1-unit steps until "match" is reported. Then, starting from a "match" position, the examiner moves back toward the "no match" position. Three or four such runs are made at each end of the matching range. For the dichromat, the full red–green range is examined in larger (10-unit) steps. The examiner must adjust the yellow test field luminance at each red–green mixture. In the Pickford-Nicolson anomaloscope, the luminance of the red primary is greater than that of the green primary. To the normal observer, the mixture field changes in both hue and luminance as the knob is varied. Adjustment of the radiance of the yellow test field on each trial is needed for both protanopes and deuteranopes. For the anomalous trichromat, large steps on the red–green scale are used to establish the gross range of anomalous settings. The ends of the matching range are then established using small steps and the method of limits as described for normal trichromats.

The Engelking-Trendelenburg equation is examined in a similar manner. In evaluation of the Pickford-Ląkowski equation, the matching range is the statistic of importance. Examination of the matching range is obtained using the method of limits as described for the Rayleigh match. The equation is primarily for acquired color vision defects. In congenital tritan defect, the dichromat may not necessarily accept the full matching range on either Engelking-Trendelenburg or Pickford-Lakowski equations.

The scale units may be reported as is or may be converted to statistical or jnd units.

PRACTICAL ASPECTS OF ANOMALOSCOPE TESTING

There are a number of features of anomaloscope testing that deserve emphasis. These include initial setting of norms for the instrument, the use of color names, and the use of the Trendelenburg adaptation screen.

Establishing norms. When an anomaloscope is purchased or introduced into a laboratory or clinic, the first step is to establish norms for the instrument. Matching ranges are established for all of the normal observers who are working in the laboratory or clinic; others may be invited also to participate. Such an informal set of norms will probably serve to establish a clinical norm for the Rayleigh equation. A more formal survey with matched age groups will be necessary for the Pickford-Lakowski equation. Once norms are established, the examiner is better equipped to deal with occasional "peculiar" matches.

In the Rayleigh equation, the yellow luminance settings accepted by congenital red–green defectives and by achromats are characteristic and diagnostic of the defect. Graphs showing the yellow test settings on the Nagel model I anomaloscope as a function of red–green mixture are shown in Chapter 7 (Figs. 7.17 and 7.20). It is important for the examiner to obtain the appropriate normative information on dichromats and achromats so that the characteristic settings are easily recognized. The examiner should be alert to the occasional patient who sets or accepts "impossible" luminance settings, e.g., turning the yellow test to very high levels to match the red primary and then claiming a color match exists. This type of behavior can occur with children and is indicative of poor attention or cooperation.

Using color names. Both normal and color-defective observers can and do use color names reliably. However, caution is in order. The examiner should let observers use their own terminologies and should not tell observers what the colors are. For example, if the green primary and yellow test are presented in a Rayleigh match, the examiner should not ask, "Do you see the green on the top and the yellow on the bottom?" but "What color do you see on the bottom?" There are two reasons for this practice. First, normal trichromats may see the Rayleigh test field as orange or yellow-orange. Introducing a color term to a normal (or anomalous) trichromat may involve the unwary examiner in an unnecessary argument about color terminology. Second, the dichromat may not see these two colors but may see the color pair as green and red, or yellow and red, or as the same color and may be perturbed or confused by the examiner's assertion.

Color terms used by dichromats and many anomalous trichromats depend on the luminance relation between the two halves of the field. In the Rayleigh equation a protanope may see a dim test field as red but if the radiance is raised may say, "Now the red has switched sides." Reports such as these indicate improper luminance relations. The skilled examiner can make use of such reports to set a proper luminance balance. If such reports occur, the yellow test luminance should be carefully checked *before* the red–green scale is changed. Thus color names can be very helpful to the examiner in abbreviating the testing procedure.

The Trendelenburg screen.   The Trendelenburg adaptation screen was proposed by Drescher and Trendelenburg (1926) to allow the observer to maintain a neutral state of adaptation during testing with the Nagel anomaloscope. The Trendelenburg screen is not used during testing with the Pickford-Nicolson anomaloscope. The difference is essentially that the Nagel uses telescope-view mode and the Pickford-Nicolson uses direct-view mode. With the Nagel the observer places an eye at the aperture and stares down the tube. The color fields appear in a dark surround, and the observer adapts to the stimulus array. With the Pickford-Nicolson, the observer is in a lighted room and remains adapted to the ambient illumination. Using the Nagel anomaloscope, matches of normal trichromats are not usually affected by the state of chromatic adaptation (see Chapter 7 for a description of minor color abnormalities). However, matching ranges of color-defective observers are affected by adaptation state. If a careful examination of the R–G matching range is required using a Nagel anomaloscope, the Trendelenburg screen should be used.

Types of Anomaloscopes

There are a multitude of anomaloscope designs. In the modern anomaloscope the primary and test lights are obtained either by using prisms to select narrow radiation bands from a white light source or by using colored filters. There have been many designs of anomaloscopes, and many researchers construct their own instrument. The design and manufacture of an anomaloscope is sufficiently complex that few models are available commercially; of the five anomaloscopes surveyed by Willis and Farnsworth (1952), none are available today.

The concept of a clinical instrument specifically designed to detect color-matching abnormality dates to Nagel's (1907b) design, which used a direct-view spectroscope to isolate the three wavelength bands used by Lord Rayleigh. Nagel (1907b) termed the instrument "an anomaloscope." The model II Nagel anomaloscope had adjustments to select test and primary wavelengths, and there was a set of apertures to control field size. It was possible to set up the Engelking-Trendelenburg equation in addition to the Rayleigh equation. The problems with the Engelking-Trendelenburg equation led to its discontinuance. The modern version of the Nagel (model I) has only the Rayleigh equation and no field size variation beyond that occurring when field of focus is adjusted. The Trendelenburg adapation screen is an integral part of the instrument. The only other anomaloscope in commercial production currently is the Pickford-Nicolson anomaloscope, which uses broadband filters. There are three equations available, the Rayleigh equation, an equation similar to the Engelking-Trendelenburg equation, and the Pickford-Lakowski equation. Field size can be varied, and the instrument is direct view rather than telescopic view. The direct-view mode is easier to use with children and with persons with reduced visual acuity.

A filter anomaloscope made in the U.S.S.R. (the AN-59 anomaloscope) has been described by Rautian 1961) and Mailáth (1972). Recently, there has been interest in new designs for a reasonably priced and versatile anomaloscope. Prototypes have been described by Eichengreen (1974), Roth, Renand, and Víenot (1974), Moreland and Young (1974), and Piantanida (1976). One of the best of the designs appears to be the Moreland Universal Anomaloscope, of which six have been manufactured as of this writing. The Moreland design incorporates narrow-band radiations using interference filters, variation in field size, and a wide array of possible equations.

THE NAGEL MODEL I ANOMALOSCOPE

The Nagel model I anomaloscope was designed to measure the Rayleigh equation in the general population. The Nagel anomaloscope is a constant-deviation spectroscope employing three entrance slits to select primary and test wavelengths. The instrument presents to the observer a ciruclar bipartite field. In the currently distributed instrument, the spectral yellow (589 nm) appears in the lower half-field. The radiance of the yellow half-field can be varied by means of a knob located on the right-hand side of the anomaloscope. A scale visible to the examiner indicates the radiance setting of the yellow. When this knob is adjusted, the yellow half of the field varies from dark at scale 0 to increasingly brighter yellows as the scale increases to a maximum of 80. The upper half of the field is filled with the spectral green (545 nm) and the spectral red (670nm) primary lights. The relative proportions of green and red, from all green through any mixture to all red, can be continuously adjusted by a knob on the left-hand side of the anomalscope. A scale visible to the examiner indicates the position of the red–green setting. At scale 0 the upper field appears all green (only spectral green present); as the knob is adjusted to higher numbers (increasing proportion of red to green primary in the mixture) the upper field changes continuously in appearance for the color-normal observer from green to greenish yellow, yellow, orange, and , finally, red at knob value 73 (only spectral red present). A normal observer can achieve a good color match between the two halves of the field by adjusting the red– green knob and the yellow luminance knob. The calibration is set at the factory; the normal match usually occurs between 40 and 50 units of red and 15 of yellow.

Features of the anomaloscope are summarized in Table 5.5. The primary and test wavelengths are narrow-band radiation of high spectral purity that are specified by their peak wavelengths and half-widths (Chapter 1). The peak wavelengths are 589 nm for the yellow test field, 545 nm for the green primary, and 670 nm for the red primary, although there may be minor variation from one instrument to another. A spectroscope may be used to check the wavelength bands. The half-width pass bands (Chapter 1) range from 6.5 to 16 nm (Pokorny, Moreland, & Smith, 1975). At the normal match the field luminance is approximately 5 cd m^{-2}. The red and green primary lights have approximately equal luminance. The observer views the bipartite field through a telescope view. A focusing barrel on the telescope tube allows for minor adjustments. These are accompanied by a 10 percent variation in the field size. The field size in the Nagel ranges from 1.8° to 2°. On the front panel below the telescope tube is Trendelenburg adapting field to present a uniform adapting field (illuminant A). The test should be run in darkness or semidarkness.

There is a booklet distributed by the manufacturer, Haag and Streit, that describes the apparatus and the testing procedure (written by Linksz). For clinical screening purposes the data are expressed as anomalous quotients. For theoretical purposes it may be necessary to perform a precise calibration of a given insturment. The amount of yellow test field and the ratio of green to red primary fields are achieved by moving slits in the optical path. The slit mechanisms are quite delicate and will slip if the instrument is

Table 5.5
Summary of Nagel Features*

	Nominal (nm)	Calibrated (nm)
Primaries†	545	537 (6.5)
	670	666 (16)
	589	589 (9)

Instrument scale reading at normal match
Mixture scale: 40–47
Test scale: 13–18
Field luminance: 2–5 cd m^{-2}
Field size: 1.8°–2° (depending on focus)

*Current production model.

†Peak wavelength and half-width are given for the relative energy output of each narrow radiation band (calibration reported by Pokorny, Moreland, & Smith, 1975). See Chapter 1 for definitions.

handled roughly. The Nagel anomaloscope should be placed where it will not be disturbed. If the slits are displaced, the midmatch position and/or yellow brightness setting will vary. The anomalous quotient may still be used, but it may not be valid to compare the data to those of other instruments, since the spectral distribution of the primaries may have been affected.

Anomaloscope data on observers with normal color vision were reported by Willis and Farnsworth (1952) and Schmidt (1955b) for the Nagel model II anomaloscope and by Helve (1972a) for the Nagle model I anomaloscope.

Norms for the Nagel Model I anomaloscope.   Helve (1972a) tested 186 normal observers selected from 1200 conscripts (median age 21–22 years). Matching ranges and midmatching points were evaluated under neutral adaptation. The distributions of matching ranges and midmatching points are shown in Fig. 5.7, where the percentage distributions are shown for raw scale units. The distribution of matching ranges is skewed with a modal value at 3 scale units. The distribution of midmatching points is peaked and symmetrical with a mean value near 40 scale units. Similar data are shown for deuteranomalous and protanomalous trichromats for comparison. The diagnosis of anomalous trichromacy and some theoretical aspects of the midpoint and matching ranges are discussed in Chapter 7.

When converted to anomalous quotients, the total range of the midmatching points for normal observers was 0.80–1.20 (total range of all matches was 0.65–1.30). In previous studies of the midmatching point using the Nagel model II, Schmidt (1955b) reported a range of 0.45–2.00 and Willis and Farnsworth (1951) a range of 0.72–1.41.

THE PICKFORD-NICOLSON ANOMALOSCOPE

The Pickford-Nicolson anomaloscope was designed to measure the Rayleigh equation, an equation similar to the Engelking-Trendelenburg equation, and the Pickford-Lakowski equation in the general population. The Pickford-Nicolson anomaloscope is a filter anomaloscope that uses broadband filters to provide primary and test wavelengths. These broadband stimuli are specified by their dominant wavelength and excitation purity (see Chapter 2). Some features of the pilot model of the anomaloscope (Pickford & Lakowski, 1960) are summarized in Table 5.6. There is variation in different instruments because of variation in the color filters (Lakowski, 1971). The instrument presents the observer with a circular bipartite field. The test field appears in the left half, its radiance varied by means of a knob with a scale on the top of the instrument. When the knob is adjusted the test field varies from dark at scale 0 to increasingly brighter test fields until its maximum at 82. In the right half the primary mixture appears. The relative proportion of the primaries may be adjusted continuously and the mixture read from a scale on the top of the instrument.

For the Rayleigh match, a 585 nm (0.955 excitation purity) test is matched to a mixture of 555 nm (0.717 excitation purity) and 642 nm (0.99 excitation purity). At scale 0 the mixture field appears to the color normal observer all red and as the scale value is increased changes continuously (red, orange, yellow, yellow-green, green) to 80. The normal match is at 36–39 and the yellow field is at 20. The luminance of the red primary is greater than that of the green primary. The field luminance is 8.6 cd m^{-2}. For the Engleking-Trendelenburg equation, a 496 nm test (0.43 excitation purity) is matched to a mixture of 555 nm (0.717 excitation purity) and 470 nm (0.937 excitation purity). At scale 0 the mixture field appears green and changes continuously from green through pale blue-greens and greenish-blues to blue at scale 80. The normal match occurs at 45–49, and the desaturated blue-green test field is set at 40. The field luminance is 5.58 cd m^{-2}. For the Pickford-Lakowski equation a white test (near illuminant A) is matched to a mixture of 585 nm (0.955 excitation purity) and 470 nm (0.937 excitation purity). At scale 0 the mixture field appears yellow and changes continuously to white and then blue at scale 80. The normal match occurs at 36–41, and the white brightness value is about 25. The field luminance is about 7 cd m^{-2}.

The experimenter sets up the equation that is required. The correct filter pair is inserted into the mixture field. A shutter (controlled with a knob on top of the instrument) controls the total radiance of the mixture fields. This shutter is usually in the open position and is never adjusted during the test procedure. A filter pair is also used in the test field to provide desaturation of the test. For the Rayleigh and Engleking-Trendelenburg equations a neutral-density filter is used with the 585 nm or 495 nm test filter. By using a knob on the top left the experimenter can fix the amount of desaturation. In the pilot model the desaturation knob was at 60 for the Rayleigh match and 67 for the Engel-

Table 5.6
Summary of Pickford-Nicolson Features

Equation	Rayleigh	Engelking-Trendelenburg	Pickford-Lakowski
Primaries*	555 nm (0.717)	470 nm (0.937)	470 nm (0.937)
	642 nm (0.99)	555 nm (0.717)	585 nm (0.955)
Test*	585 nm (0.955)	496 nm (0.43)	Illuminant A
	Instrument scale readings at normal match		
Mixture ratio	36–39	45–49	36–41
Test luminance	20	40	25
Field luminance	8.6 cd m^{-2}	5.58 cd m^{-2}	6.85 cd m^{-2}
Field size (at 1 m)	20′–3°		

*The dominant wavelength (and excitation purity in parentheses) are given for each broadband filter (see Chapter 2 for definitions). Illuminant A is output of tungsten lamp (see Chapter 1 for definition).

As reported by Pickford and Lakowski (1960).

king-Trendelenburg match. For the Pickford-Lakowski match the white provided by illuminant A is made slightly reddish by using the 642 nm filter to adjust the color balance and was at 43. For any of the three equations, once the desaturating knob is set it is not changed again during the experimental procedure.

The color fields appear on a diffusing screen at the front of the instrument. By use of apertures (5–50 mm diameter) various-sized circular bipartite fields or even two small circles may be presented. The field size is determined by viewing distance; distances up to 2 m may be used. Usually the observer is at 1 m, giving a range of about 20' to almost 3° depending on the aperture.

The testing procedure detailed by Pickford (1951; 1957; Pickford & Lakowski, 1960) may be followed. The examiner makes all adjustments for the observer (who probably cannot reach the knobs). The matching ranges are carefully examined. Ambient illumination provided by the room or window light is allowed, provided that no source of illumination is directed at the viewing screen. Maximal illumination on the desk or table holding the instrument should be no more than 100 lux. The experimenter sits at the front side of the instrument close enough to adjust the knobs and in position to view the screen and point at the bipartite field if necessary. The data are obtained as arbitrary scale numbers. They may be converted to statistical units (standard deviations) or jnd units. Anomalous quotients may be calculated but cannot be compared with AQs derived from other Pickford-Nicolson anomaloscopes or from the Nagel anomaloscope. Precise calibrations were reported by Pickford and Lakowski (1960) for the pilot model and by Lakowski (1971) for his model. Further calibration is not required for screening purposes but would be necessary for experimental work.

Norms for the Pickford-Nicolson anomaloscope. Lakowski (1971) has presented norms for over 124 observers with normal color vision assessed in the Pickford-Nicolson anomaloscope. The Rayleigh, Engelking-Trendelenburg, and Pickford-Lakowski equations were evaluated. Figure 5.8a shows the midmatching points reproduced from their paper and Fig. 5.8b shows the matching ranges in jnd scale units. The midmatching points show peaked, symmetric distributions for all three equations. The matching ranges are asymmetric for all three equations.

OTHER TESTS*

Lantern Tests

Lantern tests were developed primarily as vocational color vision tests to assess signal recognition in military, aviation, and transport services. Vocational testing is required because an individual's capacity to perform a particular task is not necessarily evaluated by a screening test for defective color vision. Lantern tests are of two types, those that show pairs of lights together and those that show single colors. In the former group only red, white, and green colors are used, and a statistical treatment is applied to the results (Paulson, 1968). There are anomalous trichromats who are considered to have sufficient color vision for "routine duties." If prolonged dark adaptation is used, the examination comprises a threshold or visibility test. In this case normal trichromats are allowed a certain number of errors, and a statistical treatment is again applied to determine pass/fail criteria (Sloan, 1944). In general, lanterns that display single colors contain a

---

*Contributed by Jennifer Birch, M. Phil.

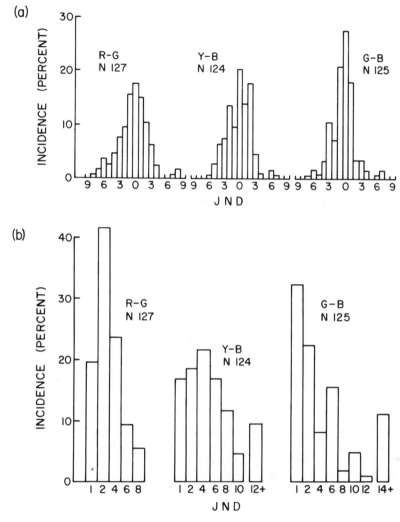

Fig. 5.8. Norms for the Pickford-Nicolson anomaloscope. (a) Histogram showing percentage distributions of midmatching points for normal subjects (16–60 years of age). Abscissa indicates jnd units, with zero representing the most frequent ratio. (b) Histogram showing percentage distribution of matching ranges. [From Lakowski, R., *British Journal of Physiological Optics*, 1971, 26, 166–182 (reproduced with permission of the British Optical Association).]

greater range of colors, including yellows, and, in some cases, glasses to simulate different weather conditions. Some lanterns are mechanized, and the speed and sequence of the color presentation is critical to the success of the test.

Lovibond Color Vision Analyzer

The Lovibond color vision analyzer is a self-luminous instrument designed both for screening and for disgnosis of the type and degree of any color defect (Dain, 1974). The instrument contains a display of 27 colors derived from Tintometer glass filters and representing a complete hue circle. The colors subtend approximately 1° and are placed in random order in a circle together with a neutral glass. An identical neutral of equal subtense is placed at the center of the circle. The subject must choose from the circle those colors that appear identical to the central color; there is provision for altering the luminance of the central neutral and for desaturation of the entire display by superimposing varying amounts of white light (equivalent to standard illuminant C). The format is therefore one of demonstrating isochromatic lines through the neutral point, and unique pairs of colors should be chosen in protan, deutan, and tritan defects. This choice is maintained at different levels of desaturation in different degrees of defect. Only dichromats accept diagnostic colors at full saturation, and simple anomalous trichromats choose diagnostic colors only at moderate levels of desaturation. The test therefore demonstrates isochromatic lines of different length that are equivalent to different degrees of defect.

Accurate screening and the establishment of the degree of the defect depend very heavily on the desaturation device. Although very good results have been obtained in the initial trials, it appears that the mechanical construction of the desaturation control is weak, and it is therefore difficult to set a suitable level of desaturation for screening so as to maintain the repeatibility of the scale results for anomalous trichromats. Moreover, because the isochromatic lines of congenital protan and deutan subjects are close together the protan and deutan diagnostic colors are adjacent in the hue circle, and both may be selected as a match by the color defective. The test distinguishes between normal and congenital red–green color-defective observers but does not differentiate well between protan and deutan observers (Ohta, Kogure, & Yamaguchi, 1978). No data are available for the use of the color vision analyzer in the study of acquired defects.

Chromagraph

Gunkel and Cogan (1977) devised a clinical instrument to assess the size of the achromatic area. In this instrument colors are produced by addition of three broadband spectral lights. These are balanced to give an achromatic percept and can be adjusted from neutral to various hue percepts. Data are reported on a perceptual hue circle. The task is to map the size of the achromatic area. They reported an achromatic area that is small and roughly symmetrical in normal observers. Observers with defective color vision show either enlarged neutral area, sector defects (red, green, yellow, or blue), or band defects (red–green, blue–yellow).

USING COLOR VISION TESTS*

Color vision tests are used for a wide variety of purposes. Some of these include rapid screening of congenital red–green defects for military or transport purposes and classification of discrimination ability within the population of congenital red–green defects for job assignment purposes within the military. Another use for screening involves recognition and diagnosis of congenital disorders for psychophysical or genetic study. In the eye clinic, screening is used for recognition and differentiation of congenital and acquired disorders and for the classification of acquired disorders in patients with eye disease. Finally, in education and industry screening is used for vocational orientation or aptitude in professions depending on visual judgement.

Color vision tests are usually used with observers who are not familiar with the

*Contributed by Paul Kinnear, Ph.D., A. J. L. G. Pinckers, M.D., Joel Pokorny, Ph.D., Vivianne C. Smith, Ph.D., and Guy Verriest, M.D.

specific test or testing procedure. The observers may be nervous about the testing situation or may not understand the explanation of the test. Thus test results may be biased by cognitive or emotional factors. Further, the majority of color vision tests were designed for use with young adults with normal visual acuity. The performance elements of some tests may be beyond the capabilities of some patients, notably individuals with visual, motor, or intellectual handicaps, the elderly, and the very young. There are several precautions that can help reduce variation due to such problems.

Establishing rapport with the patient.   Unfamiliarity with the testing situation and high anxiety can lead to erratic test results. An occasional patient may even be uncooperative. The clinician must spend several minutes explaining why the patient is being treated and putting the patient at ease in his or her presence.

Use of a test meaningful to the patient.   A patient is more likely to cooperate in a difficult test such as the anomaloscope if he or she has already performed a test that has seemed meaningful, such as arranging colors (e.g., 100-hue test) or naming colors (e.g., Dvorine naming discs).

Administering standard tests in a uniform way.   It is vital that the same procedure and conditions be used always for administering standard tests such as the 100-hue test or pseudoisochromatic plates. This then allows comparisons to be made between data collected by clinicians in other clinics or even by the same clinician on different occasions. Normally the procedure and conditions are given in the test manuals. Variations in instructions to the patient are especially liable to bias responses, but other conditions, such as the level and type of illumination and the state of adaptation of the eyes, are also important.

Use of an appropriate psychophysical method with complex apparatus.   Great care must be taken to control procedure and method when equipment such as adaptometers, anomaloscopes, and perimeters are used to assess visual function. There are established psychophysical methods for evaluation of dark adaptation and static perimetric thresholds. Procedures for use with anomaloscopes are detailed above.

Evaluation of Congenital Defects

The existence of the X-chromosome linked disorders was recognized at the end of the 18th century. In the 19th century there were major disasters with loss of life in the shipping and railroad industries attributed to the failure of engineers to recognize a color signal. These incidents mark the beginning of an era in which persons with congenital red–green defects were excluded from positions as pilots or engineers in commercial air, sea, and rail transport and similar duties in the armed forces. The tests that were developed were practical and empirical. While the anomaloscope remains the only clinical method for precise diagnosis of the presumed genetic entities, many tests have been devised for quick, cheap, and efficient screening of the color-defective population. Screening tests are used mainly to identify individuals who may eventually require more extensive color testing, and their usefulness is in the identification of such individuals rather than the exact diagnosis of the color defect. Screening tests are easy to administer and score and are of modest cost.

DIAGNOSIS OF RED–GREEN DEFECTS

The anomaloscope is the most convenient instrument for diagnosis and classification of the presumed genetic entities of dichromacy and simple and extreme anomalous trichromacy. Anomaloscope examination is time consuming, and only a trained person can use the anomaloscope. A further problem is that commercially available anomaloscopes are very expensive.

The test must include a full examination of the matching range. It is inappropriate to allow one or two matches. In the past, many examiners determined only the quotient of anomaly on the basis of one or two matches without investigating the matching range. A further problem is that protanomaly and deuteranomaly have been classified in severity on the quotient of anomaly (especially in Germany). This procedure is unsound (Verriest, 1960a; see also Hurvich, 1972), there is no correlation between the quotient of anomaly and the matching width. The aspect of color vision deficiency that is most important in daily and professional life is the extent or severity of chromatic discrimination loss. This factor may be assessed by the error score on the FM 100-hue test, by matching widths on the color matches, or by specific field tests that replicate the color task.

RAPID SCREENING OF RED–GREEN COLOR DEFECTS

Rapid screening of red–green color defects may be necessary for military and transport purposes or in schools or industry. The most effective single test is one of the validated plate tests designed for this purpose: the Ishihara, the AO HRR, or other series of pseudoisochromatic plates, which detect about 96 percent of the cases confirmed by anomaloscope. The most common way is to rely on a single test or even a few selected plates.

There are difficulties associated with this procedure, however. Some normal subjects read the "normally not readable" digits of the Ishihara; on the other hand, some normal subjects will misread certain plates. The distinction between normal color vision and deuteranomalous vision with good discrimination by pigment tests (Chapter 7) remains an unsolved problem. Observers with minimal deuteranomaly will pass plates 12 and 13 of the Ishihara (6th ed.) and plates 3–20 of the AO HRR (1st ed.).

CLASSIFICATION OF CHROMATIC DISCRIMINATORY ABILITY

In some applications it is important not only to screen for congenital red–green color defects but also to classify the defect according to chromatic discriminatory ability. A test battery may be used with or without anomaloscope examination. An example of such a battery is that designed at the U.S. Naval Submarine Laboratory (Paulson, 1974). The battery includes use of a set of plates, a lantern, and ranking tests; it is accomplished in a brief period. The battery allows recognition of 95 percent of all congenital red–green color defectives and separation of color defectives into three categories of individuals, those showing "mild," "moderate," and "severe" loss of chromatic discrimination. The "mild" and "moderate" categories tend to include predominantly simple and extreme anomalous trichromats; the "severe" category includes individuals who are extreme anomalous trichromats and dichromats. The correlation is not absolute, since chromatic discriminative ability varies widely among anomalous trichromats (see Chapter 7).

RECOGNITION OF CONGENITAL BLUE–YELLOW DEFECTS AND ACHROMATOPSIA

Recognition of congenital blue–yellow defects requires use of one or more of the tests designed for this purpose. These include the AO HRR, Tokyo Medical College, Stilling, Velhagen plates, and Farnsworth F_2 plate. Since normal observers with heavy ocular pigmentation may miss the green symbol on the F_2 plate and appear to be incomplete tritanopes, the F_2 plate should be used in conjunction with another test. Further, failure to perceive the blue symbol usually seen by normals and tritans is indicative of congenital red–green defect. The Farnsworth Panel D-15 and the FM 100-hue tests are important in recognition of blue–yellow defects.

For recognition of complete achromatopsia the Sloan achromatopsia test or the FVS plates may be used. The anomaloscope reveals the characteristic scotopic matching. A very simple and effective test is to present a deep red color chip pasted on a white cardboard: it will typically be named black by complete achromats. The Farnsworth Panel D-15 and FM 100-hue tests are important because they reveal a scotopic axis and a characteristic error accumulation of 400 or more errors on the FM 100-hue test. Incomplete achromatopsia shows many similarities to the complete form, with high error accumulations on the FM 100-hue test. The X-chromosome–linked recessive incomplete achromat gives results similar to those of complete achromats on the Rayleigh equation but shows residual color discrimination on other tests, showing a deutan tracing on the Farnsworth Panel D-15. Autosomal recessive incomplete achromats may make a Rayleigh match displaced to red. With a small field the match enlarges on the scotopic axis. These observers show a scotopic axis on the Farnsworth Panel D-15 or the FM 100-hue test.

Evaluation of Acquired Color Vision Defects

The detection and classification of the acquired color vision defects may be accomplished by use of an anomaloscope combined with a test measuring chromatic discrimination. In addition, 8–10 percent of affected males may have a concomitant congenital color defect, and the examiner should be alert to this possibility.

USE OF THE ANOMALOSCOPE IN ACQUIRED COLOR VISION DEFECTS

An anomaloscope is used for measurement of the Rayleigh, Eng-elking-Trendelenburg, and Pickford-Lakowski equations. The position and width of the Rayleigh equation allow differentiation of the type I and type II acquired color vision defects. The brightness matches allow a gross estimate of the luminous efficiency function in the long-wavelength range. Figure 5.9 shows typical Rayleigh match results on the Nagel model I anomaloscope in acquired color vision defects. The Engel-king-Trendelenburg and Pickford-Lakowski equations are useful in evaluating the type III acquired color defect. Evaluation of a Rayleigh equation shifted to red requires special care. A red-shifted match may occur not only in protanomalous trichromacy (Chapter 7) but also in incomplete achromatopsia of autosomal recessive inheritance (Pokorny, Smith, & Newell, 1978; 1979) or in pseudoprotanomaly (Pokorny, Smith, & Ernest, in press). Screening tests and the FM 100-hue test or Farnsworth Panel D-15 are necessary adjuncts.

The Nagel anomaloscope is not an ideal instrument for evaluation of acquired color

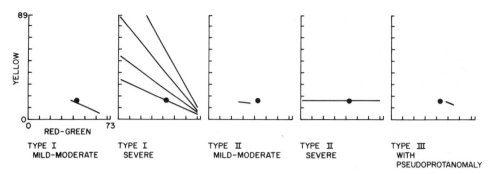

Fig. 5.9. Typical Rayleigh matches on the Nagel model I anomaloscope in acquired color vision defects.

vision defects, since the small field size and telescope view are difficult for observers with reduced visual acuity. Additionally, the Pickford-Nicolson anomaloscope or other equivalent is more useful than the Nagel anomaloscope in acquired color vision defects, since this anomaloscope allows determination of other equations (Lakowski, 1972).

EVALUATION OF DISCRIMINATION

The FM 100-hue test is the most sensitive clinical test to establish the deterioration of chromatic discrimination or a minimal defect of chromatic discriminative ability. The test reveals a faint blue–yellow defect with its characteristic monopolar bulge and can be used to trace the course of the defect during followup. A disadvantage of the FM 100-hue test is that it is rarely performed well by children under 12, presents difficulties to an observer with visual acuity of 0.2 or less, and is too difficult for the elderly or dull patient.

When the FM 100-hue error score exceeds 400–800, the examiner may prefer to use the Farnsworth Panel D-15. The Farnsworth Panel D-15 can be given to people with reduced visual acuity (as low as 0.1), and is easier for children and elderly patients. If there are no major errors on the standard Farnsworth Panel D-15, the Lanthony Desaturated Panel D-15 may be given. The AO HRR test may also be helpful in differentiating red–green from blue–yellow acquired color defects. The Lanthony New Color Test was recently developed for study of acquired color vision defects. The New Color Test allows the examiner to follow the decline in saturation discrimination typical of the type II acquired red–green defect. The New Color Test can be used for both young children (8 years and older) and elderly patients and can be used even with severe reduction in visual acuity.

The nature of the foveal acquired color vision defect can be explored by specialized psychophysical techniques described in Chapter 6. Furthermore, peripheral color vision may also be disturbed and can even be solely affected in some ophthalmic diseases.

Screening for Professional Purposes

Several occupations require a minimal level of competence in discriminating colors. The screening of candidates for such occupations is best performed by means of tests reproducing as closely as possible the conditions of color discrimination encountered on the job. For example, the ability to recognize color signals is best assessed by means of a lantern equipped with the same filters as those used in the signal equipment. The ability to sort samples of cotton, rice, diamonds, pearls, oils, and so on is best assessed by a trial performance using real materials, taking care to ensure that the trial is conducted under similar conditions (e.g., similar spectral stimuli and level of illumination) as would prevail in the job situation. Likewise, the ability to discriminate electrical resistors by means of their color-coded bands can be evaluated by a trial test with resistors. In this case it is worth pointing out first, that electronic means of assessing resistors are becoming increasingly common in electronic workshops, thus eliminating the color discrimination problems for the color-defective person (except in the case of damaged resistors where other means of identification must be sought). Second, filters or other devices are available to assist congenital color defectives with visual identification of resistors.

Some indications of chromatic discriminative ability may be given by tests, such as the FM 100-hue test, Dimmick's color aptitude test, or even the Burnham-Clark-Munsell color memory test (when color memory is involved). Furthermore, many authors (Walraven & Leebeek, 1960; Lakowski, 1968b; Ichikawa, Hukami, & Majima, 1969; Voke, 1978) have studied correlations between results of practical tests and results of clinical tests (such as the AO HRR, the Pickford-Nicolson anomaloscope, or the FM 100-hue test) and showed that the aptitude for a specific task can be inferred, with more or less accuracy, from the results of common clinical tests (Verriest & Hermans, 1975).

Choice of a Test—Test Batteries

Many examiners decide on a test battery to fulfill their specific needs. Choice of a test battery reflects not only the requirements to be fulfilled but also the availability of tests, the personal experience of the examiners, and the time available for testing.

A number of batteries have been proposed. Paulson (1973) discussed the battery used in the U.S. Naval Submarine Laboratory. This battery allows rapid evaluation of chromatic discriminative ability. Verriest (1968) proposed a battery (Table 5.7) for evaluation of congenital defects that includes the Ishihara, the F_2 plate, the AO HRR, the Farnsworth Panel D-15, the Lanthony Desaturated Panel D-15, and the Nagel model I anomaloscope. The Lanthony Desaturated Panel should be used when the Standard Farnsworth Panel D-15 gives normal results or shows only minor errors. Still less time consuming is to use selected plates from the 6th Ishihara and AO HRR tests (e.g., plates 5–7, 12, and 13 from the Ishihara 6th edition and plates 1, 2, 3, 6, and 11–15 of the AO HRR). This battery allows a good differentiation of protanomaly, protanopia, deuteranomaly, deuteranopia, incomplete X-chromosome-linked achromatopsia, and complete achromatopsia. The FM 100-hue test was not included because it is time consuming and does not aid the differential diagnosis.

Pinckers and Baron (1978) proposed a battery for diagnosing acquired color vision defects in the ophthalmology clinic. The battery shown in Table 5.7 includes the AO HRR, the Lanthony New Color Test, the F_2 plate, the Ishihara, FM 100-hue test, and both the Nagel and Pickford-Nicolson anomaloscopes.

Unfortunately, these tests are not universally available. In a research laboratory, available tests may be supplemented by specially designed tests such as those described in Chapter 6. The minimal requirement (Table 5.8) for the ophthalmology clinic should include a screening test, the Panel D-15 or Lanthony New Color Test, the FM 100-hue test, and an anomaloscope. If the screening test does not include blue–yellow plates, the F_2 plate may be added.

Table 5.7
Test Batteries for Congenital and Acquired Color Defects

Test Battery for Congenital Color Defect*	Test Battery for Acquired Color Defect†
Full version	**Initial screening**
Ishihara (16- or 24-plate editions)	AO HRR
F_2	Lanthony New Color Test—box 6/4
AO HRR	If box 6/4 failed, do box 6/8
Standard Panel D-15	If box 6/4 passed, do the Desaturated Panel
Lanthony Desaturated Panel D-15 (if Standard Panel is normal, retest with Desaturated Panel)	**Red–green defects revealed by initial screening**
Nagel model I anomaloscope	Ishihara
	FM 100-hue
Abbreviated version	Nagel model I anomaloscope
Ishihara 6th Edition—plates 5, 6, 7, 12, 13	**Blue–yellow defects revealed by initial screening**
AO HRR—plates 1, 2, 6, 7, 11–16	F_2
Standard Panel D-15	FM 100-hue
Lanthony Desaturated Panel D-15 (it Standard Panel is normal, retest with Desaturated Panel)	Pickford-Nicolson anomaloscope
Nagel model I anomaloscope	

*Recommended by Verriest (1968).
†Recommended by Pinckers and Baron (1977).

130

Table 5.8
Minimal Requirements for Color Vision Evaluation

A screening test (include F_2 plate if no B-Y plates)
Farnsworth Panel D-15 and Lanthony Desaturated Panel D-15 or
  Lanthony New Color Test
FM 100-hue test
Appropriate illuminant (approximately standard illuminant C)
  for pigment tests
An anomaloscope

Special Problems of Testing

Color vision tests were designed by adults for use with adults with normal visual acuity. Some adults—e.g., the illiterate, those speaking foreign languages, or the elderly—can offer special problems to the examiner; testing of children requires special attention. The testing of a suspected malingerer or concealer may similarly offer problems. The general rule is to use common sense and to perform a test only if it is clear (1) that the patient understands the procedure and (2) that the test can be performed using appropriate technique.

TINTED GLASSES AND HARD CONTACT LENSES

It is imperative that color testing not be performed on patients wearing tinted glasses or tinted contact lenses. Tinted glasses are easily identified, but tinted contact lenses may not be noticed; all patients should be asked if they wear such a correction. Some contact lens wearers also have regular clear glasses; in this case an appointment should be made for a future date and the patient told to wear the glasses rather than the contact lenses.

The majority of screening tests can in fact be performed with glasses or contact lenses removed. Refractive error of myopes is often reduced on first removing the hard contact lens. Refractive errors of several diopters should not cause difficulties for screening plates. If necessary, a hand-held ophthalmic lens for screening plates or ophthalmic trial spectacle for arrangement tests may be used. The Nagel model I anomaloscope has adjustment for focus.

ILLITERATES

The Ishihara test icludes tracing patterns for illiterates; the symbols on the AO HRR may be traced, as may the numerals on other plate tests. Arrangement tests should offer no particular difficulty. Anomaloscope examination may prove difficult unless the purpose of the test is understood.

Illiteracy is relatively rare in American and European countries with compulsory universal grade-level education. Illiteracy may, however, be encountered in less developed countries, especially by researchers interested in genetic studies. The problem of illiteracy may then be compounded by language difficulties. Provided some mutual understanding is reached, tracing of screening plates is still appropriate.

FOREIGN LANGUAGE–SPEAKING ADULTS

Foreign language–speaking adults may similarly offer problems to the examiner if no translator is available. With good will and by mimicry and sign language a foreign language–speaking individual may be tested on screening plates. The patient should either trace the symbols with a brush or write the symbol or numeral on an adjacent piece of blank paper (not the scoresheet). Alternatively, a matching technique ("appariement") may be used in which drawn or cutout outlines of the figures are prepared for the subject to point at or superimposed on the plate. Arrangement tests and anomaloscope examination require a better level of communication.

ELDERLY PATIENTS

With respect and consideration, elderly patients should offer no problems in testing. Two specific problems may arise caused by loss of manual dexterity or by the use of bifocals. With poor manual dexterity, as in arthritic patients, the arrangement tests become difficult. The patient may drop the chips, becoming embarrassed or impatient with the task. Again, the solution is common sense; perform only tests that are necessary for diagnosis and within the patient's ability. Bifocal prescription may offer a problem in anomaloscope testing. The patient may have trouble finding the field in the telescope view of the Nagel anomaloscope or may be puzzled as to which part of the bifocal to use. In some cases removing the glasses and using the telescope adjustment may be all that is needed. In other cases the patient may prefer a hand-held positive ophthalmic lens (+2 to +3 D) rather than the regular bifocal glasses. It is important to ensure that the dividing line of the bipartite anomaloscope field appears clear. The Pickford-Nicolson anomaloscope should offer fewer difficulties to bifocal wearers.

TESTING CHILDREN

Children under age 12 years offer special problems in color testing, since many of the tests require intellectual abilities that develop at different ages; i.e., screening tests require knowledge of alphabet or numerals, arrangement tests require the concept of serial ordering. The situation is even more difficult in the case of retarded children.

With increased use of color coding in school materials, it is of growing importance to identify congenital color defects in young children. Many observers with a congenital color defect retain memories of being treated as "stupid" or "troublemakers" because they had difficulties making color discriminations that were immediately evident to color normals. Color tests may also be helpful in identifying hereditary retinal disease in children.

There are two tests designed especially for children: the Guy's Hospital color vision test and the Matsubura test. The Guy's Hospital color vision test contains design flaws that make it ambiguous and confusing to adults (and thus presumably equally confusing to children) (Alexander, 1975). The Matsubura test contains symbols of items familiar and important in Japanese culture (e.g., cherry blossoms) but not necessarily familiar to American or European children. To date, neither test has received full validation in an American or European population.

Although a review of the literature revealed rather variable results in testing young children (Alexander, 1975), it is possible to test children successfully with adult tests such as the AO HRR and the Ishihara. Care is needed to match the task to the age, attention span, and intellectual development of the child. It is important to give careful instruction to ensure that the child understands what to do. Such instruction should not contain reference to color names or color differences, which the color-defective child may not understand. By their very nature color tests are frustrating and difficult for color defectives; this point must be remembered when dealing with color-defective children.

Preschool and kindergarten children (3–5 years old).   Today, with increased use of preschools and educational television, many children of 3–5 years know alphabet letters, the numerals from 1 to 10, and simple geometric shapes as well as the concept of "same"/"different."

Young children may be tested with the AO HRR test (Alexander, 1975). If necessary, the examiner may even draw the three symbols—triangle, circle, and square—on a sheet of paper (technique of "appariement") and ask the child, "Do you see any of these shapes on the color plate?" The child who says, "Yes," then points to the quadrant of the plate where the picture appears and then to the matching symbols on the page that were seen on the plate. It is important to practice the procedure with the demonstration plates and to make certain that the child knows the three geometric shapes.

The AO HRR is preferable to the Ishihara or Dvorine with young children even if they know some numerals, since many children of this age will confuse certain numerals and will not be sure how to identify a double-digit number. For example, shown a plate containing "26" the child may say "6" or "2" or even "9", not knowing that the combined symbol is called "twenty-six." An alternative is to use the tracing patterns designed for illiterates, although not all young children have the necessary manual dexterity to perform an accurate tracing.

First- and second-grade children (6–8 years old).   Many children of 6–8 years can perform the screening tests. However, few children in this age range understand the concept of serial ordering or have the attention span necessary to complete a sorting test such as the Panel D-15 (Adams, Balliet, & McAdams, 1975; Cohen, 1976). A 6-year-old may start the Farnsworth Panel D-15 correctly, put in five chips, and then suddenly put two favorite colors together.

In addition to the plate tests, a limited amount of information may be obtained from 6–8-year-olds on an anomaloscope. The Pickford-Nicolson anomaloscope has the advantage that both child and examiner can point to one or other side of the vertically split field, eliminating the need to describe what is seen. The Nagle anomaloscope has a disadvantage in that some children have difficulty aligning themselves to see the field in the telescope view. The examiner should set both the color mixture and brightness and ask the child, "Do you see a circle of color or can you tell that there are two colors in the circle?" The tester must present matches that have obvious brightness difference (green primary and yellow turned dim), matches representative of a normal trichromat, and matches of the common red–green defects.

Third- through sixth-grade children (8–11 years). Children of ages 8–11 can usually perform the screening tests and the Panel D-15. They will perform the anomaloscope match provided that the examiner sets the color mixture and watches carefully how the child sets the yellow brightness, setting it also if necessary. Children of ages 8–10 can perform the FM 100-hue test; however, many become bored after one or two boxes, with a consequent performance decrement. It is advisable to give a 2–3-min informal rest period after the second box.

Mentally retarded.   Color vision screening among mentally retarded boys reveals a high incidence of defect, 20–30 percent of males (Salvia, 1969; Salvia & Ysseldyke, 1971a, b) with poor intertest correlations. Analysis of the data showed that the high rates represent failure of screening plates by mentally retarded boys with normal color vision defined by anomaloscope. The problems are evident in AO HRR, Dvorine, and Ishihara. Plate tests are not suitable for screening in the mentally retarded population. Arrangement tests such as the FM 100-hue test and Farnsworth Panel D-15 (Salvia, 1969) also offer difficulties and may reveal high incidences of color defect. Salvia and Ysseldyke (1971a, b) reported an incidence of 8.7 percent for congenital red–green color defects when the Pickford-Nicolson anomaloscope was used. Provided that the examiner is confident that the subject understands the anomaloscope test, this test may be used for evaluation of color vision in the mentally retarded population.

MALINGERING AND CONCEALING

Two problems that arise occasionally include the person with normal color vision who demonstrates a color vision defect (either by malingering or due to hysteria) and the person with a color vision defect who wants to obtain a report of normal color vision (concealment). The malingerer is more difficult to detect.

Malingering and hysteria. Malingering can occur in connection with the assessment of financial compensation after an accident, avoiding full blame in motor accidents (Desvignes & Legras, 1973), and avoiding government service, especially with regard to defense. Hysteria reflects a psychological basis such as the need for attention. The line between malingering and hysteria is a narrow one. An example of a pointer toward psychological problems is when a person reports symptoms of pain caused by certain colors.

An obvious way of revealing malingering or hysteria is to use tests such as visual fields or electroretinography. Generally, a battery of tests is used, in which case the observer tends to produce atypical or contradictory results.

The ignorant malingerer may claim to be unable to read all pseudoisochromatic plates, even the first (demonstration) plate of the Ishihara series, thus being exposed immediately if visual acuity is not much reduced, since even the complete achromat can read these plates. The same person will arrange such tests as the Panel D-15 or the FM 100-hue test haphazardly and give inconsistent answers when being tested with an anomaloscope. The more knowledgeable malingerer might try to simulate one of the deficiencies of color vision by learning beforehand appropriate responses for the Ishihara and color-sorting tests. Skilled examiners should be prepared by giving plates out of order or even by producing tests that they do not usually use.

The most difficult cases are those where there exists some kind of congenital or acquired defect on which color malingering or hysteria is superimposed. When the subject is knowledgeable the examiner can even believe a "new" color vision defect has been discovered. A color vision specialist must be extremely careful before diagnosing extraordinary color vision defects. Cases of hysterical symptoms superimposed on congenital color defects have been reported by Kalberer (1971a) and Pickford (1972). A comparison of the color vision test results and other visual functions such as visual acuity, dark adaptation, and especially the visual field enables the alert specialist to recognize these cases.

Concealment. A person deliberately trying to conceal a color vision deficiency usually wants to be accepted for a job in which normal color vision is a prerequisite, such as in shipping or air transport. In many cases the subject has a good chance if the correct answers are provided by a color normal and learned by heart, e.g., for the Ortho-Rater transparency or for a small series of Ishihara plates. Some subjects can learn to put the Farnsworth Panel D-15 caps in the correct order. Other subjects help themselves in reading more correctly the pseudoisochromatic plates by wearing tinted glasses or an X-chrom contact lens (neither method makes color vision normal, but such filters may help a patient to pass a pseudoisochromatic color vision test).

Just as in the case of the malingerer, the skilled examiner should be able to expose the concealer's bluff by presenting material out of order or using an unusual test that the concealer would not have learned. The AO HRR test can be changed in orientation and subjects asked to trace the digits with a brush (Verriest & Hermans, 1975; Perdriel, Lanthony, & Chevaleraud, 1975). It is virtually impossible to conceal successfully on an anomaloscope test.

Paul Kinnear, Ph.D.

Marion Marré, M.D.

Joel Pokorny, Ph.D.

Vivianne C. Smith, Ph.D.

Guy Verriest, M.D.

6

Specialized Methods of Evaluating Color Vision Defects

PSYCHOPHYSICAL TESTING*

While clinical tests are more than adequate to diagnose and classify color vision defects, special psychophysical techniques extend our information about color vision defects and offer the promise of analysis of acquired color vision defects. The psychophysical techniques discussed below include spectral sensitivity, chromatic discriminative ability, specialized colorimetric techniques, and the Stiles-Crawford effect. A number of investigators have adapted the static perimeter for evaluation of spectral sensitivity at absolute threshold, or with achromatic or chromatic background fields, and for evaluation of colorimetric purity. These studies are discussed below (Perimetry).

Spectral Sensitivity

There are many methods to evaluate spectral sensitivity, each yielding a characteristic function. Some of these functions include the absolute threshold of vision, heterochromatic measurements, which yield the relative luminous efficiency function, and increment thresholds.

ABSOLUTE THRESHOLD

The absolute threshold is the least energy at which the presence of a monochromatic test light is detectable on a criterion percentage of trials.

Techniques. The optical system allows presentation of a test light of specified size and duration. The stimulus is centered entirely within the rod-free fovea, where cone

---

*Contributed by Joel Pokorny, Ph.D., and Vivianne C. Smith, Ph.D.

density is greatest; for example, a circle subtending 40' visual angle may be pulsed for 20 msec. The subject who has been in the dark for 10–15 min. before the experiment begins is asked to report when the flash is seen as the energy of the test light is varied.

The energy required to elicit a response at the visual threshold is greatest for short and long wavelengths, and for foveal fixation of small test objects is at a minimum at about 550 nm. Individual absolute threshold functions for normal observers show variability of up to 0.3 log unit in the height of their maxima (Hsia & Graham, 1957). The absolute threshold method allows for absolute comparisons of sensitivity between individuals. Threshold spectral sensitivity functions obtained from a given individual are repeatable from day to day, with variability of 0.1–0.2 log unit. Differences between observers are of the order of 0.1–0.3 log unit. The individual function may show irregularities or shoulders that are reproducible both within and between observers. These shoulders depend on experimental technique.

When a small stimulus is centered on the fovea, the absolute threshold is measured for cone photoreceptors. For retinal areas outside the fovea, the absolute threshold can be measured for rods (λ_{max} near 505 nm) and for cones (λ_{max} near 550 nm). Using an extrafoveal test light, as the energy is raised from a minimum value a dim gray is seen first (rod mediated). With a further increase in energy, the gray increases in brightness until the cone threshold is reached. The interval between the appearance of the achromatic rod response and the chromatic cone response is known as the photochromatic interval. The transition from rod to cone vision is not abrupt and depends on many factors. The fact that the rod and cone systems have different spectral maxima means that a change in illumination near the rod-cone transition level results in a shift (the Purkinjé shift) in the relative brightness of different portions of the spectrum. It was Purkinjé who first noted that at dawn red colors appeared dark, dimmer than blue colors, although at full daylight the reds appeared very bright, even brighter than the blues.

At the fovea it is possible to assess an absolute threshold for light perception and a threshold for color perception (Graham & Hsia, 1969). The difference between the threshold for light and color is called the foveal achromatic interval. The foveal achromatic interval varies with wavelength in a manner similar to a colorimetric purity function being greatest in the yellow and least at the spectral extremes.

Clinical applications. Measurements of absolute threshold spectral sensitivity are important in ascertaining sensitivity loss. Overall sensitivity loss may be an indication of a neutral absorption system. Sensitivity loss for short wavelengths usually occurs in absorption defects such as brown nuclear cataract. Sensitivity loss for long wavelengths is frequently related to receptoral disease. Measurement of absolute threshold spectral sensitivity may reveal participation by rods; since the absolute threshold depends critically on the retinal area stimulated, it is important to know the preferred fixation of any observer with reduced visual acuity. Absolute threshold spectral sensitivity has been widely studied in observers with congenital color vision defects. Some of these data are discussed in Chapter 7. Absolute thresholds using perimetric techniques are discussed below (Perimetry). The Zanen photometer (Zanen, 1959; 1972; Zanen & Vazquez, 1962) has been used to assess the foveal achromatic interval in ophthalmic disorders. Zanen (1972) has emphasized that elevation of the chromatic thresholds can occur in patients with optic nerve disorders and has shown (1974) how these types of threshold measurements are of assistance in differentiating patients with acquired and congenital color vision defects.

HETEROCHROMATIC MATCHING MEASUREMENTS

Methodologies used to obtain spectral sensitivity functions by matching spectral lights to a reference light presented at a radiance above threshold include heterochromatic brightness matching, heterochromatic flicker photometry (HFP), and minimally distinct border (MDB). In these methods a comparison stimulus is present and the data are expressed relative to the peak sensitivity of the observer. Thus the techniques do not allow comparison of absolute sensitivities of different observers. For example, an absorption system represented by a neutral-density filter that attenuates both the standard and comparison lights 50 percent would not appreciably alter the sensitivity function obtained using matching techniques; however, such a filter would uniformly displace an absolute threshold function by 0.3 log unit. Only relative sensitivity losses are revealed by the methods.

Techniques.   The techniques of deriving brightness matching, flicker photometry, and minimally distinct border were described in Chapter 2. The HFP and MDB spectral sensitivity functions are narrower in shape than the brightness matching function. The HFP spectral sensitivity function shows interindividual variation that has been studied by several investigators. Verriest's (1970a) data are shown in Fig. 6.1. The normalization technique constrains variability at the peak; with midspectrum normalization, interobserver variability is greatest in the short-wavelength region of the spectrum and is attributed to individual differences in the lens absorption function and the macular pigment density. Interobserver variability in the long-wavelength region of the spectrum has customarily been attributed to individual differences in the relative proportions of the

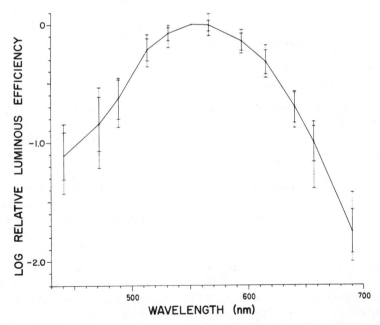

Fig. 6.1.   Log relative luminous efficiency measured by HFP showing interobserver variability. The solid bars indicate 2 SD and the dotted bars indicate the total range of observations.   [From Verriest, G. *Nouvelle Revue d'Optique Appliquée*, 1970, *1*, 107–126 (reproduced with permission of Masson & Cie).]

populations of MWS and LWS cone receptors (Durup & Piéron, 1943; De Vries, 1947; Crone, 1959; Rushton & Baker, 1964; Adam, 1969).

Clinical applications.   The heterochromatic methods are widely used in observers with congenital color vision defects, as described in Chapter 7. Brightness matching and heterochromatic flicker photometry (HFP) have been used in acquired color vision defects (Verriest, 1970b). Both techniques will reveal luminosity loss at specific wavelength regions. For example, brightness matching was used by Gibson, Smith, and Alpern (1965) to demonstrate a relative long-wavelength sensitivity loss in a case of digitoxin toxicity. The HFP technique was used by Verriest (1969) in retinal and optic nerve disorders. Verriest (1970b) has reviewed and summarized both the earlier studies (using methods other than HFP) and his own HFP studies of relative luminous efficiency in acquired color vision defects.

Despite considerable interobserver variability, Verriest's (1970b) results using the HFP technique may be generally summarized as follows: In type I acquired color vision defect the luminous efficiency function may be normal. The first changes with moderate loss are to a mixed photopic/scotopic function and eventually, in severe loss, to a purely scotopic function. In type II acquired color vision defect the luminous efficiency function usually appears normal; however, in severe cases scotopization can occur, giving a mixed photopic/scotopic luminosity efficiency function. In type III acquired color vision defect the relative luminous efficiency function is usually within normal limits. A selective short-wavelength loss is observed in senile nuclear cataract.

A particular advantage of the HFP method at retinal illuminances above 100 td is the use of alternation rates of 15–20 Hz. At these rates rods are relatively insensitive to temporal alternation. The HFP technique therefore allows evaluation of residual cone function in incomplete achromatopsia (Smith, Pokorny, & Newell, 1978; 1979) and disorders that are accompanied by scotopization.

INCREMENT OR FLICKER DETECTION ON ACHROMATIC BACKGROUNDS

A technique developed by King-Smith and his associates (King-Smith, 1975; King-Smith & Carden, 1976; King-Smith, Kranda, & Wood,1976) requires that the observer detect the presence of flicker in a temporally alternating spectral light presented on a 1000 td white background.

Techniques.   The optical system allows for a centrally viewed target presented on a larger background field. The temporal alternation of the spectral light is set at a fixed rate, and the observer increases its radiance until the central field appears to flicker or pulsate. The spectral sensitivity function is the relative radiance at which each spectral light first seems to flicker. The spectral sensitivity is obtained at two alternation rates, one and 25 Hz. When the stimulus is in rapid temporal alternation at 25 Hz, the flicker detection spectral sensitivity shows a single maximum at 560 nm and resembles a conventional luminous efficiency function obtained by HFP. When the spectral light is in slow temporal alternation at one Hz, the flicker detection spectral sensitivity has three maxima, 450, 525, and 600 nm (Fig. 6.2).

King-Smith interprets the differences in the two functions within the framework of an opponent-process theory. He suggests that the single-peaked function represents achromatic luminance processing, mediated by large-diameter nerve fibers of the ganglion

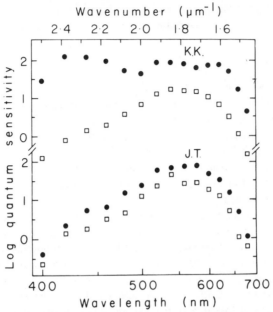

Fig. 6.2. Spectral sensitivity curves determined for detection of 1° 200-ms foveal test flash (●) and 20 Hz flicker (□) on white (3200 K) background of 1000 td. Upper set of data points are for a normal observer; lower set of data points are for an observer with an (unspecified) acquired color vision defect. [From King-Smith, P. E., Kranda, K., & Wood, I. C. J. *Investigative Ophthalmology,* 1976, *15,* 584–587 (reproduced with permission of the Association for Research in Vision and Ophthalmology).]

cell layer and geniculate pathways. For slow temporal alternation, he suggests that chromatic opponent signals mediated in a slow fiber system dominate the response. Fast and slow systems have been described in many species. In particular, Gouras (1969), working with rhesus monkeys, has described fast and slow systems linked to achromatic and chromatic activity (see Chapter 3).

In an alternative technique, chromatic detection on a high-radiance white background is required, as described, for example, by Sperling and Harwerth (1971). The technique was further developed as a specialized clinical technique by Verriest and Uvijls (1977a, b), who adapted a Tübinger perimeter for the purpose (see below, Perimetry).

Clinical applications. Detection of flickering chromatic stimuli on white backgrounds was used by King-Smith, Kranda, and Wood (1976) to demonstrate a selective loss of color opponency, as shown in the lower curves of Fig. 6.2. There are several advantages of this technique in the study of color defect. Flicker detection on white backgrounds allows an estimate of absolute sensitivity loss. The fast temporal alternation gives information similar to that of HFP; rod activity can be suppressed by choice of a sufficiently high alternation rate. At low alternation rates the technique allows evaluation of the chromatic opponent activity and is therefore particularly suited to the study of optic nerve disorders. Zisman, Bhargava, and King-Smith (1978) have used the technique to study optic neuritis. Sperling, Piantanida, and Garrett (1976) have used the

increment threshold technique to study an observer with an unusual color defect, and
Harwerth and Levi (1977) measured increment threshold spectral sensitivity in amblyopic
eyes.

INCREMENT DETECTION ON CHROMATIC BACKGROUNDS

In the 1930s Stiles (1939) devised an ingenious way of studying chromatic
mechanisms by measuring their detection on chromatic backgrounds. The rationale for the
experiment is that it is often possible by a suitable choice of background wavelengths to
depress the sensitivity of one mechanism so that the sensitivity of a second mechanism,
less sensitive than the first, may be revealed. This rationale saw its first use in the
separation of cone and rod activities in the parafoveal and peripheral retina. The increment
thresholds (Fig. 6.3a) measured as a function of field luminance trace a duplex function
that reflects rod response to test wavelength λ at zero or low radiance backgrounds and
cone response at higher radiance backgrounds (Stiles, 1949). Such curves are called
threshold versus radiance (tvr; previously called the threshold versus intensity, tvi) curves;
each branch traces a characteristic path. A 500-nm backgound may be used to isolate the
photopic mechanism at high background radiances, since the rod response is rendered
insensitive by the background light.

Stiles (1939) realized the potential applicability of the technique to separate the
spectral sensitivities of foveal cone mechanisms. The choices of wavelengths for test and
background fields and radiance of the background field proved enormously more
complicated, and the experiment involved many hours of psychophysical observation.
Stiles obtained foveal tvr curves (Fig. 6.3b) for various combinations of background and
test (Fig. 6.3c) wavelengths (Stiles, 1949). Some of the tvr curves were duplex, some
triplex. For each branch Stiles (1939) was able to identify the spectral sensitivities of
mechanisms to which he later gave the atheoretical nomenclature π mechanisms. Each
mechanism was defined by its characteristic spectral sensitivity.

Techniques.   The technique involves measurement of the increment threshold for a
small monochromatic light flashed upon a continuously presented chromatic background.
The increment threshold may be measured using methods similar to those described for
the absolute threshold. Variables include the spectral composition of the background (μ)
and the test field (λ) and the radiances of the background field (M_μ) and of the test field
(N_λ). Precise radiometric calibration is required.

Formally, it is possible to use two methods to derive the spectral sensitivities of
possible cone mechanisms. In the test sensitivity method, the test wavelength is changed
while background wavelength and radiance are fixed. Referring back to Fig. 6.3, the test
sensitivity at background wavelength 500 nm at zero radiance would yield the rod
function, while at high radiance it would yield the cone function. The π mechanisms are
more complicated, and a given π mechanism is isolated for only a limited wavelength
range. The second technique used to define the spectral sensitivity of the π mechanisms is
the field sensitivity method in which test wavelength λ is fixed and the wavelength and

---

Fig. 6.3.   (See p. 143.) Threshold versus radiance (tvr) curves obtained by Stiles.   (a) Parafoveal
data showing the separation of rods and cones.   (b) Foveal data showing the effect of varying the
background wavelength.   (c) Foveal data showing the effect of varying the test wavelength.

[From Stiles, W. S. *Documenta Ophthalmologica,* 1949. *3.* 138–165. (reproduced with permission
of W. Junk. BV).]

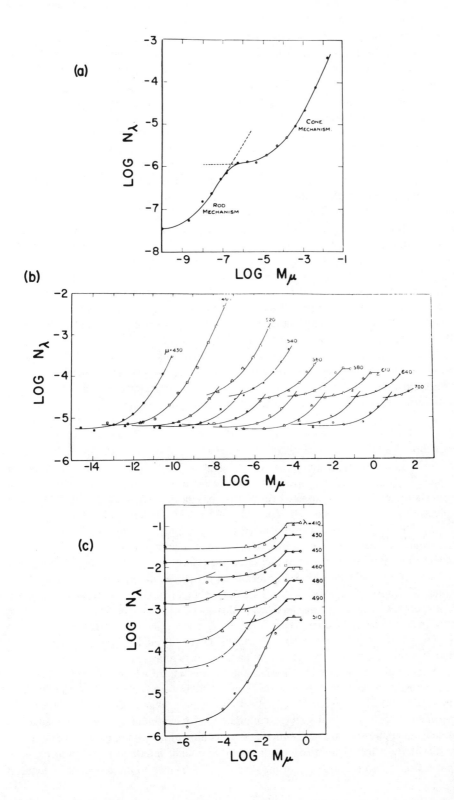

radiance of μ are varied. The experimenter seeks the radiance of the background necessary to raise the test threshold tenfold (one log unit) above its zero background sensitivity. If for a given choice of μ the increment function is duplex, then tenfold field sensitivities are obtained for both branches either by direct measurement or by the use of a template for the increment sensitivity function. The procedure is then repeated for many values of μ. The advantage of the field sensitivity method is that it allows determination of the spectral sensitivity of the π mechanism over a wide wavelength range. Enoch (1972) and Marriott (1976) have reviewed methodology and data of the Stiles two-color threshold experiment.

A total of seven foveal mechanisms have been defined, three (π_1, π_2, and π_3) having sensitivity peaks in the short-wavelength region of the spectrum, two in the middle-wavelength region (π_4, π'_4), and two in the long-wavelength region (π_5, π'_5) (Stiles, 1959). Figure 6.4 shows the relative field sensitivities of the π_1, π_3, π_4, and π_5 mechanisms plotted as the logarithm of quantal energy as a function of wave number. The π mechanisms are to a first approximation independent, but analysis (Boynton, 1963) suggests that the π mechanisms demonstrated by field sensitivities may not represent the spectral sensitivities of isolated cone receptors. Enoch (1972) stated ". . . the two-color increment threshold method provides curves which certainly are substantially influenced by cone pigments, but a large number of intervening physical, chemical, and neural interactive events probably limit conclusive interpretations."

The test sensitivity technique was further developed by Wald (1964). Test thresholds were measured across the spectrum in the presence of one of three very intense background lights of fixed radiance. This method is comparable to that of measuring spectral sensitivity after an intense bleach of the visual photopigments.

Clinical applications.   Both the Stiles (1939) and Wald (1964) techniques have been used in the study of congenital color vision defects. These data are described in Chapter 7. Marré derived a specialized clinical version of the Wald technique (the Wald-Marré technique discussed below) that has been widely used in patients with acquired color vision defects. De Vries–de Mol (1977; De Vries–de Mol, Went, Van Norren, & Pols, 1978) used increment threshold sensitivity on chromatic backgrounds to distinguish the heterozygote female carrier of congenital red–green color defect. Sandberg and Berson (1977) have measured the tvr curves in retinitis pigmentosa, and Sandberg, Rosen, and Berson (1977) measured tvr curves in vitamin A deficiency with chronic alcoholism. Their data indicate that in retinitis pigmentosa both blue (π_1 or π_3) and longer-wavelength cone mechanisms (either π_4 or π_5) were abnormal at 10° from the fovea. In comparison, the blue (π_1) cone mechanism was selectively affected in vitamin A deficiency with chronic alcoholism. Pearlman, Owen, Brounley, and Sheppard (1974) reported tvr curves in a family with a dominant cone dystrophy.

In general, the two-color threshold technique is sufficiently complex that few investigators have attempted its study in acquired color vision defects. A word of caution is in order. Use of increment detection on chromatic backgrounds requires meticulous experimental technique and precise calibration of the stimulus. Normative data are essential. In application to eye disorders, interpretation of the data may prove complex. If test sensitivity is used with a fixed-radiance background, failure to isolate a mechanism might reflect reduced sensitivity of the disputed mechanism to the test light or reduced

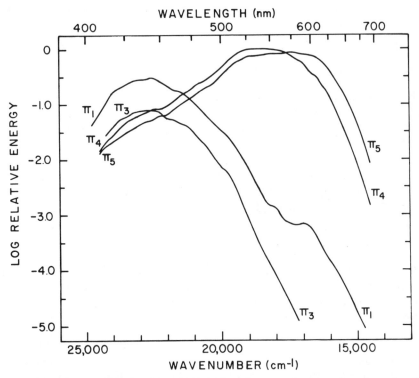

Fig. 6.4. Log relative quantal field sensitivities of the π mechanisms plotted as a function of wave number.

sensitivity of the other mechanisms to the background light. In this event it would be necessary to measure the full tvr curve, as done, for example, by Sandberg and Berson (1977) and Sandberg, Rosen, and Berson (1977).

A different clinical application of the increment detection technique was developed by Boynton and Wagner (1961). An advantage of this technique is that it does not necessitate precise radiant energy calibration of the test and background fields. It is based on the observation that a normal trichromat shows selective chromatic adaptation. The threshold for a long-wavelength test light is raised more when it is presented on a homochromatic background than when it is presented on a heterochromatic background. Boynton and Wagner (1961) termed the phenomenon the heterochromatic threshold reduction factor (HTRF). Dichromats with congenital red–green defects do not show this selective adaptation phenomenon when test and background are greater than 540 nm. Anomalous trichromats also show a severely reduced HTRF compared with normal trichromats. The HTRF can therefore distinguish normal trichromats from observers with congenital red–green defects. Further, by plotting the thresholds for a long-wavelength test (R) on a midspectrum background (G), called condition (R * G), against the thresholds for a midspectrum test (G) on a long-wavelength background (R), called condition (G * R), the subtypes of color defectives may be distinguished in a scatter plot. Ikeda and Urakubo (1968) and Ikeda, Hukami, and Urakubo (1972) developed Boynton and Wagner's (1961) idea by refining the test to allow a flicker rather than increment detection task. These authors noted that the HTRF technique distinguishes the color-defective observer from the normal and may be helpful in detecting the female heterozygote carrier of color defects, at least for carriers of one of the protan defects.

Chromatic Discriminative Ability

The common laboratory methods of evaluation of chromatic discriminative ability involve the measurement of the smallest perceptible wavelength or purity difference. Wavelength discrimination and colorimetric purity discrimination represent two special cases of chromatic discriminative ability. In fact, any chromaticity can be taken as the origin, and discrimination can be evaluated in all relevant directions. Chromatic discrimination for a diverse set of origins has been reported for normal trichromats by several investigators (e.g., Wright, 1941; MacAdam, 1942; Brown, 1957; Wyszecki & Fielder, 1971). Yet another method of evaluating chromatic discriminative ability is the method of color naming.

WAVELENGTH DISCRIMINATION

A person with normal color vision can distinguish about 150–200 variations of hue in the spectrum. Discrimination varies with spectral region. Wavelength discrimination refers to the ability of an observer to detect differences in wavelength.

Techniques. In a representative wavelength discrimination experiment the observer views two fields, one filled with light of a standard wavelength (that is, a narrow spectral band of light) and the other with light of a comparison wavelength. Both fields must be variable in spectral comparison and radiance. Usually, monochromators are used to control wavelength composition of the fields.

In the step-by-step method both fields are initially of identical spectral composition and radiance (isomeric fields). The wavelength of the comparison field is changed in small steps (one nm or less) until the observer reports that the fields do not appear to be of the same hue. It is important to adjust the radiance of the comparison field following each change in the comparison field so that the discrimination is not made on the basis of a brightness difference. The size of the wavelength difference at which the observer reports that the two fields cannot be equated by adjustment of the radiance of the comparison field is called the wavelength discrimination step, $\Delta\lambda$. The procedure is repeated for many standard wavelengths in the visible spectrum. Some experimenters scale in only one direction (e.g., to longer wavelengths); others scale in both directions and average the results.

In an adjustment procedure the experimenter initially sets the two fields to be different in wavelength. The observer is asked to adjust the wavelength and radiance of the variable field until the fields appear the same. The procedure is repeated many times, and the measure of discrimination is taken as the standard deviation of the matching wavelength. The step-by-step method is more rapid but requires an absolute calibration of wavelength. The adjustment procedure is time consuming but more accurate, with somewhat less dependence on criterion changes from the observer.

A wavelength discrimination function showing the value of $\Delta\lambda$ as a function of the standard wavelength for a 3° field of 16 td shows characteristic peaks and valleys (Fig. 6.5a) (Pokorny & Smith, 1970). From 440 to 650 nm the $\Delta\lambda$ values range from 1 to 6 nm , showing a number of peaks and valleys; relative minima occur at 590, 490, and 440 nm,

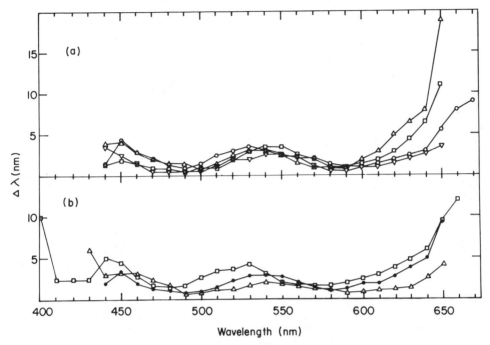

Fig. 6.5. (a) Wavelength discrimination functions obtained from four observers. (b) Comparison of the average wavelength discrimination function (●) with the functions of Bedford and Wyszecki (□) and Wright and Pitt (Δ). [From Pokorny, J., & Smith, V. C. *Journal of the Optical Society of America,* 1970, *60,* 562–569 (reproduced with permission of the Optical Society of America).]

and relative maxima occur at 450 and 530 nm. At the ends of the spectrum, below 430 and above 650 nm, wavelength discrimination deteriorates rapidly and Δλ values rise above 6 nm. Other investigators showed similar functions (Fig. 6.5b). The long-wavelength end of the spectrum is called unitonal in the European literature.

Wavelength discrimintion deteriorates when the luminance or the field size is decreased. With sufficient reduction in field size at moderate light levels, the discrimination function is similar to that occurring in tritanopia (McCree, 1960); reduction in luminance for moderate sized fields results in a generalized loss of discrimination (Weale, 1951; McCree, 1960).

Clinical applications. Wavelength discrimination functions have been measured in observers with congenital color defects and are fully described in Chapter 7. Grützner (1971) and Lakowski (1971) reported wavelength discrimination in minor color abnormalities (Chapter 7). In acquired color vision defects, wavelength discrimination has been reported by Cox (1961b), Grützner and his colleagues (Grützner, 1963b; 1966; Aulhorn & Grützner, 1969; Grützner & Schleicher, 1972), Marré (1973), and Scheibner and Thanberend (1974) for patients with optic nerve disorders and glaucoma. In a disorder accompanied by a mild defect, Δλ thresholds are elevated at all spectral wavelengths. In optic neuritis with a severe type II acquired red–green defect, measurable Δλ steps may be obtained at only two spectral regions, one near 480–500 nm and one near 590 nm (Grützner, 1966; Marré, 1973). Marré (1973) has discussed the relation between the wavelength discrimination function and results using the Wald-Marré adaptation technique. Wavelength discrimination functions have been assessed in patients with retinal disorders by Grützner (1961; 1962), Cox (1961b), Marré (1973), and Pearlman, Owen, Brounley, and Sheppard (1974). These functions show elevated thresholds for all wavelengths (Grützner, 1961). In some patients the $\Delta\lambda$ functions may resemble those of observers with congenital blue–yellow defects (Cox, 1961b); in others discrimination is more affected at the short-wavelength region (Cox, 1961b; Marré, 1973). Marré (1973) reviewed studies of wavelength discrimination in acquired color vision disorders.

COLORIMETRIC PURITY DISCRIMINATION

Adding white to a spectral color desaturates that color; the mixture color appears paler than the spectral color. The term colorimetric purity, p_c, has been defined for mixtures of a spectral color and white as the ratio $p_c = L\lambda/(Lw + L\lambda)$, where $L\lambda$ is the luminance of the spectral color and Lw is the luminance of the white. Colorimetric purity discrimination refers to the ability to discriminate two chromaticities that vary only in the ratio $L\lambda/(Lw + L\lambda)$. Colorimetric purity discrimination usually refers to the measurement of least colorimetric purity (Δp), the minimal amount of spectral light that allows a mixture of colorimetric purity p_c to be distinguished from a specified white. The index of saturation is the reciprocal of the least colorimetric purity.

Techniques. In a representative experiment a standard and a variable field, which may vary in colorimetric purity, are presented side by side in a bipartite field. Although the standard field may have any colorimetric composition, the usual procedure is to measure the first step from white, Δp_c. In this case the standard field is a specified white of fixed luminance Lw; the variable field must be variable in purity. As with wavelength discrimination, the step-by-step method may be used. Initially, both fields are identical whites of equal luminance. The experimenter adds some amount of spectral light, $L\lambda$, to the variable field, maintaining the total luminance $(L\lambda + Lw)$ constant and equal to that of the standard field. The observer reports when the fields first appear different, that is, when the variable field is perceptibly tinged with color. An alternative procedure is the adjustment procedure, in which the variable field is set at a discriminable value of p_c and the observer adjusts its purity until both fields are of equivalent appearance.

Reciprocal colorimetric purity thresholds measured by Priest and Brickwedde (1938) are shown in Fig. 6.6; the highest values occur in the blue, decreasing steadily to a minimum in the yellow, and then increasing again in the red. The colors with the greatest saturation—blues and reds—are those for which only a small amount of $L\lambda$ is necessary to make a white appear tinged with color. Similarly, successive purity discriminations can be obtained—for example, a pink from a red-tinged pink. Such experiments indicate that there are more discriminable steps between white and the spectral radiation for spectral hues that appear highly saturated (blues and reds) than there are for spectral hues (yellows) that appear less saturated. Kaiser, Comerford, and Bodinger (1976) review data from these and other methods of estimating the saturation of spectral lights.

Clinical applications. Measurements of discrimination steps for colorimetric purity have been made for red–green and blue–yellow congenital defects (Chapter 7). Marré (1973) reported colorimetric purity discrimination for acquired color vision defects accompanying retinal disorders. These functions show either an overall decrease of purity discrimination for all wavelengths or a pronounced decrease at short wavelengths.

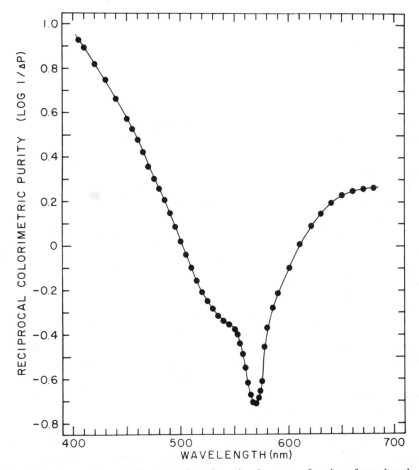

Fig. 6.6.   Log reciprocal of least colorimetric purity shown as a function of wavelength.

COLOR NAMING

Color naming is one of the oldest techniques for evaluation of color defect but is only rarely used today. A major difficulty in color naming procedures is that observers may use idiosyncratic color names, making their responses uninterpretable. Modern technique requires use of high-purity stimuli. Further, the color names must be restricted to those four or five basic terms—e.g., blue, green, yellow, red—that show good agreement in the normal population.

Technique.   There are three variants of the basic color naming procedure; all involve repeated presentations of spectral stimuli. The observer responds to each stimulus with color names from a restricted set of terms. In the first procedure (Beare, 1963) only one name is allowed on each presentation. The experimenter sums and plots the frequency with which each color name is used. In a second procedure, one or two color names are allowed and the experimenter assigns arbitrary point values to the responses (Boynton & Gordon, 1965). For example, if one color name is used, it receives three points; if two are used, the primary name receives two points, the secondary name one point. Cumulative point distributions are plotted for each name. In the third variant, the observer directly estimates the chromatic distribution of a stimulus using proportions—e.g., a 490-nm light may be called 50 percent blue and 50 percent green (Sternheim & Boynton, 1966). Proportions for each color name are averaged over trials. The color naming functions obtained with the three techniques are generally equivalent and demonstrate the reliability with which normal observers assign terms from a restricted set of color names to brief monochromatic flashes. Blue is used for spectral stimuli between 400 and 520 nm, green for those between 460 and 570 nm, and yellow for those above 520 nm; red is used in two spectral regions, between 400 and 450 nm and above 570 nm. The regions of overlap occasionally seen between red and green (at 460 and 570 nm) and yellow and blue (at 520 nm) result from the observer on different trials identifying the predominant color as having different secondary components (for example, on different trials 460 nm might be identified as a slightly reddish blue or a slightly greenish blue).

Smith (1971) derived an Index of Nameable Color Differences (INCD) from color naming data and showed that the INCD gives an estimate of chromatic discriminatory ability similar to that of wavelength discrimination. Graham, Turner, and Hurst (1973) offered an alternative derivation. Boynton and Scheibner (1967) have shown how a perceptual color space may be derived from color naming data using a Kruskal multidimensional scaling technique.

Clinical application.   Studies of color naming in observers with congenital color defects are summarized in Chapter 7. Boynton and Scheibner (1967) derived a perceptual color space for two protanopes using multidimensional analysis. Smith, Pokorny, and Swartley (1973) have described techniques allowing analysis of which color terms are necessary and sufficient for the deuteranomalous trichromat. This procedure is time consuming and has not been used extensively for other color defects. Smith (1973) has described the INCD in tritan defect.

Color naming was used by Köllner (1912) and subsequently by François and Verriest (1957b) to study acquired color vision defects. More recently, Smith, Cole, and Isaacs (1973) described color naming in autosomal dominant optic atrophy. François and Verriest (1957b) found that in acquired red–green color defect the distinction between yellow-orange and red for wavelengths above 570 nm deteriorates, and wavelengths near 495 nm (normally reported as green) appear desaturated. In advanced defect the spectrum is reported as blue below 495 nm and ranging from pale to dark yellow above 495 nm, with a neutral zone at 495 nm. The neutral zone gradually widens to include the wavelength range 435–600 nm. Pale blue below 435 nm and pale yellow above 600 nm are the remaining color sensations. In acquired blue–yellow defects the initial changes are for yellows to appear pink, and the short-wavelength distinction between violet and blue is lost. With moderate defect a neutral zone appears at 550–560 nm. Above 560 nm spectral wavelengths are reported as pink ranging toward red at long wavelengths. Below 460 nm spectral wavelengths are reported blue, green, or even white. In severe defect the neutral zone widens to include the wavelength range 470–589 nm; wavelengths below 470 nm are reported as pale blue and those above 610 nm are reported as pink.

Colorimetric techniques

Full-spectrum colorimetry is rarely performed in normal or color-defective observers. Full-spectrum colorimetry for observers with congenital color vision defects is described in Chapter 7. Few laboratories have used full-spectrum colorimetry in acquired color vision disorders. Clinical screening includes use of the anomaloscope (Chapter 5). Some special matches do have use in analysis of color defect and are further considered here.

THE ANALYTICAL ANOMALOSCOPE

The analytical anomaloscope was described first by Baker and Rushton (1963) and more fully by Mitchell and Rushton (1971b).

Techniques. The primaries and test wavelengths may be those for a conventional anomaloscope, but the primary energies are adjusted in radiance to one of two possible analytical modes: the red and green primary energies are matched either for protanopic sensitivity (protan mode) or for deuteranopic sensitivity (deutan mode). In the Baker and Rushton (1963) experiment a protanope set the R and G primaries equal in luminance for the protan mode and a deuteranope set the R and G primaries equal in luminance for the deutan mode. In the protan mode the protanope sets the radiance of the yellow test field for a match to any arbitrary R-G mixture. Now, all possible R-G mixtures are also color matches to the yellow test field for protanopes. Normal and protanomalous trichromats need not adjust the radiance of the yellow test field from the protanope's setting, except for possible minimal adjustments reflecting interobserver variability in receptor or ocular media absorptions. The trichromat achieves a match simply by adjusting the ratio of red to green in the R-G mixture.

Similarly, in the deutan mode, once the deuteranope sets the radiance of the yellow test field for one R-G mixture, all R-G mixtures are a color match for deuteranopes. Normal and deuteranomalous trichromats need only adjust the R-G mixture to find their matches.

The anomaloscope in analytical mode is a "single-knob" instrument. Once the mode and yellow radiance are set, the observer need only adjust the R-G mixture knob and matching ranges are quickly established. It may be noted that the Nagel model I anomaloscope is close to deutan mode, since the primaries are set at approximately equal luminance for normal trichromats (and also for deuteranopes). With the Nagel anomaloscope, deuteranopes set similar or identical radiances of the test field for all R-G mixtures. Normal and deuteranomalous trichromats also usually do not need to make major adjustments of the yellow test field from the deuteranope's setting. In contrast, protanopes, protanomalous trichromats, and achromats do make major adjustments of the yellow radiance knob at different R-G settings of the Nagel anomaloscope.

The analytical anomaloscope may also be used with a series of test wavelengths. The test radiance will then vary with test wavelength. In the protan mode the test radiance set by protanope, normal, or anomalous trichromat is determined by the spectral luminous efficiency curve of the protanope; in the deutan mode the test radiance set by deuteranope, normal, or deuteranomalous trichromat is determined by the spectral luminous efficiency curve of the deuteranope (Mitchell & Rushton, 1971b).

Clinical application. In the study of matching ranges of anomalous trichromats there is an obvious time saving to have the anomaloscope in the appropriate mode, since the observer need not adjust the Y control. There is also an important theoretical advantage pointed out by Pokorny, Smith, and Katz (1973) and Pokorny and Smith (1977): In the analytical modes the signals generated by photopigment absorptions are linear functions of the fraction of long-wave primary in the match. In consequence, match width is independent of match midpoint, allowing interobserver comparisons of both the widths and the midpoints. This fact is correct also for match widths of normal and deuteranomalous trichromats measured on the Nagel anomaloscope (Pokorny & Smith, 1977).

For use in color vision evaluation the deutan mode offers the following advantages: (1) For normal trichromats and deutan observers, who are the most frequent type of color-defective observer, the deutan mode allows "single-knob" control (varying only the R-G control); the Y control set at the deuteranopic setting will require little or no manipulation. (2) Protanopes and achromats make unique, easily recognized brightness matches. (3) With optic nerve disorders observers can still make matches by varying only the R-G control knob.

EXTENDED RAYLEIGH MATCHES

The extended Rayleigh match was devised by von Kries (1897) as a technique to differentiate a color defect caused by an absorption system from a color defect caused by an alteration system.

Technique. The technique involves presentation of a bipartite colorimetric field with fixed primaries, green and red. The primaries used for the Rayleigh match (545 and 670 nm) are a convenient choice. Four or five test wavelengths are chosen in addition to the sodium line (589 nm) used for the Rayleigh match; for example, 560, 575, 589, 600, and 620 nm might be used. The midmatching point and range are measured using techniques described in Chapter 5. The anomalous quotient (AQ) for each wavelength is calculated and plotted as a function of wavelength. In an absorption system, AQ is displaced but shows no dependence on wavelength. In an alteration system, AQ shows systematic changes with wavelength. As an example of an alteration system, Fig. 6.7 shows data of François and Verriest (1957b) comparing extended matches of normal trichromats with those of two deuteranomalous trichromats.

A different although mathematically identical procedure is to calculate all AQs relative to the normal match at 589 nm and then plot the difference in log AQ (or ratio of AQs) between the normal and affected eyes. The effect of an absorption system on the color match is to multiply the normal match ratio by the factor T_{670}/T_{545}, where T_{670} is the transmittance factor for the absorption system at the 670 nm primary and T_{545} is the transmittance factor at the 545 nm primary. The log (G/R) ratios at the matches are not affected by the transmittance factors for the test wavelengths. In an absorption system the matches plotted as $\log[(G_\lambda/R_\lambda)/(G_{\lambda N}/R_{\lambda N})]$ are displaced uniformly by the factor log (T_{670}/T_{545}); however, in an alteration system the photopigment spectra differ from those of normal—the matches and the log G-R ratios vary with test wavelength.

Clinical application. The extended Rayleigh match has been used with variable success in the study of pseudoprotanomaly accompanying the type III macular color defect. The extended Rayleigh match has been studied in central serous choroidopathy by Jaeger and Nover (1951) and Smith, Pokorny, and Diddie (1978). In such a disease it is possible to compare the normal and affected eyes in the same individual. Smith, Pokorny, and Diddie (1978) showed that two observers with only minimal acuity loss made matches consistent with an alteration system (Fig. 6.8). The data suggested that the visual photopigments were in reduced effective optical density due to receptor disorientation. Receptor disorientation was proved by an abnormal Stiles-Crawford effect. The third

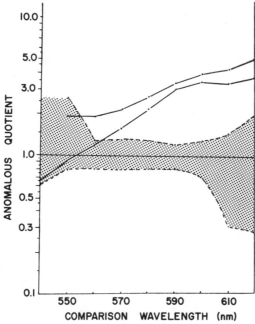

Fig. 6.7. Example of extended Rayleigh matches. The anomalous quotients are plotted as a function of test wavelength. The stippled area shows the matches of normal trichromats. The lines show color matches made by two deuteranomalous trichromats. (Redrawn from François & Verriest, 1957).

observer, with a more severe visual acuity reduction in the affected eye, made variable matches that did not distinguish between an absorption and an alteration system, a finding similar to that of Jaeger and Nover (1951). The difficulty lies in the precision of color matching and the fact that pseudoprotanomaly involves only a minimal displacement of the Rayleigh match. Further, some small absorption effects may accompany the pseudoprotanomaly if serous fluid is coursing among the photoreceptors. Although the technique is powerful, the results may be equivocal in observers with pseudoprotanomaly, especially if reduced chromatic discrimination results in poor matching precision.

Full-spectrum color matching was used by Alpern, Bastian, Pugh, and Gras (1976) in a study of hypercupremia. To analyze the data they compared the differences in the ratio of the red and green color-matching function; i.e., their analysis was similar to that of the extended Rayleigh match. Since their sample included more than 20 wavelengths over a full spectral range, they were able statistically to demonstrate that the visual effects of hypercupremia can be accounted for by an absorption system even though the data showed considerable variability.

COLOR MATCH AREA EFFECT

Color matches change with the size of the field of view (Horner & Purslow, 1947; 1948; Pokorny & Smith, 1976).

Technique. The effect can be demonstrated by measuring the Rayleigh equation for different field sizes. The log(*G/R*) ratio decreases systematically as the field of view increases. Pokorny and Smith (1976) termed the phenomenon the color match area effect. The change occurs because the effective optical density of the visual photopigments is reduced as the field of view enlarges. The color matches represent an average of the stimulated photoreceptors, and the color match area effect reflects the changing dimensions of the photoreceptors, since the enlarging field of view includes greater proportions of parafoveal cones.

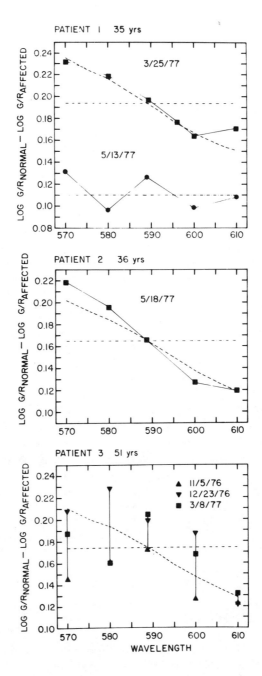

Clinical application. The color match area effect depends on the normal good alignment of photoreceptors in the young eye. Therefore the effect is a sensitive test of the normal architecture of the macula. The color match area effect has been studied in a variety of acquired and heredity chorioretinal diseases (Smith, Pokorny, Ernest, & Starr, 1978; Pokorny, Smith, & Ernest, in press).

NEUTRAL ZONE DETERMINATION

The neutral zone refers to those spectral wavelengths that are exactly matched to white. The existence of a spectral neutral point or zone is diagnostic of dichromacy and indicative of a severe form of color deficiency.

Techniques. The classical technique of neutral point determination involves presentation of a bipartite colorimetric field. In one half, a white, preferably the equal-energy white or a high–color temperature white, is presented. In the other, a continuous range of spectral wavelengths is presented. The observer's task is to locate those spectral wavelengths that after radiance adjustment match the white exactly. For a trichromat there are none; for a dichromat a group or range of wavelengths does match the white. In congenital stationary disorders there are just a few wavelengths, and it is customary to refer to a neutral point. In protanopia and deuteranopia the neutral point wavelengths are near 500 nm; in tritanopia they are near 570 nm. The exact spectral location of the neutral point depends on the reference white, varies with macular pigment density, and shows interindividual variability.

A drawback of the classical technique is that a monochromator is necessary in order to ensure a sufficient range of wavelength variation. Further, the observer must adjust both wavelength and radiance to achieve the match. To demonstrate dichromacy, it is only necessary to show the existence of a neutral point. A filter anomaloscope and appropriate filter pairs may be used for this purpose. For example, in congenital red–green dichromacy the neutral point is in the blue-green. The appropriate blue-green wavelength can be matched either to the equal-energy white or to a purple, a mixture of a blue primary and a red primary. Further, any white and any blue-green can be matched to a mixture of blue and red primaries by the dichromat. To demonstrate the existence of a neutral point in a color defective using a filter anomaloscope, primaries of red and blue—e.g., 450 and 650 nm—are used. The test color may be a white (preferably high color temperature) or a blue-green (e.g., 500 nm). The observer follows a typical anomaloscope procedure,

---

Fig. 6.8. (See p.154.) Extended Rayleigh match series for three patients with central serous choroidopathy. The ordinate shows the difference between log *(G/R)* for the normal eye and log *(G/R)* for the affected eye; the abscissa shows the test wavelength. The dashed lines are predictions based on a reduced effective optical density hypothesis; the solid line is the prediction for an absorption system. The upper panel shows data for patient 1 using a 2° field for the normal eye and an 8° field for the affected eye. The middle panel shows data for patient 2 using an 8° field for normal and affected eyes. The lower panel shows data for patient 3 using a 2° field for the normal eye and an 8° field for the affected eye.

[From Smith, V. C., Pokorny, J., & Diddie, K. R. *Modern Problems in Ophthalmology;* 1978, *19*, 284–295 (reproduced with permission of S. Karger AG).]

adjusting the blue-red ratio and the test field luminance to achieve a match. To demonstrate the existence of a neutral point in tritanopia, using a filter anomaloscope, the primaries may be green and red (e.g., the Rayleigh primaries 545 and 670 nm). The test color may be equal-energy white or a blue (e.g., 450 nm). The observer follows the typical anomaloscope procedure, adjusting the green to red ratio and luminance of the test color to achieve a match.

Clinical application.   The classical neutral point technique was used extensively by Grützner (1963a; 1966), whose studies have been summarized in the Handbook of Sensory Physiology (1972). Grützner (1966) noted that when a neutral zone occurs in acquired color vision defects it is usually a broad neutral zone, in contradistinction to the narrow neutral points of the congenital dichromacies.

Acquired color vision defects are usually accompanied by loss of purity discrimination, extending from the white point. Only after progression to very severe defect does a true spectral neutral zone occur. It is therefore useful in acquired color vision defects to have a measure of this enlarging neutral zone. This type of measurement may be accomplished with a filter anomaloscope, e.g., the Pickford-Lakowski equation, available on the Pickford-Nicolson anomaloscope (see Chapter 5). This equation allows determination of the width of the match of white to a mixture of blue and yellow. The match width is a sensitive measure of purity discrimination loss in acquired color vision defects (Lakowski, 1972).

Stiles-Crawford Effect

A pencil of light that enters the center of the pupil parallel to the long axis of the photoreceptors is more effective visually than light entering at the edge of the pupil at an angle to the long axis. A light entering on or near the optic axis appears brighter than an equivalent light entering at the edge of the pupil (Stiles & Crawford, 1933). This effect is called the Stiles-Crawford effect of the first kind (SCE 1). If the stimulus field is colored, the color appearance of the field, when it enters the edge of the pupil, is changed in both hue and saturation. This effect is called the Stiles-Crawford effect of the second kind (SCE 2). The Stiles-Crawford effects are ascribed to the fact that the photoreceptor has dimensions close to the wavelength of light and acts as a waveguide when electromagnetic radiation is incident on the inner segment. Reviews of the data and theory of the Stiles-Crawford effect may be found in Vos (1960), Stiles (1962), Enoch (1963), Crawford (1972), and Starr (1977).

Technique.   Measurement of the SCE 1 may be accomplished by brightness-matching techniques using a maximally dilated pupil. The optical design involves the presentation of a photometric field, either a circular split field or a small circular field embedded in an annulus. One field is a standard field—the stimulus beam enters through the center of the pupil. The other field is the variable field—the position of the entry beam is variable on the eye pupil. For a given pupil entry the radiance of the variable field is adjusted to provide a brightness match to the standard field. The experimenter measures the relative radiance required to maintain a brightness match for all entry positions. When the entry beam is decentered, a spherical aberration of the eye may produce an apparent misalignment of the two halves of the photometric field. This effect may be corrected by adjustment of the position of one of the field stops or by adding spherical correcting lenses at the eye. Heterochromatic flicker photometry has also been used to determine the SCE 1 (Safir & Hyam, 1969). Matching techniques are used in the determination of the relative luminous efficiency with traverse of the pupil. The give information about the shape and centering of the Stiles-Crawford effect but not about absolute sensitivity.

To determine the absolute sensitivity of the SCE 1, it is necessary to use a threshold technique—either absolute (Stiles & Crawford, 1933), increment threshold (Crawford, 1937; Enoch & Hope, 1972a), or constant CFF (Alpern, Falls, & Lee, 1960). The optical design allows for a beam whose entry position on the pupil may be varied. The radiance of the beam at each pupil entry position is adjusted for detection. In the constant CFF technique the stimulus is presented in rapid temporal alternation and at a given luminance appears to flicker. The luminance is adjusted until the stimulus field appears fused or steady.

Frequently, the variable beam is adjusted on only one meridian, usually the horizontal meridian. Some investigators, however (Dunnewold, 1964; Enoch, 1959a), have measured the Stiles-Crawford effect on multiple meridians.

Figure 6.9 shows data of Stiles and Crawford (1933) using techniques of brightness matching and absolute threshold with a foveally viewed 2° field. The data are presented as the logarithm of luminous efficiency (inverse of threshold luminance) plotted against the position of the entry beam on a given meridian in the pupil. The maximal luminous efficiency occurs near the center of the pupil; luminous efficiency decreases smoothly on either side of the maximum.

Stiles and Crawford point out that the data for the central ±3 mm may be fitted by a parabola of the form

$$\log \eta = p^2 \, (d - d_o),$$

where η is the relative luminous efficiency, p is a parameter of the curve, d is the displacement in millimeters on the pupil, and d_o is the displacement for which $\log \eta$ is maximal. The relative efficiency of light drops rapidly as the entry beam is decentered; the loss is approximately 50 percent (0.3 log unit of density) within a ±3 mm displacement of the entry beam from its center position. Each millimeter of displacement on the plane of the pupil represents an angle of about 2.5° at the outer segment. For foveal measurements the parameter p takes on values ranging from 0.45 to 0.7 in normal observers. The value d_o is at or close to the observer's visual axis. Figure 6.9 is for foveal cones.

Measurement of SCE 1 in the parafovea reveals a narrower function than the foveal function, peaking near the optic axis. The narrower parafoveal SCE function reflects the changing dimensions of the photoreceptors. The central peak reflects the observation that the long axis of the photoreceptors is oriented toward the exit pupil of the eye (Laties & Enoch, 1971; Enoch & Laties, 1971; Enoch & Hope, 1972a; 1972b).

With pupil entrance positions beyond ±3 mm, the function flattens (Safir & Hyams, 1969), and in persons with an eccentric peak to the Stiles-Crawford effect a pronounced flattening can be seen (Safir, Kulikowski, Kuo, & Edgerton, 1972; Wijngaard & Van Kruysbergen, 1975).

It has been difficult to measure a Stiles-Crawford type 1 effect for the rods using angles obtainable through the pupil. The functions usually show little change in luminous

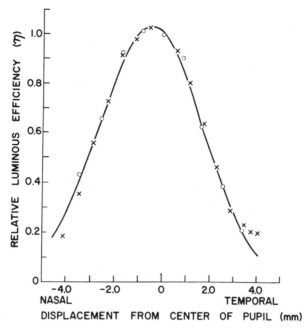

Fig. 6.9. Relative luminous efficiency (η) of light entering the eye pupil at different points for foveal vision. $\times$, measurements by photometric matching method (Stiles & Crawford, 1933); O, measurements by brightness threshold method (Crawford, 1937); curve $\eta = 1.04e^{-0.108(r + 0.47)}$ [From Crawford, B. J. In D. Jameson & L. M. Hurvich (Eds.): *Handbook of sensory physiology,* Vol. VII/4. Berlin, Springer-Verlag, 1972 (reproduced with permission of Springer-Verlag).]

efficiency with pupil entry. However, when the measurements are corrected for the path lengths through the lens a small Stiles-Crawford effect for rods does in fact exist (Weale, 1961; Vos & Van Os, 1975) and has been measured by Daw and Enoch (1973) and Van Loo and Enoch (1975).

When the stimulus is a spectral radiation, decentering the pupil causes not only a decrease in luminous efficiency but also a change in hue and saturation (SCE 2). For wavelengths above 550 nm the hue change is to longer wavelengths and there is slight desaturation. Between 500 and 550 nm the hue change is to shorter wavelengths and there is an increase in saturation. Below 500 nm the hue change is again to longer wavelengths and there is minimal change in saturation.

Alignment of the observer: There are four methods for aligning the observer's eye in the optical equipment: (1) The dilated pupil may be centered on the optic axis of the apparatus (Stiles & Crawford, 1933; Vos, 1960; Vos & Huigen, 1962; Dunnewold, 1964; Enoch, 1969a; Enoch & Hope, 1972a). (2) The observer may align himself to eliminate asymmetric chromatic fringes (due to chromatic aberration of the eye) when viewing a bichromatic mixture field (Wright, 1946). (3) The observer may align visually to maximize his or her Stiles-Crawford effect (Vos, 1960; Vos & Huigen, 1962). (4) The corneal reflex may be used to align the eye with the optic axis of the apparatus (Enoch, 1957; Safir & Hyams, 1969; Starr, 1977). Alignment by centering on the dilated pupil has the disadvantage of enlarging both interobserver variability and daily intraobserver variability in the measured value of d_0. This effect occurs because the pupil does not always dilate symmetrically. The effect will be small for maximal mydriasis but will interfere with precise estimation of the locus and variation of d_0. Self-alignment of the observer precludes evaluation of d_0. The techniques of centering on the pupil and of self-alignment may be used for procedures when precise evaluation of d_0 is unnecessary.

When the observer's fixation is aligned with the optic axis of the apparatus, measurement of d_0 may be made with high precision and repeatability. This technique consists of aligning the optic axis of the apparatus with its reflection from the cornea (first Purkinjé image). A small portion of the optically centered incident beam is compared visually with its corneal reflection. A telescope is used, and the experimenter may if necessary maintain a continual monitor of the corneal reflex during the experimental procedure. With this method of alignment the measured value for d_0 is rarely at 0 but tends to occur about 1 mm into the superotemporal quadrant.

Clinical application.   Measurement of the Stiles-Crawford effect has been accomplished in congenital color vision defects. The Stiles-Crawford effect of the first kind has been measured in dichromats (Starr, 1977) with the aim of establishing the role of optical density of the photopigments in the shape of the $\log\eta$ function. Studies of the Stiles-Crawford effect of the second kind in anomalous trichromats are described in Chapter 7.

The Stiles-Crawford effect of the first kind has been an important tool in the study of achromatopsia. Alpern, Falls, and Lee (1960) established that the rapid-adapting receptors of the complete achromat have Stiles-Crawford properties of the cone photoreceptors. Measurements of the Stiles-Crawford effect in X-chromosome–linked recessive incomplete achromacy were made by Alpern, Lee, Maaseidvaag, and Miller (1971), who found a receptor class with Stiles-Crawford properties of cones but spectral sensitivity of rods. Daw and Enoch (1973) preformed a similar experiment in an X-chromosome–linked recessive achromat, but the directional sensitivy of the rhodopsin-containing receptor was that of rods.

Measurement of the Stiles-Crawford effect of the first kind is growing in use as a clinical tool in acquired color vision defects. The Stiles-Crawford effect was first used clinically by Enoch and his associates (Enoch, 1957; 1959a; 1959b; 1967; Fankhauser, Enoch & Cibis, 1961; Fankhauser & Enoch, 1962; Benson, Kolker, Enoch, Van Loo, & Honda 1975) and by Dunnewold (1964). Enoch (1967) and Enoch, Van Loo, & Okun (1973) have emphasized that an abnormal Stiles-Crawford effect may show recovery. More recently, the technique has been applied by Pokorny, Smith, and their associates (Smith, Pokorny, Ernest, & Starr, 1978; Smith, Pokorny, & Diddie, 1978; Pokorny, Smith, & Johnston, 1979; Pokorny, Smith, & Ernest, in press).

The Stiles-Crawford effect reflects the physical characteristics of the photoreceptors and is critically dependent on the normal good orientation of the visual photoreceptors. The reasons for using the Stiles-Crawford effect as a special psychophysical test in acquired color vision defect are that it can reveal a disease process that causes disorientation of the photoreceptor layer and that it can follow the recovery of orientation following reattachment surgery (Fankhauser, Enoch, & Cibis, 1961; Enoch, Van Loo, & Okun, 1973); it can also follow the resolution of central serous choroidopathy (Smith, Pokorny, & Diddie, 1978). Figure 6.10 shows the Stiles-Crawford effect in an observer with central serous choroidopathy in the left eye (visual acuity 0.67). In the acute phase

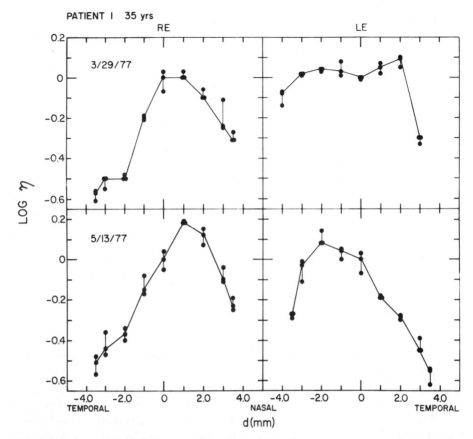

Fig. 6.10. Stiles-Crawford effect of the first kind for a 35-year-old observer with central serous choroidopathy: log relative luminous efficiency (η) plotted as a function of pupil entry position. The upper panel shows data obtained in the acute phase; the lower panel shows data obtained 1 month after laser treatment [From Smith, V. C., Pokorny, J., & Diddie, K. R. *Modern Problems in Ophthalmology,* 1978, *19,* 284–295 (reproduced with permission of S. Karger AG).]

the normal right eye showed a normal well-peaked and centered Stiles-Crawford effect; the abnormal left eye showed an abnormal Stiles-Crawford effect. One month later, following resorption of fluid, a peaking Stiles-Crawford effect was obtained in the affected eye.

WALD-MARRE APPROACH TO MEASUREMENT OF THE
THREE PRIMARY COLOR VISION MECHANISMS (CVMs)*

The measurement of visual thresholds for colored stimuli under conditions of selective chromatic adaptation opens the possibility of isolating, representing, and measuring quantitatively the three primary color vision mechanisms (CVMs). The Wald-Marré approach examines psychophysically the function of the visual pigments in a circumscribed retinal area and the alterations, between receptor and cortex, that these functions undergo in pathologic states. Wald (1964; 1966) developed the selective chromatic adaptation technique, which is the basis for the approach, in order to

*Contributed by Marion Marré, M.D.

demonstrate the action spectra of the three visual pigments in the living human eye. He also examined congenital color-defective photopigment action spectra with this technique for the first time. Marré (1969; 1970; 1972a; 1973) and Marré and Marré (1972) extended this technique to give quantitative measurements of abnormalities of the three CVMs in acquired color vision defects. The technique of selective chromatic adaptation has also been used in electrophysiology to separate the inputs of the three cone types at various levels of visual processing (DeValois, 1970; Gouras, 1970).

The Wald-Marré approach differs from the two-color threshold technique of Stiles (1939) with its monochromatic adaptation by using bright and well-defined although broadband adaptation lights that selectively desensitize two of the three CVMs. It also differs from King-Smith's (1976) method of flicker detection on white backgrounds. The spectral sensitivity curves yielded by the latter method show maxima at 450, 525, and 600 nm. These were interpreted as resulting from color-opponent systems. The maxima of the CVM sensitivity curves of the Wald-Marré approach lie at about 440, 545, and 570 nm. They approximate the absorption maxima of the three visual pigments and were therefore assumed to represent the three primary CVMs.

Principle of the Method

A very bright, defined chromatic adaptation light is of such a spectral composition that two of the three CVMs are presumed to be highly desensitized. In this way the third CVM is isolated, and its sensitivity can be measured by means of increment thresholds.

APPARATUS

The apparatus used for measurement of CVMs consisted of two light paths combined in Maxwellian view (Fig. 6.11). The first one provided one of the three chromatic adaptation lights as a steady background of 20°. The light sources were two tungsten halogen lamps rated at 6 V/20 W (for additive color mixture). Color glass filters (Schott/Jena) were used to obtain the three adaptation lights: (1) GG 14, opaque to wavelengths up to 500 nm, for isolating the blue mechanism [for simplicity, the three CVMs are described by the terms "blue," "green," and "red," although it is known that it is not appropriate to associate color names with CVMs (DeValois, 1970)]; (2) BG 12 + OG 2, opaque to wavelengths between 470 and 560 nm, for isolating the green mechanism; and (3) BG 12 + ORWO No. 76 (gelatin filter) opaque to wavelengths longer than 560 nm, for isolating the red mechanism. The three selective chromatic adaptation lights were of equal photometric retinal illuminance, about 1500 td. A fixation stimulus composed of four concentric circles, leaving open the central visual test field of 1.2°, facilitated steady fixation even in diseased eyes with eccentric fixation. The second light path was used to present monochromatic test pulses of variable radiance. The target size was 1.2°, and the light source was a halogen lamp rated at 24 V/140 W. A series of interference filters was used, and the resulting energy for the lamp-filter combinations was calculated. Radiance could be continuously varied by five neutral-density filters and two neutral-density wedges. Stimulus presentation time was 50 msec.

METHOD

The observer fixated the center of the chromatic background for 3 min before threshold measurements were begun. Monochromatic test flashes of graduated radiance were then presented on the chromatic background within the center of the fixation

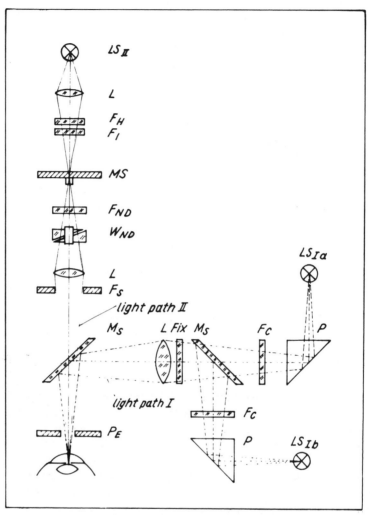

Fig. 6.11. Arrangement of the apparatus (Maxwellian view). Fᴄ, color filter; Fₕ, heat-absorbing filter; Fɪ, interference filter; Fɴᴅ, five neutral-density filters in logarithmic steps; Fix, fixation arrangement; Fs, field stop; L, lens; LSɪₐ,ɪᵦ,ɪɪ, light sources; Ms, semitransmitting mirror; MS, motor shutter; P, prism; Pᴇ, exit pupil (3 mm); Wɴᴅ, neutral-density wedges. Light path I provides selective chromatic adaptation lights for a steady background. Light path II gives monochromatic test flashes of variable intensity for increment threshold measurements.

arrangement. Increment thresholds were measured in steps of 10–20 nm across the wavelength range relevant for the adaptation condition and in wider steps across the remaining spectrum. The ranges of wavelengths carefully explored were chosen so that at their extremes the sensitivity of the CVM in question was only a few percent of the absolute sensitivity of the fovea (Wald, 1964). The ranges explored were for the blue mechanism 402–497 nm; for the green mechanism 475–601 nm; and for the red mechanism 497–649 nm. After examination of each CVM, a 15-min rest was given. All three CVMs could be measured in one session of about 2½ hours. Additionally, the absolute retinal sensitivity could be measured by means of absolute thresholds after a 30-min dark adaptation.

REPRESENTATION AND CALCULATION

The logarithm of the relative sensitivity of the three CVMs is plotted against wavelength in Figs. 6.12 and 6.13. The mean difference between the normal curve (logS_N) and the pathologic one (logS_P) over the wavelength range λ_I . . . λ_{II} allows calculation of the reduction factor N/P (Mierdel P. G.: Unpublished communication). This mean difference can be calculated as

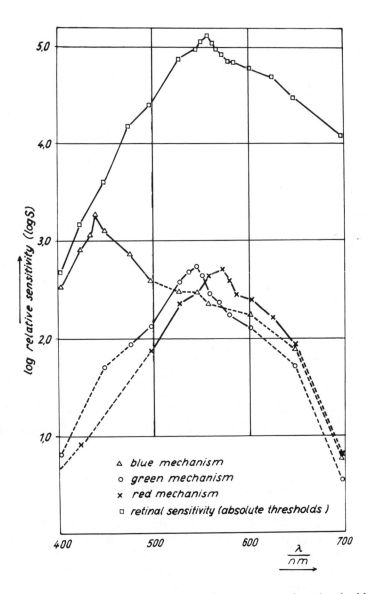

Fig. 6.12. Representation of the three CVMs. Mean curves of twelve healthy normal trichromatic eyes of the age group 20–40 years. For quantitative calculation the following wavelength ranges are chosen (continuous lines): blue mechanism, 402–497nm; green mechanism, 475–601 nm; red mechanism, 497–649 nm.

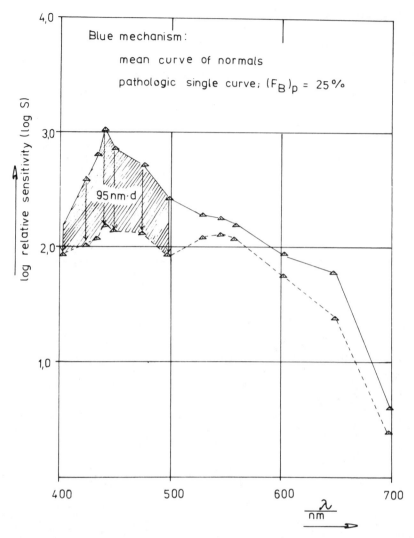

Fig. 6.13. Example of a pathologic blue mechanism $(F_B)_P$ in a case of tapetoretinal degeneration.

$$\frac{1}{\lambda_{II} - \lambda_I} \int_{\lambda_I}^{\lambda_{II}} (\log S_N - \log S_P)\, d\lambda = d, \qquad (6.1)$$

where the range of $\lambda_I - \lambda_{II}$ is 402–497 nm for the blue mechanism, 475–601 nm for the green mechanism, and 497–649 nm for the red mechanism. The difference d goes to the factor N/P after a change to linear scale,

$$N/P = 10^d. \qquad (6.1a)$$

The integral is numerically calculated over the range $\lambda_I \ldots \lambda_{II}$ according to the wavelength steps of the used interference filters. The calculation may be carried out by means of a computer, or by hand as follows (Table 6.1):

Table 6.1
Sample Calculation of a Pathologic Blue Mechanism

Measured Values

λ_i (nm)	$\log S_N$ (mean)	$\log S_P$
402	2.17	1.91
424	2.59	2.03
434	2.80	2.07
440	3.02	2.20
449	2.85	2.13
475	2.70	2.11
497	2.43	1.92

Calculation

$\lambda_{i+1} - \lambda_i$ (nm)	(1) $\dfrac{(\log S_N)_i + (\log S_N)_{i+1}}{2}$	(2) $\dfrac{(\log S_P)_i + (\log S_P)_{i+1}}{2}$	(1) − (2)	$(\lambda_{i+1} - \lambda_i)[(1) - (2)]$
22	2.38	1.97	0.41	9.02
10	2.70	2.05	0.65	6.50
6	2.91	2.14	0.77	4.62
9	2.94	2.17	0.77	6.93
26	2.78	2.12	0.66	17.16
22	2.57	2.02	0.55	12.10
				56.33

$d = 56.33/95 = 0.5929;\quad N/P = 10^{0.5929} = 3.92;\quad$ i.e., $F_B = 100/3.92 = 25.5\%$.

165

$$d = \frac{1}{\lambda_{II} - \lambda_{I}} \sum_{i=1}^{h-1} (\lambda_{i+1} - \lambda_i) \left(\frac{(\log S_N)_i + (\log S_N)_{i+1}}{2} \right.$$

$$\left. - \frac{(\log S_P)_i + (\log S_P)_{i+1}}{2} \right), \tag{6.2}$$

where λ_i is the wavelength of the i interference filter $(i = 1, \ldots, n)$, $\lambda_I = \lambda_I$, and $\lambda_{II} = \lambda_n$. The function of the pathological CVM can be obtained by

$$F_{CVM}(\%) = \frac{100}{N/P}. \tag{6.3}$$

Figure 6.13 illustrates the difference between a normal and a pathologic blue mechanism (for observers of similar age).

NORMAL VALUES

Table 6.2 presents the normal ranges of the three CVMs in two age groups. The asymmetry of the standard deviations results from the logarithmic values of the measurements. Table 6.3 shows the relative values of three CVMs of two normal eyes at different eccentricities in the central visual field. The CVM values for foveolar fixation were set to 100 percent. With increasing eccentricity the sensitivity of the blue mechanism increases and the sensitivities of the green and red mechanisms decrease, with the sensitivity of the red mechanism decreasing somewhat more than that of the green. From these data two normal CVM patterns can be derived: (1) the foveolar CVM pattern as examplifed by the mean values with standard deviations of normal trichromatic eyes; (2) the normal CVM pattern with varying eccentricity, measured by varying the position of the test flash relative to the fixation area.

CVMs in Congenital Color Vision Deficiencies

Wald and Brown (1965) and Wald (1966) reported relative sensitivity curves of "the blue, green, and red receptors" in 20 deutans, 8 protans, and 3 tritans. In deutans the examinations revealed normal "blue and red receptors," but all attempts to measure the "green receptor" yielded only the "red receptor" with depressed sensitivity. Corresponding results were found with the "red receptor" in protans and with the "blue receptor" in tritans. Anomalous trichromats gave results similar to those of dichromats. The examination method could not distinguish between the two types of color defects. Only in a very unusual case of a deuteranomalous tritanope did Wald (1966) succeed in isolating an abnormal "green receptor" with low sensitivity and a spectrum displaced

Table 6.2
Normal Ranges of the Three CVMs (%) (Foveal Fixation)

Age Group (years)	n	Blue Mechanism	Green Mechanism	Red Mechanism
10–39	12	61–164	82–122	71–142
40–59	12	67–145	70–141	69–147

Table 6.3
CVM Values of Two Normal Trichromatic Eyes at Different Retinal Eccentricities (%)

Eccentricity (Related to the Fovea)	Temporal			Nasal			Above			Below		
	B	G	R	B	G	R	B	G	R	B	G	R
1° U.T.	113	70	48	131	68	50	160	106	74	118	101	63
E.B.	117	63	63	126	69	43	181	99	85	191	91	68
2° U.T.	122	48	30	156	53	38	198	79	55	115	61	64
E.B.	173	53	35	178	50	28	181	87	67	296	68	57
4° U.T.	134	41	26	227	41	28	221	37	26	163	69	54
E.B.	220	43	28	202	36	34	217	65	51	324	57	46
6° U.T.	188	29	19	207	29	24	250	25	20	183	36	29
E.B.	257	34	25	206	28	24	237	53	40	340	50	37

The CVMs in foveal fixation equal 100 percent.

toward red. Marré (1969) confirmed Wald's results in protanopia, protanomaly, deuteranopia, and deuteranomaly.

CVMs in Acquired Color Vision Deficiencies

Quantitative measurement of the three primary CVMs reveals three patterns in acquired color vision defects (Table 6.4). These pathologic patterns are dependent on the fixation mode of the diseased eye and can be directly derived from the two normal CVM patterns. Further, the data correspond approximately to the Verriest classification (Chapter 4) of acquired color vision defects.

THE THREE CVM TYPES OF ACQUIRED
COLOR VISION DEFECTS

CVM type I. The blue mechanism is distinctly more reduced than the green and red mechanisms. Two stages can be quantitatively differentiated. In the initial stage, Ia, the blue mechanism is disturbed but green and red mechanisms are still normal. In the advanced stage, Ib, all CVMs are diminished, but the blue mechanism much more so than the other two (Table 6.5). CVM type I can be derived from the normal foveolar CVM pattern. Stage Ia corresponds to the Verriest type III acquired blue–yellow defect and stage Ib to the type III defect with concomitant red–green defect.

CVM type II. The blue mechanism shows values higher than or equal to those of the green and red mechanism. Two stages can be quantitatively distinguished. An initial stage, IIa, in which the blue mechanism is distinctly higher than the other two (the blue mechanism is often equal to or greater than the normal foveolar value, while the green and red mechanisms are reduced below the normal foveolar value), and an advanced stage, IIb, in which all CVMs have apprximately equal values and are clearly reduced below the normal foveolar values (Table 6.6). CVM type II can be derived from the normal eccentric CVM pattern. Stage IIa corresponds to the Verriest type I or II acquired red–green defects, stage IIb to those defects with concomitant blue–yellow defect.

CVM type III. All three CVMs are reduced to values below 25 percent of the normal sensitivity with the blue mechanism somewhat more depressed than both the others (Table 6.7). CVM type III is the endpoint of progression of acquired color vision defects. It develops from both CVM types I and II. It corresponds to defects of anarchic character.

CVM type II develops only in diseased eyes with a fixation outside the foveola. If the eccentric CVM pattern found by varying fixation area in normal observers is compared to the CVM type II pattern, the sensitivity of the blue mechanism is more reduced than those of the red and green mechanisms, in CVM type II as well as in CVM types I and III. The characteristic pathologic CVM patterns of CVM type II (as well as the classical description, "acquired red–green defect") result from the fact that in eccentric vision the blue mechanism exhibits higher sensitivity and the green and red mechanisms exhibit lower sensitivity than in foveolar fixation and, further, from the (questionable) practice of referring all acquired defects to normal color vision in foveolar fixation.

Table 6.4
Three CVM Types of Acquired Color Vision Defects

Type	Stage	Data Related To:			Corresponding Classic Type
		Normal Foveal CVM Pattern	Normal CVM Pattern of the Fixation Area Used	Fixation Mode	
I	Ia	/B/</G/, /R/	B↓; G, R normal	Enlarged foveal (exclusively)	B-Y defect
I	Ib	/B/</G/, /R/	B↓↓; G, R↓	Foveal, para-foveal-macular	B-Y defect with accompanying R-G defect
II	IIa	/B/>/G/, /R/	B normal,↓↓↓; G, R normal,↓	Parafoveal, parafoveal-macular, extramacular (never foveal)	R-G defect
II	IIb	/B/~/G/, /R/	B↓↓; G, R↓		R-G defect with accompanying B-Y defect
III	—	/B/</G/, /R/	B↓↓↓; G, R↓↓	Enlarged foveal, parafoveal-macular, extramacular	Anarchic

169

Table 6.5

CVM Type I of Acquired Color Vision Defects in Retinal and
Optic Nerve Diseases

Diagnosis	Visual Acuity	B (%)	G (%)	R (%)	Fixation Mode
Stage Ia					
Chorioretinal central serous	0.8	27	99	77	Foveal
Tapetoretinal degeneration	0.5	48	80	81	Enlarged foveal
Senile macular degeneration	0.5	2	105	77	Enlarged foveal
Thrombosis	0.3	2	70	72	Foveal
Optic atrophy	0.8	15	75	92	Foveal
Optic atrophy	0.5	5	69	84	Foveal
Stage Ib					
Chorioretinal central serous	0.6	2	47	61	Enlarged foveal
Chorioretinal degeneration	0.5	10	39	38	Parafoveal
Thrombosis	0.3	2	41	43	Enlarged foveal
Myopia	0.2	2	36	44	Upper macular border
Neuritis	0.8	28	59	54	Unsteady foveal
Optic atrophy	0.5	2	30	36	Macular
Optic atrophy	0.3	2	43	64	Foveal nystagmus

DEPENDENCE OF THE CVM TYPES OF ACQUIRED COLOR
DEFECTS ON THE FIXATION MODE IN RETINAL DISEASES
AND OPTIC NERVE DISEASES*

In eyes with acquired color vision defects and preserved foveolar fixation we find
exclusively CVM type I (stage a or b), irrespective of whether the retina or the optic nerve
is affected (Table 6.5). In diseased eyes with a fixation area peripheral to the perifovea,
we find mostly CVM type II (stage a or b), again in both retinal and optic nerve diseases
(Table 6.6.). The situation is somewhat more complicated when the fixation area lies
outside the foveola but within the fovea, parafovea, or perifovea. Then, retinal diseases
and optic nerve diseases show different results. Retinal diseases develop nearly
exclusively type Ib patterns, while optic nerve diseases develop type IIa or IIb patterns in
the majority of cases and type Ib patterns in a smaller number of cases. CVM type III, the
final form, can appear in retinal and optic nerve diseases concomitant with enlarged
foveolar fixation areas or with all kinds of fixations outside the foveola, but especially in
cases with peripheral fixation.

Terminology of the central retina (Spitznas, 1975). Foveola: 20′ (in the center of the fovea); fovea: 0°–3°
eccentricity (diameter 6°); parafovea: 3°–5.3° eccentricity; perifovea: 5.3°–11.3° eccentricity. *Terminology of
the fixation mode.* Foveolar: steady fixation with the foveola, normal case of fixation; parafoveolar: outside the
foveola but within the fovea; parafoveal: outside the fovea but within the parafovea; perifoveal: outside the
parafovea but within the perifovea; peripheral: outside the perifovea; eccentric: all kinds of fixation outside the
foveola.

Table 6.6
CVM Type II of Acquired Color Vision Defects in Retinal and
Optic Nerve Diseases

Diagnosis	Visual Acuity	B (%)	G (%)	R (%)	Fixation Mode
Stage IIa					
Myopia	0.2	188	60	50	Disc-macula
Juvenile macular degeneration	0.2	54	31	31	Upper macular border
Optic atrophy	0.5	90	88	60	Parafoveal
Optic atrophy	0.5	91	12	16	Macular
Optic atrophy	0.2	51	40	40	Macular border
Stage IIb					
Juvenile macular degeneration	0.25	27	33	32	Upper macular border
Chorioretinal degeneration	0.1	50	48	43	Extramacular
Neuritis	0.8	58	50	60	Macular
Optic atrophy	0.5	46	44	43	Macular
Optic atrophy	0.2	27	25	29	Parafoveal

Figure 6.14 clearly demonstrates the dependence of the pathologic CVM types I and II on the fixation mode in the two eyes of a patient with excessive myopia. The right eye showed parafoveal-perifoveal fixation and therefore a CVM type Ib pattern. For the left eye, a peripheral fixation area was used (between perifovea and optic disc), and a CVM type IIa pattern was observed.

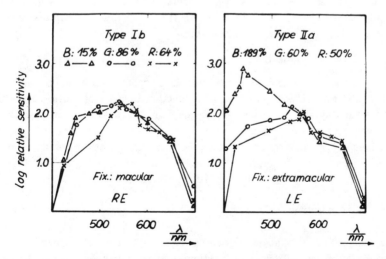

Fig. 6.14. Different CVM types of acquired color vision defects in a case with bilateral excessive myopia. The right eye with macular fixation shows CVM type Ib, the left eye with extramacular fixation CVM type IIa.

Table 6.7

CVM Type III of Acquired Color Vision Defects in Retinal and
Optic Nerve Diseases

Diagnosis	Visual Acuity	B (%)	G (%)	R (%)	Fixation Mode
Chorioretinal degeneration	0.3	0	19	23	Enlarged foveal
Thrombosis	0.3	1	24	24	Enlarged foveal
Choroidal rupture	0.04	1	14	16	Parafoveal
Choroiditis	0.25	0.4	10	18	Foveal/macular
Optic atrophy	0.8	3	9	15	Macular/nystagmus
Optic atrophy	0.1	1	11	13	Parafoveal
Optic atrophy	0.5	2	22	16	Parafoveal
Neuritis	0.5	1	10	14	Macular

PROGRESSION OF THE CVM TYPES OF ACQUIRED COLOR VISION DEFECTS

CVM type I.   As a rule, development of CVM type I patterns progresses from a normal foveolar CVM pattern to stage Ia, later to stage Ib, and finally to CVM type III (this kind of progression is typically found in retinal diseases if the fixation area lies within the fovea, parafovea, or perifovea). A transition to CVM type II from CVM type I may occur if fixation becomes peripheral in retinal diseases or if it becomes parafoveolar, parafoveal, perifoveal, or peripheral in optic nerve diseases.

CVM type II.   The CVM type II pattern may develop from CVM Type Ia or Ib but also from a normal eccentric CVM pattern. CVM IIa patterns may progress to IIb and then to type III.

All CVM types and stages of color vision defects can recover in the reverse order during the healing process. Köllner (1912) observed similar progressions using color naming tests. He described a blue–yellow defect that can combine with a red–green defect and lead to total color blindness. Furthermore, he found a progressive red–green blindness that progressed to total color blindness.

Evaluation of the Method

Although the technique of selective chromatic adaptation does not result in complete isolation of the three CVMs, it allows the function of each of the three CVMs to be evaluated separately. The quantitative measurement and method of analysis of the three CVMs renders possible qualitative determination and quantitative measurement of acquired color vision defects and enables us to measure these disturbances during the course of disease. Furthermore, the method provides essential insights into the pathophysiologic rules of acquired color vision defects.

COLOR ADAPTOMETRY*

The shape of the dark adaptation curve for a white centrally located test light large enough to cover regions of the retina including both rods and cones is well known. After the subject has spent about 8 min in the dark the curve forms a plateau indicating the

---

*Contributed by Paul Kinnear, Ph.D.

transition between the photopic and scotopic phases of dark adaptation, and the cone threshold is reached. Thereafter the curve shows a rapid phase of increasing sensitivity before finally reaching the rod threshold after a total of about 30–40 min in the dark. Apart from the psychophysical method used in dark adaptation, the following variables are important in determining the shape of the curve: (1) preadaptation conditions: duration, luminance, and spectral composition; (2) test conditions: size, position on retina (eccentricity), spectral composition.

In this section the effects of using different spectral compositions for the preadaptation and the test lights will be discussed. The rationale for using colored lights is that the relative states of adaptation of rods and cones can be altered, which in turn will lead to differing rod–cone interactions in the course of dark adaptation. If a deficiency of rods or cones exists, these interactions will be upset and show up in the adaptation curves. In addition, the relative dark adaptation processes of the various cone mechanisms can be altered in order to reveal one or more of the mechanisms more clearly.

There has been a long history of manipulating colored adaptation fields and test stimuli in dark adaptation. Mandelbaum and Mintz (1941), using six colored adaptation fields and violet, green, and red test stimuli, observed very little differences among all of the dark adaptation curves obtained under the various combinations of adaptation field and test stimulus. Auerbach and Wald (1955) used much more intense adaptation fields and found that there were marked differences in the shapes of the dark adaptation curves for test stimuli of different wavelengths. Individual curves often had two or three plateaus and when plotted with other curves crossed each other once or even twice. Adaptation with orange light had the effect of reducing the sensitivity temporarily of the long-wavelength mechanisms, thereby producing an enhancement of the short-wavelength mechanism, and vice versa for blue adaptation. When deuteranopes were adapted to orange light, the subsequent curve for a test stimulus of 436 nm showed only one early plateau instead of the two found with normal observers, which suggested that the deuteranopes were missing a mechanism, presumably the green one. The adaptation curves of protanopes were consistent with their lack of a red mechanism.

Wald (1960), using a white preadaptation light and then alternately yellow (dominant wavelength 570 nm) and violet (460 nm) test lights, demonstrated the rod–cone relation across the retina and the effect of macular absorption around the fovea. With central positioning of the 0.75° test fields the adaptation curves followed the typical cone pattern, with the violet curve running parallel to the yellow curve and about 1.2 log units above it. As the test stimulus is moved further away from the fovea, the exaggerated difference due to the macular pigment is lost and the curves cross at increasingly earlier times. The rod threshold for violet is about 0.8 log unit *below* that for yellow, and the cone threshold for violet is 0.5 log unit *above* that for yellow. At 10° below fixation the crossover time occurs after about 12 min in the dark after an initial adaptation of 6 min to white light of luminance 8000 cd m^{-2}. With these results in mind it is interesting to examine the situation when patients considered to be achromatic (and hence lacking cone function) are used.

Most typical achromats do appear to have receptors other than rods, as shown by the fact that the dark adaptation curve after light adaptation consists of at least two phases. Sloan (1954; 1958) and Auerbach and Kripke (1974) have demonstrated photopic phases in the early stages of dark adaptation mediated by receptors that appear to have the same spectral sensitivity as rods. For example, Auerbach and Kripke (1974), using an adaptometer of their own design, examined five achromats and found evidence of three plateaus at certain areas of the retina during the photopic phase of dark adaptation and also the usual scotopic plateaus. Only one eye was light and dark adapted; the other eye was used for the fixation point when peripheral regions of the retina were being tested. Patients were adapted to white light of 32,000 lux for 3–5 min and then tested by means of the method of limits using 50-msec exposures of a 1° field. By combining the data from various test wavelengths from 420 to 680 nm, the authors found that the threshold curves for all of the plateaus fitted the 1951 CIE, $V'\lambda$ function; they concluded that their achromats had different kinds of cones but that they contained rhodopsin rather than the usual cone pigments and that the multiple plateaus suggested different rates of adaptation. In short, their data revealed receptors in part of the retina that were active immediately after the adaptation light had been turned off (i.e., with cone kinetics) and yet having a spectral sensitivity resembling that of rods. The "moral" of their work is that great care has to be taken in interpreting what mechanism may be responding at various phases of dark adaptation.

Another clinical application of color adaptometry has been with glaucomatous eyes. Lakowski, Drance, and Goldthwaite (1976) used a modified form of the Wald two-color procedure. They preadapted and then tested with the same color (either 493 or 583 nm), and then they repeated the procedure with the other color, taking care in both cases to equate the preadaptation and test lights for photopic vision. Their adaptation conditions were such that dark adaptation proceeded rapidly, with the crossover of the two curves occurring after only about 5 min for persons with normal vision. The results from patients with glaucoma typically showed evidence of damage to both photopic and scotopic vision because the thresholds for both the yellow and blue-green tests were elevated from normal. The damage seemed to be worse for the scotopic function, however; the crossover of the two curves occurred at a time much later than normal. The authors feel that their method is a valuable way of testing rod and cone function in eyes at risk and are currently extending their work by using three instead of two test wavelengths (Lakowski & Creighton, 1976).

It is one matter to be able to record the psychophysical results of dark adaptation; it is another to interpret their meaning. Electrophysiologic work (e.g., Brown & Murakami, 1968) has demonstrated the complex manner of the neural interactions between rods and cones. The relationship between neural and photopigment events is complex, and readers interested in this topic are advised to read Barlow (1972). Nevertheless, it seems to be a promising field because of the possibilities it holds for clinical assessment of rod and cone function.

COLOR PERIMETRY*

Testing of peripheral color vision is subject to two major difficulties—there is a fairly rapid decrease of visual acuity with eccentricity, and there is a rapid increase of the phenomena of local adaptation (Troxler's effect). For eccentricity greater than 30°, the usual pseudoisochromatic plates and color arranging tests are inadequate, even with steady fixation (Verriest & Metsälä, 1963), while color matching becomes very difficult. Thus perimetric methods are necessary for the study of peripheral color vision in the clinical setting.

Moreover, modern methods of color perimetry described below allow us to assess color vision mechanisms both foveally and peripherally, which is of paramount importance from both theoretical and practical points of view.

___

*Contributed by Guy Verriest, M.D.

The Past—Color Perimetry Using Pigmented Objects

Before the Goldmann perimeter became available, the visual field was examined by means of pigmented colored objects (initiated by Aubert, 1857) and was extensively applied in clinical ophthalmology in two more or less distinct ways: (1) to provide less intense objects for measurement of the central isopters in barrel-stave perimetry and in campimetry—Rönne (1911) so distinguished "relative" defects (for the colored objects) from "absolute" ones (for the white objects)—and (2) to demonstrate acquired color vision defects in peripheral vision—Köllner (1912) showed that in tests when the patient is asked to name the perceived color, chorioretinal diseases are characterized by a selective contraction of the isopter for a blue object, while diseases of the optic nerve are characterized by a selective contraction of the isopters for green and red objects. This second method was improved in different ways: (1) by using colors that Hess (1889) showed to be invariant in hue when presented at different eccentricities; (2) by presenting colored objects on a gray background of the same lightness, as advocated by Engelking and Eckstein (1920) and Ferree and Rand (1924); (3) by comparing the threshold for recognizing the color of a target with the threshold for detecting the presence of the target independently of its color and thereby determining the photochromatic interval [Wilbrand and Saenger (1913) noted that optic nerve diseases could be characterized by an increase of the photochromatic interval]; and (4) by comparing the local adaptation times for colored and white objects (Cibis, 1948) (this method is used in a simplified form of scotometers, often used for diagnosing tobacco amblyopia).

The peripheral relative luminous efficiency function was estimated by means of another method of Engelking, called *Peripheriewerte*. Dots of five different colors are pasted on pieces of gray cardboard of increasing lightnesses. These are viewed in the (nearly achromatic) temporal extreme periphery of the visual field, and for each color the gray of the same lightness is found. Abnormal subjects are compared with normal ones. The same materials can be used for other experiments, e.g., for the measurement of local adaptation phenomena.

Modern Trends—Increment Thresholds for Colored Objects

Soon after the introduction of the Goldmann perimeter, Dubois-Poulsen's book (1952) so discredited perimetry performed with pigment colors that such methods were almost entirely abandoned. Accordingly, the rebirth of color perimetry depended on the use of colorimetrically defined or nearly monochromatic targets, as used in the normal eye by Wentworth (1930).

The pioneer work was that of the Belgian ophthalmologist Jules Zanen (1953), who determined the achromatic and chromatic static absolute foveal thresholds for monochromatic objects and showed that chorioretinal diseases were characterized by an increase of achromatic thresholds, especially for long wavelengths, while optic nerve diseases were characterized by an increase of the photochromatic interval. However, his measurements were restricted to foveal vision, and his apparatus was never commercially available.

INCREMENT THRESHOLDS ON ACHROMATIC BACKGROUNDS

Verriest (1960b; 1963) initially used the color targets of the kinetic Goldmann perimeter for the study of congenital and acquired color vision defects. Subsequently, Verriest and Israel (1965) used a static Goldmann perimeter equipped with broadband blue, green, and red filters calibrated for relative spectral energy outputs. They studied the age factor in foveal and peripheral achromatic increment threshold sensitivities of normal subjects and subjects with congenital defects of color vision. Results obtained by using the same method in ocular pathology were published by François, Verriest, and Israel (1966), who showed that (1) type III acquired blue–yellow defect is characterized by a lowering of the sensitivity to the blue object and sometimes also by a lowering of the sensitivity to the red one; (2) type I acquired red–green defect is always characterized by a relative increase in sensitivity to the blue object and decrease in sensitivity to the red object, just as in congenital typical achromatopsia; and (3) type II acquired red–green defect does not affect the relative sensitivities to the three colored objects, except at the spatial locations defining the borders of the defect, where the sensitivity to the blue object was often enhanced. It was concluded that static perimetry with colored objects is very useful for the differential diagnosis of many ocular diseases.

During this period, static increment threshold perimetry by means of two colored objects (e.g., blue and red) was used in the United States to obtain "rod" and "cone" retinal profiles, the rods being more sensitive to the blue object and the cones to the red one (Goodman, Ripps, & Siegel, 1963; Gunkel, 1967). The physiologic background of this method was investigated by Sloan and Feiock (1972), who showed that the white light increment thresholds of the normal cone and rod receptor systems are approximately equal for the rather low background luminances of modern projection perimeters, and thus both receptor systems can be easily differentiated by means of colored objects. For example, an eye suffering from cone degeneration with a normal field for a white object may have a pathologic field for a red object (Fig. 6.15).

The Tübinger perimeter, despite its lower maximal background luminance (only 3.18 cd m^{-2}), is more convenient than the Goldmann instrument for static increment threshold perimetry using colored objects not only because it is better suited for static measurements but also because it can be ordered with a series of nine interference filters giving narrow-band test stimuli and even with some selective filters for controlling the chromaticity of the background. Nolte (1962; 1974) studied normal retinal profiles with the Tübinger perimeter and noted a central scotoma for shorter wavelengths, a finding also reported by Verriest and Israel (1965). In order to express results not only as profiles but also as increment threshold spectral sensitivity curves, it is necessary to measure relative energies for all the targets, a task achieved independently by Verriest, Padmos, and Greve (1974) and by Kitahara and Ichikawa (1975).

Verriest and Kandemir (1974) showed that by using the Tübinger perimeter the increment threshold spectral sensitivity curves of normal subjects on white backgrounds do not resemble the smooth unimodal standard CIE $V(\lambda)$ relative luminous efficiency function but present several peaks. The normal curves of Verriest and Kandemir are characterized by peaks for the 451-, 528-, and 600-nm filters, and these peaks have been identified with opponent color vision mechanisms (King-Smith, 1975). Verriest and Kandemir (1974) showed that peripheral spectral sensitivity curves include mesopic features at the background luminance of 3.18 cd m^{-2}, and they accordingly increased it to 10 cd m^{-2}. The central scotoma for lights of shorter wavelengths is much less evident at this level and thus appeared to be also a mesopic feature. Curves obtained in the congenital color deficiencies by Verriest and Uvijls (1977a) showed that the red peak is missing in protanopia, the green peak is broader and shifted to longer wavelengths in deuteranopia, and the blue peak missing in tritanopia (Fig. 6.16). Using a background luminance of 10 cd m^{-2}, Verriest and Uvijls (1977a, b) studied the age factor in normal

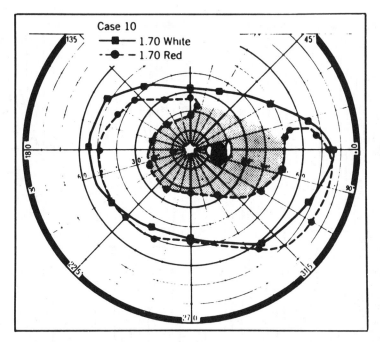

Fig. 6.15. Comparison in a case of selective cone impairment of the visual fields for a white test object and for a red object that are equally luminous to a normal eye. Tübinger perimeter. [From Sloan, L.L., & Feiock, K. *Modern Problems in Ophthalmology,* 1972, *11,* 50–62 (reproduced by permission of S. Karger AG).]

subjects, demonstrating not only prereceptoral but also retinal factors. In a comparison of the data of 120 pathologic eyes with normal eyes allowing for age (Fig. 6.16), the spectral sensitivity curves of affected retinal areas were found to be reduced selectively as follows: (1) in juvenile macular degeneration and in progressive cone dystrophies the sensitivities for the longer wavelengths are selectively lowered, and scotopic luminosity curves can be obtained; (2) in central serous retinopathy the sensitivities for the shorter and for some intermediate wavelengths are selectively lowered; (3) in some cases of pigmentary retinopathy the sensitivities to the shortest wavelengths are selectively lowered; and (4) in some cases of optic nerve disease there is apparent enhancement of the sensitivities to the shorter wavelengths (Fig. 6.16). In other diseases spectral sensitivity is reduced uniformly. Moreover, the method proved to be a more sensitive test than static perimetry with white objects. Foveal measures were more sensitive than a traditional battery of color vision tests (Ishihara, F_2 plate, AO HRR, Farnsworth Panel D-15, and anomaloscope). Similar measurements made with foveal stimuli are described above and show that pathologic conditions can give rise not only to depression of one color vision mechanism but also to a reduction or, on the contrary, to an increase of the opponency between the mechanisms.

Hansen (1974a) showed that chloroquine retinopathy is characterized by a decrease in sensitivity to red in the pericentral scotoma, and Hansen, Larsen, and Berg (1976) again demonstrated peripheral scotopization of vision in progressive cone dystrophy. Marmion (1977) showed that in exudative diabetic retinopathy, static perimetry with color objects is a more sensitive test than the FM 100-hue test.

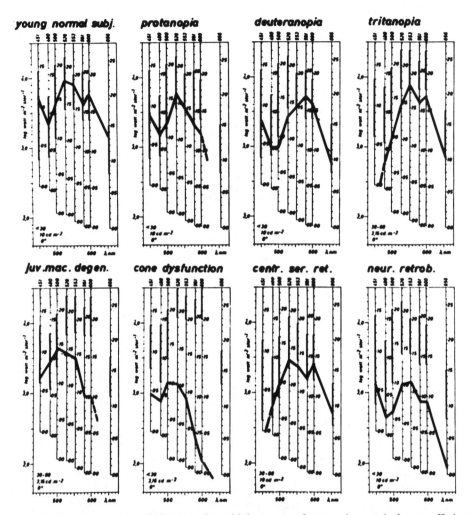

Fig. 6.16.   Increment threshold spectral sensitivity curves of a normal eye and of eyes suffering from congenital and acquired color vision defects; 116′ diameter, circular foveal 500-nsec stimulus against an A-white 10 cd m^{-2} background. Tübinger perimeter.   [From Verriest, G., & Uvijls, A. *Documenta Ophthalmologica*, 1977, *43*, 217–248 (reproduced with permission of W. Junk BV).]

Most recently, two-color absolute thresholds have been used by Massof and Finkelstein (1979) to differentiate subgroups of patients with retinitis pigmentosa. These authors showed that some retinitis pigmentosa patients have selective loss of rod vision throughout the entire retina while others showed concomitant rod and cone sensitivity losses. A third group showed a regional loss of rod sensitivity in the central 10° to 15°.

INCREMENT THRESHOLDS ON CHROMATIC BACKGROUNDS

In comparison to measurements on a white background, the use of colored backgrounds allows at least the partial isolation of retinal CVMs (above, Wald-Marré approach).

At the Second Symposium of the International Research Group on Color Vision Deficiencies in Edinburgh, several authors independently described foveal and peripheral Stiles π functions (above, Psychophysical Testing), using specially adapted commercial perimeters. Hansen used the Goldmann perimeter (1974b) and found an aberrant green mechanism with a peak at 500 nm in two cases of cone dystrophy (1974c); he also studied cases of chloroquine retinopathy (1974a) and pigmentary retinopathy (1977), which are characterized by an early loss of the blue π_1 mechanism. Greve, Verduin, and Ledeboer (1974) used the Tübinger perimeter and found that a blue object (448 nm) on a yellow background provided the most significant difference between normal eyes and those with macular edema. Vola, Leprince, Langle, Cornu, and Saracco (1978) have used the Tübinger perimeter to study π functions in optic neuritis. Moreland, Maione, Carta, Barberini, Scoccianti, and Lettieri (1977), using the Goldmann perimeter, showed the π_5 mechanism may be selectively involved in degenerative fundus diseases and refined the method for determining Westheimer functions for the monochromatic targets.

TECHNICAL ASPECTS

The determination of increment thresholds for monochromatic objects on white or colored backgrounds is a developing research field that is extremely promising not only for the assessment of the mechanisms of the acquired color vision defects but also for purely clinical purposes. However, its application outside the research laboratory using commercially available perimeters is subject to three major difficulties: (1) achieving a sufficiently high background luminance in order to avoid rod intrusion in peripheral studies and to promote selective chromatic adaptation; (2) achieving even higher test luminances in view of the use of narrow-band interference filters and of the high background luminances; and (3) calibrating the relative radiances of the test objects in order to plot the increment threshold spectral sensitivity curves. Taking into account the technical paper of Lakowski, Wright, and Oliver (1977) and as a result of an inquiry within the Research Group on Color Perimetry of the International Perimetric Society, Verriest (1978) wrote a list of concrete requirements for submission to manufacturers of commercially available perimeters. These requirements are already fulfilled in experimental perimeters (Verriest, G., Personal communication).

Modern Trends—Other Methods

We will subdivide recent papers on other methods in color perimetry into two groups—(1) new methods of examination and (2) revivals of older methods with newer technical means.

NEW METHODS

Hokama (1968) and Yokoi (1971; 1972) showed that the assessment of the flicker fusion frequency for colored objects using the Tübinger perimeter enabled retinal diseases to be differentiated from optic nerve diseases. The colored objects of the Tübinger perimeter were also occasionally used for measuring spatial summation (Conreur & Meur, 1966) or early adaptation (Conreur, Meur, & Zanen, 1966). Finally, Verduyn-Lunel and Crone (1974; 1978), by modifying the Goldmann perimeter, and Drum (1976), by modifying the Tübinger perimeter, developed special techniques for determining foveal and peripheral achromatic and chromatic sensitivities. The method developed by

Verduyn-Lunel and Crone (1974; 1978) provides an easy way of determining colorimetric purity thresholds at any retinal location.

REVIVED TECHNIQUES

Kinetic perimetry with colored objects for determining achromatic and chromatic isopters is still practiced. The Goldmann perimeter was used in this way by Maione and Carta (1967; 1972) and by Israel and Galan (1971). Liuzzi and Bartoli (1975) even contend that pathologic defects are better recognized if the kinetic Goldmann perimeter is equipped with a laser source of highly monochromatic coherent light. However, Israel and Verriest (1977) showed that the normal spreads of the achromatic and chromatic kinetic isopters are very large in the Goldmann perimeter. Carlow, Flynn, and Shipley (1977) demonstrated that the extent of the chromatic isopter depends on the saturation of the target colors.

Grützner, Born, and Hemminger (1976) showed that the color naming of a 1° stimulus at different locations up to 10° on the horizontal meridian allows the recognition of heterozygotes for congenital dichromacy.

Frisen (1973) and Dannheim (1977) reintroduced the very simple and effective diagnosis of neuroophthalmic syndromes by means of the subjective differences in apparent saturation of a suprathreshold color target presented in the various quadrants of the visual field.

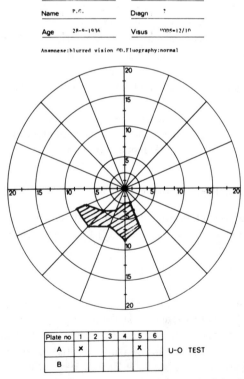

Fig. 6.17.   Drawing on a visual field chart of the paracentral color vision defect stated by means of the Umazume-Ohta test plates. (Figure supplied by A. J. L. G. Pinckers.)

The old method of scotometry (assessment of a scotoma by the disappearance of the color attribute of a target) has been reintroduced by the Umazume-Ohta central scotometric plates, now commercially available and in growing use as a clinical test of paracentral color vision (Ohta, 1972; Pinckers, 1976a). The Umazume-Ohta test consists of six plates, each plate presenting the same pattern of desaturated dots of known chromaticities. The defects can be drawn on a visual field chart (Fig. 6.17); in order to avoid drawing on six different charts, one notes the numbers of the plates disclosing any defect and draws only the largest defect. Graphic representation in followup examination is possible if the defect remains within the 18° central area. No information concerning false-positive or negative results is yet available. Plates 1 and 2 are sensitive to acquired blue–yellow defects, plates 3 and 4 to acquired type I red–green defects, and plates 5 and 6 to acquired type II red–green defects. Plate 5 proves to be the most sensitive even in conditions other than those affecting the optic nerve. In a followup examination of a retrobulbar neuritis the test seemed to be as effective as the FM 100-hue test (Pinckers, 1976a). Matsuo, Ohta, Endo, and Kato (1972) have presented a new test combining the principles of the Umazume-Ohta plates with that of the Amsler grids and allowing, like the original Umazume-Ohta plates, the testing of color vision from 0° to 18° eccentricity.

Joel Pokorny, Ph.D.
Vivianne C. Smith, Ph.D.
Guy Verriest, M.D.

7
Congenital Color Defects

The congenital color defects include the red–green defects, the blue–yellow defects, and the achromatopsias. The inheritance, incidence, and types of color vision for these defects are summarized in Table 7.1. The most common congenital defects are the X-chromosome–linked red–green defects, which occur in 8 percent of the European male and 0.4 percent of. the European white female population (4–5 percent of the total European white population). The blue–yellow defects are rarer, occurring equally in both sexes in about 1 in 15,000 to 1 in 50,000 (0.002–0.007 percent) of the population. The achromatopsias are another rare group of disorders in which there is a profound disorder of color sense. These disorders occur in about 1 in 30,000 (0.003 percent) of the population (Krill, 1977).

THE RED–GREEN DEFECTS

Observers with red–green color defects have normal visual acuity but an abnormality of color vision. Two qualitatively different forms of defect are recognized. The protan defects include a dichromatic form, protanopia, and a trichromatic form, protanomaly (protanomalous trichromacy). Color confusions of protanopes and protanomalous trichromats are qualitatively similar, justifying the inclusive term "protan" (Farnsworth, 1947). Deutan defects include a dichromatic form, deuteranopia, and a trichromatic form, deuteranomaly (deuteranomalous trichromacy). Color confusions of deuteranopes and deuteranomalous trichromats are qualitatively similar, justifying the inclusive term "deutan" (Farnsworth, 1947). Full-spectrum colorimetry, spectral sensitivity, and wavelength and colorimetric purity discrimination functions all have been described in the literature. Some major features of red–green color deficiency are summarized in Table 7.2. The red–green defects have X-chromosome–linked heredity and are attributed to the activity of two sets of alleles, one governing a protan series of defects and one governing a deutan series of defects. Color matching, using the anomaloscope to measure the Rayleigh match, allows differentiation of the various defects.

Table 7.1
Inheritance and Incidence of the Congenital Color Vision Defects

Type	Inheritance	Incidence (%)	Type of Color Vision
Red–green defects	X-chromosome-linked recessive	8–10 (males)	
Protanopia		1	Dichromatic
Deuteranopia		1	Dichromatic
Protanomaly		1	Trichromatic
Deuteranomaly		5–6	Trichromatic
Blue–yellow defects			
Tritan defect (tritanopia and incomplete tritanopia)	Autosomal dominant	0.002–0.007	Dichromatic and trichromatic
Tritanomaly	?	?	Trichromatic
Achromatopsias			
Complete, with reduced visual acuity	Autosomal recessive	0.003	Monochromatic
Incomplete, with reduced visual acuity	Autosomal recessive X-chromosome-linked recessive	? ?	Dichromatic and trichromatic Dichromatic
Complete, with normal visual acuity	?	0.000001	Monochromatic

Table 7.2
Characteristics of Red–Green defective Vision

Characteristic	Normal	Protanopic	Deuteranopic	Protanomalous	Deuteranomalous
Number of primaries required for color mixture	3	2	2	3	3
Neutral point, i.e., wavelength of spectral stimulus that matches white	None	494 nm	499 nm	None	None
Reduced luminous efficiency at long wavelengths	No	Yes	No	Yes	No
Wavelength of the maximum of the relative luminous efficiency curve	555 nm	540 nm	560 nm	540 nm	560 nm
CIE chromaticity of the confusion point (dichromats only)	None	$x_p = 0.7365$ $y_p = 0.2635$	$x_d = 1.400$ $y_d = -0.400$	None None	None None
Minimum of $\Delta\lambda$ function (best discrimination)	590 nm	490 nm	495 nm	490 nm (plus other relative minima)	495 nm
Minimum of colorimetric purity	570 nm	494 nm (neutral point)	499 nm (neutral point)	494 nm	499 nm

Partially based on material reported by Wyszecki and Stiles (1967), Vos and Walraven (1971), and Verriest (1970).

Scientific analysis of dichromatic subjects with red–green defect originated with Dalton's (1798) report of his own color defect. Seebeck (1837) subdivided observers with red–green defects into two types, characterized by reduced and by normal sensitivity to long-wavelength light; von Kries (1897) called them, respectively, protanopes and deuteranopes. Recognition of X-chromosome–linked anomalous trichromacy in 1881 is credited to Lord Rayleigh. He discovered two major subtypes of anomalous trichromacy now called protanomalous and deuteranomalous trichromacy. Comprehensive reviews of the genetic aspects of red–green defects are given by Bell (1926), François and Verriest (1961a), Waardenburg (1963), and Franceschetti, François, and Babel (1974).

Dichromacy

Dichromacy occurs in 2 percent of the European male population and in less than 0.03 percent of the European female population. The two different forms of dichromacy, protanopia (1 percent) and deuteranopia (1 percent), have been recognized since the mid-19th century.

COLOR MIXTURE

Dichromatic color matching coefficients.   Dichromats require only two primaries to match spectral colors. With foveal vision, using a 1° or 2° field, the congenital red–green dichromat can match all colors by suitable mixtures of only two primaries, one usually a short-wavelength primary (below 500 nm) and one a long-wavelength primary (above 500 nm). Comprehensive modern data were collected by Pitt (1935), working in W. D. Wright's laboratory (Wright, 1946). Color mixture data have also been reported by Möller-Ladekarl (1934), Hecht and Shlaer (1937a, b), Vogt (1974), and Alpern and Pugh (1977), among others. Pitt (1935) used 460 nm as the short-wavelength (blue) primary and 650 nm as the long-wavelength (red) primary. Color matches were reported as the proportion of red and blue primaries as a function of test wavelength with WDW normalization (Chapter 2) at 494 nm. In Figure 7.1 the left panel shows data for protanopes, the right panel for deuteranopes. Recall that the test field is varying through the spectrum and to a normal observer would appear successively violet, blue, green, yellow-orange, and red; the mixture field is comprised of mixtures of blue and red and to a normal observer would successively appear blue, blue tinged with pink, purple, magenta, and red. Dichromats do not distinguish color differences that are very obvious to the normal trichromat.

The data for protanopes and deuteranopes look similar, but this is a feature of the WDW normalization at 494 nm. The actual energies (and the visual appearance) at the match used by a protanope at 494 nm are very different from those used by a deuteranope. Compared with the deuternope the protanope requires more energy at the 650 nm primary to match the 494 nm light. A true similarity of the data, however, is that for test wavelenghs above 540 nm the mixture consists primarily of the red primary, and red–green dichromats can typically match 540 nm to all wavelengths above 540 nm by simple adjustment of the relative radiances of the two wavelengths. This behavior is the basis for the oft-quoted observation that red–green dichromats confuse greens, yellows, and reds.

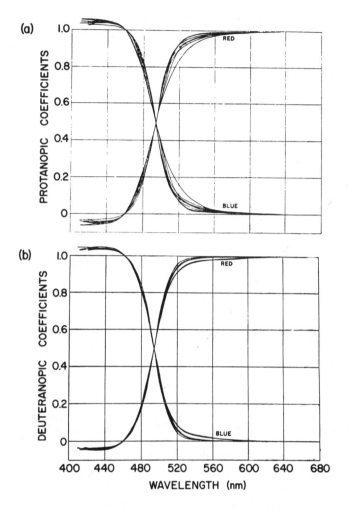

Fig. 7.1. WDW dichromatic coefficient curves measured for primaries 650 and 460 nm with normalization at 494 nm.   (a) Data for eight protanopes.   (b) Data for seven deuteranopes. [From Pitt, F. H. G. *Characteristics of dichromatic vision*. London, Medical Research Council, 1935 (reproduced with permission of the controller, HMSO Norwich, England).]

Representation in the CIE color space.   The dichromatic color-matching data can be plotted on the normal chromaticity diagram. The procedure, however, is theoretically correct only if dichromacy is truly a reduction system of normal trichromacy by either loss or collapse. A requirement for the procedure is that the dichromatic data are first renormalized. Pitt (1935) achieved the renormalization by using the measured neutral points of the dichromats, plotting the data in the WDW chromaticity space. The data can also be plotted on the *x, y* chromaticity diagram of the 1931 CIE observer (Fig. 7.2). A line is drawn connecting Pitt's primaries of 460 and 650 nm. All mixtures of the two primaries lie on this line. Suppose that for a protanope a test wavelength, 490 nm, is matched to a mixture of 0.95 of 650 nm and 0.05 of 460 nm using the dichromatic coefficients renormalized by Pitt (1935). A line—the isochromatic line—may be drawn

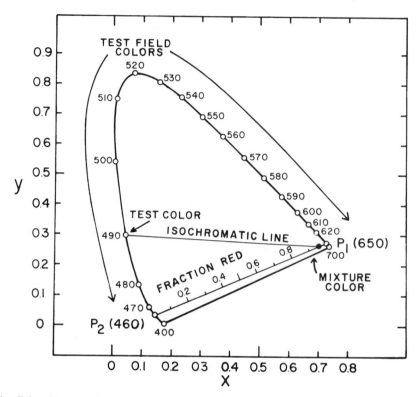

Fig. 7.2. Plotting an isochromatic line for a dichromat in the CIE chromaticity diagram. The test color wavelength is joined to the fraction red in the mixture color.

from the test wavelength at 490 nm to the point representing the matching primary mixture (i.e., 0.95 of the distance along the line joining 460 nm and 650 nm). Alternatively, Judd (1943) gives equations to convert from WDW to 1931 CIE x, y coordinates.

Sets of theoretical isochromatic lines are shown for the 1931 x, y chromaticity diagram in Fig. 7.3, the upper panel giving isochromatic lines of protanopes, the lower panel those of deuteranopes. The isochromatic lines are also sometimes called confusion lines, since they join pairs of colors that may be confused by dichromats. In principle, all colors lying along an isochromatic line are confused by the dichromat.

The isochromatic lines have proved useful in the design (Hardy, Rand, & Rittler, 1954; Birch, 1975) and evaluation (Lakowski, 1965b; 1966; 1969; 1976) of screening tests for red–green color vision defects. However, a word of caution is in order. The CIE standard observer has visual photopigments and lens and macular pigment absorptions representative of the average of a group of observers. The isochromatic lines are thus similarly indicative of those expected for an average group of dichromats whose eye media have characteristics similar to those of normal trichromats. When research is performed using a single observer, the "isochromatic" contours may curve in the diagram (von Schelling, 1950; Farnsworth, 1961) and look quite different from those of Fig. 7.3 (Halsey & Chapanis, 1952; Verriest & Gonnella, 1972; Birch, 1973). Curvature has been attributed to the effect of lens and macular pigment on viewing broadband spectra (von Schelling, 1950). Since macular pigment density varies substantially among observers, a deutan observer may misread a "protan" plate or vice versa (Birch, 1973).

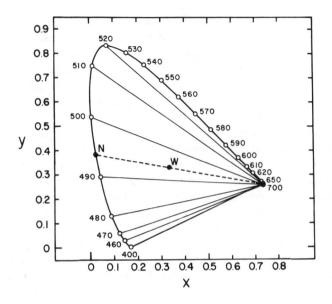

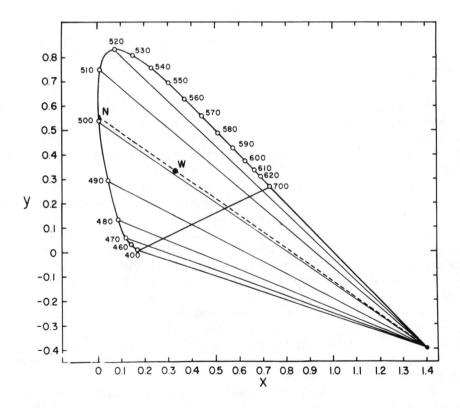

Fig. 7.3. Isochromatic lines for protanopes (upper graph) and deuteranopes (lower graph) in the CIE chromaticity diagram. The neutral point, N, for the equal-energy white is shown (dotted line), as is the copunctal point.

189

The neutral point and the achromatic point. One of the isochromatic lines of Fig. 7.3 passes through the equal-energy white. A red–green dichromat can exactly match a midspectrum wavelength (i.e., a blue-green color to a normal observer), a white, and a mixture color appearing purple to the normal observer. The spectral wavelength that matches white is called the neutral point and is further specified by the color temperature of the white light used for the match. Pitt's (1935) measurements of the spectral neutral point matched to a 4800 K white were 495.5 and 500.4 nm for five protanopes and six deuteranopes, respectively. Walls and Heath (1956) measured neutral points in dichromats using Munsell color samples. With illuminant C the mean dominant wavelength of the neutral point for 39 protanopes was 490.3 nm (range 3.3 nm); the mean dominant wavelength of the neutral point for 38 deuteranopes was 498.4 nm (range 5.8 nm). Theoretical equal-energy neutral points of protanopes and deuteranopes as calculated by Wyszecki and Stiles (1967) are 494 and 499 nm, respectively. With lower–color temperature whites the neutral points shift to longer wavelengths.

Neutral point wavelengths are also affected by macular pigment variation. Pitt's data (1935) showed considerable variation especially for the deuteranopes. The effect is most marked for measurement of neutral points using narrow-bandwidth spectral fields and is less marked for pigment colors, since both pigment colors and the neutral gray are to a large extent equivalently affected by the observer's macular pigment (Judd, as cited by Walls & Heath, 1956).

The achromatic point is the spectral wavelength that appears colorless to the dichromatic observer. Achromatic points for dichromats were assessed by Bailey and Massof (1974) and Massof and Guth (1976). Achromatic points ranged from 485 to 493 nm for protanopes and from 495 to 505 nm for deuteranopes.

The convergence point. A major feature of the isochromatic lines of Fig. 7.3 is their convergence. The convergence points are also called copunctal points. The protanopic convergence point has coordinates near $x = 0.75$, $y = 0.25$ (Nimeroff, 1970). The deuteranopic convergence shows more variability; estimates of the coordinates vary from $x = 1.08$, $y = -0.08$ to $x = 2.30$, $y = -1.30$ (Nimeroff, 1970).

An isochromatic line connects colors that appear identical to a dichromat. In reduction theory the dichromat is presumed to be lacking the mechanism that allows the normal trichromat to perceive a continuous gradation of color along an isochromatic line. The convergence point (x_{cp}, y_{cp}) of the isochromatic lines represents the locus of the missing mechanism in the CIE diagram (Judd, 1964). It is possible to derive a linear transformation of the CIE data to yield the equal-energy relative spectral sensitivity associated with the convergence point. This concept dates back to König and Dieterici (1886; 1893) and König (1897). When the procedure is performed with the assumption of a reduction system by loss of one normal mechanism for red–green dichromats, the derived sets of spectral sensitivities are called König fundamentals; with the assumption of a reduction system by fusion of a pair of normal mechanisms the derived spectral sensitivities are called Aitken-Leber-Fick fundamentals (Aitken, 1872; Leber, 1873; Fick, 1873– 1874).

Modern estimates of König fundamentals were made by Vos and Walraven (1971). In these studies the convergence point for the protanope was set at $x_p = 0.7365$, $y_p = 0.2635$, that for the deuteranope at $x_d = 1.4000$, $y_d = -0.4000$. It may be emphasized that the protanopic convergence point yields a spectral sensitivity peaking near 560 nm and closely approximates the measured relative luminous efficiency function of deuteranopes. The deuteranopic convergence point yields a relative spectral sensitivity function peaking near 540 nm and closely approximates the measured relative luminous efficiency function of protanopes. Smith and Pokorny (1972) showed that these König fundamentals had characteristics of visual pigment absorption spectra. With revised assumptions a set of fundamentals were derived [similar to those of Vos & Walraven (1971)] that could also predict color-matching data of tritanopes (Smith & Pokorny, 1975), the third class of dichromat (described below). The receptor sensitivities of Fig. 3.5 and the theoretical neutral points in Table 7.2 were all derived using König fundamentals.

SPECTRAL SENSITIVITY

The spectral sensitivity functions of protanopes and deuteranopes have been measured by absolute (Hsia & Graham, 1957; Alpern & Torii, 1968) and increment thresholds (Alpern & Moeller, 1977; Verriest & Uvijls, 1977a, b), brightness matching (Alpern, Mindel, & Torii, 1968; Alpern & Torii, 1968; Mitchell & Rushton, 1971a; Pokorny & Smith, 1972; Alpern & Moeller, 1977), heterochromatic flicker photometry (de Vries, 1948a; Crone, 1959; Verriest, 1971a; Pokorny & Smith, 1972; Miller, 1972; Smith & Pokorny, 1973a; 1975), and minimally distinct border (Tansley & Glushko, 1978). Pitt (1935) derived dichromatic luminous efficiency functions from color-matching data.

The absolute foveal thresholds of five protanopes and six deuteranopes measured by Hsia and Graham (1957) are shown in Fig. 7.4. These thresholds were obtained using a 40′ test field flashed for 10 msec. The absolute thresholds for seven normal observers are shown for comparison. The data show that compared with normal or deuteranopic observers the protanopes showed reduced spectral sensitivity for wavelengths greater than

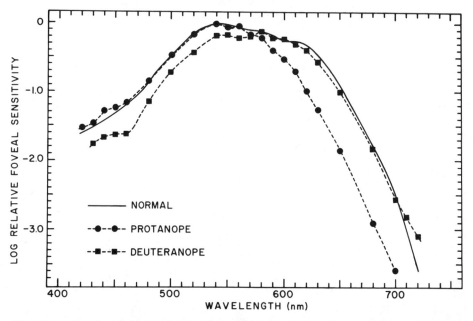

Fig. 7.4. Log foveal threshold spectral sensitivity for protanopes, deuteranopes, and normal trichromats. The protanopes show a luminosity loss in the red and the deuteranopes in the green and blue. [Data redrawn from Hsia & Graham, 1957.]

580 nm. Compared with data for normal or protanopic observers, the deuteranopes showed reduced sensitivity for wavelengths shorter than 580 nm.

Heterochromatic flicker photometry (HFP) (Verriest, 1971a; Pokorny & Smith, 1972; Smith & Pokorny, 1975) or minimally distinct border (MDB) photometry yield the relative luminous efficiency function of dichromats. The protanopic relative luminous efficiency peaks near 545 nm, the deuteranopic function near 560 nm. Comparison of absolute sensitivities is impossible; the functions are plotted to their own maxima or to the sensitivity at a given wavelength, as in Fig. 7.5, which shows average HFP luminous

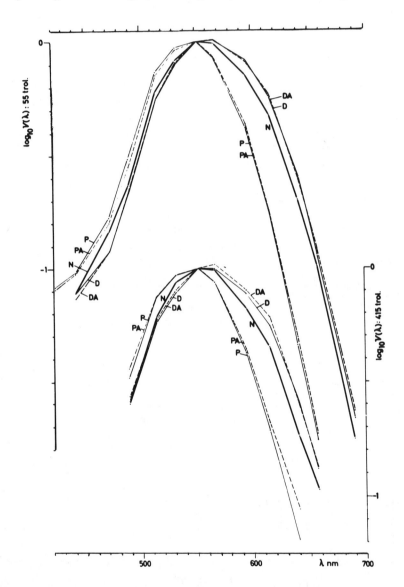

Fig. 7.5. Log relative luminous efficiency relative to 552 nm at two levels of retinal illumination for 25 normals (N), 23 protanomals (PA), 25 protanopes (P), 27 deuteranomals (DA), and 24 deuteranopes (D). Data collected using heterochromatic flicker photometry. [From Verriest, G. *Vision Research,* 1971, *11* 1407–1434 (reproduced with permission of Pergamon Press).]

efficiency obtained by Verriest (1971a). Protanopes show a long-wavelength relative luminous efficiency loss and deuteranopes show a short-wavelength relative luminous efficiency loss. The short-wavelength luminosity loss of deuteranopes is not evident for all observers (Willmer, 1949; Alpern & Torii, 1968). There is considerable interobserver variability among deuteranopes, and the sensitivity differences at short wavelengths can probably be ascribed to interobserver variation in macular pigment (Alpern & Torii, 1968; Smith & Pokorny, 1975).

Foveal and peripheral increment thresholds of 21 protanopes and of 20 deuteranopes measured by Verriest and Uvijls (1977b) are shown in Fig. 7.6, where they are compared with the results from 24 normal, 20 protanomalous, and 20 deuteranomalous subjects. These thresholds were obtained using a 1°30′ test field pulsed for 500 msec on a white background (standard illuminant A) of 10 cd m^{-2}. The dichromatic functions show two maxima, one at 450 nm, as occurs in normal observers, and one between 525 and 550 nm for protanopes and 550 and 560 nm for deuteranopes. There is no evidence of the secondary relative maximum at 600 nm that is characteristic of the normal data. The long-wavelength sensitivity loss of protanopes and short-wavelength sensitivity loss of deuteranopes is evident; moreover, the foveal increment threshold sensitivities of dichromats are reduced throughout the spectrum compared with the normal data. Toward the periphery the dichromats become relatively more sensitive and protanopes become even more sensitive than the normal trichromat for wavelengths below 560 nm.

Mitchell and Rushton (1971a) measured relative spectral sensitivity of dichromats by brightness matching for wavelengths above 500 nm at 200 and 40,000 td, the latter level calculated to bleach 50 percent of the visual photopigments. The shapes of the curves were approximately the same at the two luminance levels; those for protanopes peaked near 540–550 nm and those for deuteranopes near 560–570 nm. Miller (1972) and Smith and Pokorny (1973a) replicated this study using heterochromatic flicker photometry; their data showed that the spectral luminous efficiency curve measured at bleaching levels was slightly narrower than the low luminance function in accordance with a prediction based on self-screening of visual photopigments (Chapter 3).

In physiologic or psychophysical research an action spectrum is often measured for a given visual criterion. The absolute or increment threshold is an example of an action spectrum—the visual criterion is light perception, and we measure the radiant energy in the stimulus needed for the perception of light at each wavelength. Other examples of criteria for which an absolute energy level can be defined are equal visual acuity and equal FFF (flicker fusion frequency). When equal FFF at a high flicker rate is chosen as a criterion visual event (Heath, 1958; 1960; Collins, 1959; 1961), the spectral sensitivities show that protanopes have a long-wavelength luminosity loss compared with normals; deuteranopes have a long-wavelength luminosity gain compared with normal observers. The FFF data therefore conflict with the absolute or increment threshold data and point to the fact that different tasks involve different levels of visual processing (Graham, 1960). Pokorny and Smith (1972) measured the FFF–log I functions as a function of wavelength in normal trichromats and in protanopes and deuteranopes. These functions showed different slopes for protanopes, deuteranopes, and normal trichromats, suggesting that different temporal processing occurs in these classes of observers. In particular, deuteranopes are more sensitive at higher flicker rates. The spectral sensitivity of the action spectrum for deuteranopes thus shows a relative gain compared with protanopes or normal trichromats when the action spectrum is measured at high flicker rates compared with low flicker rates or the action spectrum at absolute threshold. Thus although the action spectrum technique is a valuable one, caution is needed in interpreting the results.

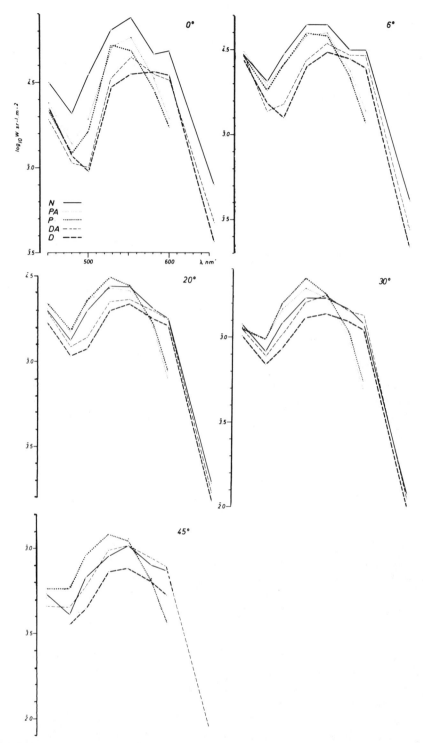

Fig. 7.6. Log relative increment sensitivity curves measured on a white background (standard illuminant A) of 10.0 cd m⁻² for 24 normals (N), 20 protanomals (PA), 21 protanopes (P), 20 deuteranomals (DA), and 20 deuteranopes (D). Data are shown for five eccentricities. [From Verriest, G., & Uvijls, A. *Atti della Fondazione Giorgio Ronchi*, 1977, *32*, 213– 254 (reproduced with permission of Fondazione Giorgio Ronchi).]

WAVELENGTH AND COLORIMETRIC PURITY

The wavelength and colorimetric purity discrimination functions of protanopes and deuteranopes were measured by Pitt (1935) using a 2° bipartite field. Others have performed similar experiments for both wavelength (Steindler, 1906; Möller-Ladekarl, 1934; Hecht & Shlaer, 1937a) and colorimetric purity (Hecht & Shlaer, 1937b; Chapanis, 1944) discrimination.

The wavelength discrimination function shown in Fig. 7.7 is U shaped with a single minimum near 500 nm. The minimum occurs near the dichromat's neutral point. Wavelength discrimination is virtually unobtainable for wavelengths above 540 nm, as predicted by the color-matching data.

The colorimetric purity discrimination function measured as the first step from white is discontinuous for dichromats. No purity step is obtained at the neutral point, since that wavelength, even with full purity, is always matched to the white. For wavelengths shorter than the neutral point, the reciprocal purity thresholds show a rapid increase as wavelength decreases (Fig. 7.8). Colorimetric purity thresholds for deuteranopes approach normal range near 470 nm. For wavelengths longer than the neutral point, the

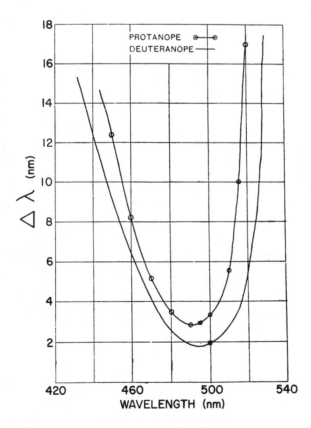

Fig. 7.7. Mean wavelength discrimination curves for the protanope and deuteranope. The average position of the neutral point is marked with an asterisk. [From Pitt, F. H. G. *Characteristics of dichromatic vision.* London Medical Research Council, 1935 (reproduced with permission of the controller, HMSO, Norwich, England).]

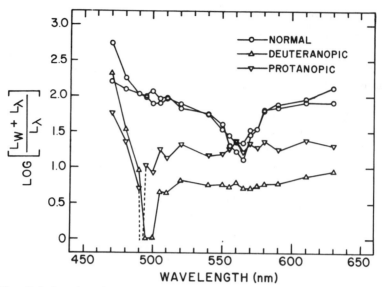

Fig. 7.8. Colorimetric purity thresholds (reciprocal log colorimetric purity) for protanopes and deuteranopes. Data for a normal trichromat are shown for comparison. [Data redrawn from Chapanis, 1944.]

reciprocal purity thresholds show a rapid rise and then level off above 520 nm, showing reduced sensitivity compared with data for normal trichromats. Above the neutral point the best purity discrimination of a dichromat is similar to the minimum at 570 nm of the normal trichromat.

LARGE FIELDS

The color-matching functions and the wavelength and colorimetric purity discrimination described for dichromats were measured using small (1° or 2°) foveal fields. When the centrally viewed field extends to 8° or more, many dichromats show evidence of an added dimension of color perception. This fact was known as early as 1905 (Nagel, 1905; 1907a; Jaeger & Kroker, 1952), although in recent years there has been little emphasis of the fact. In a recent study Smith and Pokorny (1977) noted that dichromats refuse neutral point matches and the usual dichromatic matches that allow only two primaries. Their large-field matches could be explained by assuming that large-field color vision of protanopes and deuteranopes is mediated by the receptors active in the small field plus a receptor (perhaps parafoveal rods) with a spectral characteristic similar to rhodopsin. Large-field trichromacy of protanopes and deuteranopes is dependent on the field size, a parafoveal 1.5° field does not yield trichromatic color matching (Ruddock, 1971) in protanopes and deuteranopes.

PSYCHOPHYSICAL CORRELATES OF VISUAL PHOTOPIGMENTS

Several researchers have measured the relative spectral sensitivity of dichromats either following moderate to strong chromatic adaptations (Boynton, Kandel, & Onley, 1959; Speelman & Krauskopf, 1963) or with superposition of a test stimulus on a moderate to strong chromatic background (Wald, 1966; Alpern & Torii, 1968a, b; Watkins, 1969a, b).

Wald's adaptation technique (Chapters 3 and 6) in the normal trichromat yields three overlapping functions with peaks near 442, 546, and 571 nm (Wald, 1966). These are usually termed receptor mechanisms and are assumed to be the equal-energy corneal sensitivities associated with the absorption spectra of three cone visual photopigments. In the red–green dichromat two receptor mechanisms are obtained. In protanopes one, peaking at 442 nm, is virtually identical to the SWS receptor mechanism of normal trichromats; the second, peaking at 545 nm, is virtually identical to the MWS receptor mechanism of normal trichromats. In deuteranopes one, peaking at 442 nm, is virtually identical to the SWS receptor mechanism of normal trichromats; the second, peaking at 568 nm, is virtually identical to the LWS receptor mechanism of normal trichromats. The Wald (1966) data at high adapting intensities confirmed an earlier study of Boynton, Kandel, and Onley (1959), who also found two receptor mechanisms in protanopes.

The selective bleaching technique reveals that the normal trichromat shows a selective adaptation effect; a long-wavelength background will reduce the sensitivity to a long-wavelength flash (above 600 nm) more than to a midspectral (540–570 nm) wavelength flash. Dichromats do not show this effect; a long-wavelength background reduces the sensitivity equally to all test wavelengths above 540 nm. The phenomenon was termed the heterochromatic threshold reduction factor by Boynton and Wagner (1961), who developed a color vision test—the HTRF test—based on the principle (Chapter 6). More recently, Ikeda and Urakubo (1968) and Ikeda, Hukami, and Urakubo (1972) developed a flicker version of the HTRF test.

Anomalous Trichromacy

Anomalous trichromacy occurs in 6 percent of the European male and less than 0.4 percent of the European female population. Lord Rayleigh (1881) recognized the existence of two separate forms, protanomalous trichromacy (1 percent) and deuteranomalous trichromacy (5 percent).

COLOR MIXTURE

The color mixture of anomalous trichromats was measured in the W. D. Wright laboratory (Wright, 1946) in the 1930s by Wright and his colleagues; protanomalous color mixture was reported by McKeon and Wright (1940), deuteranomalous data by Nelson (1938). More recently, Mitchell and Rushton (1971b), Vogt (1974), and Alpern and Moeller (1977) have reported color mixture data for anomalous trichromats.

A feature of the matching behavior of anomalous trichromats is considerable variability among observers. The variability is so great that data for individual observers have not been averaged to give mean sets of color mixture functions for protanomalous and deuteranomalous trichromats analogous to that available for normal observers. This variability reflects the fact that most anomalous trichromats have reduced chromatic discrimination for judgments of the redness–greenness components of spectral lights. The technique used in the Wright laboratory was to ask the anomalous trichromats to adjust the three primaries to produce a match. It is difficult to obtain an estimate of matching variance with this technique in anomalous observers, and evaluation of interindividual variability in matches depends on the match variance.

SPECTRAL SENSITIVITY

Spectral sensitivity of protanomalous and deuteranomalous trichromats has been measured at the absolute threshold of vision by brightness matching (Alpern & Torii, 1968), by heterochromatic flicker photometry (deVries, 1948a; Crone, 1959; Alpern &

Torii, 1968; Verriest, 1971a), and by increment threshold (Verriest & Uvijls, 1977a, b). Data are shown in Fig. 7.5 and 7.6. In such measurements protanomalous trichromats all show reduced sensitivity for long-wavelength light and deuteranomalous trichromats usually show reduced sensitivity for short-wavelength light. The HFP functions lie close to those of the corresponding dichromat (Fig. 7.5). Foveal increment threshold data of normal observers show a secondary long-wavelength maximum at 600 nm, which is attributed to activity of the red–green opponent channel. In protanomalous trichromats the secondary maximum does not occur possibly because it is obscured by the absolute luminosity loss. Deuteranomalous trichromats show a shoulder rather than a relative maximum (Fig. 7.6).

WAVELENGTH AND COLORIMETRIC PURITY DISCRIMINATION

Wavelength discrimination of anomalous trichromats has been measured by Pitt (1935), Nelson (1938), and McKeon and Wright (1940); colorimetric purity discrimination has been measured by Nelson (1938), McKeon and Wright (1940), Chapanis (1944), and Bouman and Walraven (1961).

Wavelength discrimination functions are shown in Fig. 7.9. All show a minimum (best discrimination) near 490–500 nm. The observers showed considerable interobserver variability. At one extreme an observer might show low $\Delta\lambda$ through the visible spectrum, not ostensibly different from those of a normal trichromat; at the other extreme an observer might give wavelength discrimination typical of a dichromat. The majority of anomalous trichromatic observers do show some discrimination loss compared with a normal trichromat.

Colorimetric purity thresholds were measured as the first step from white. The Chapanis (1944) data plotted as reciprocal colorimetric purity using a 2° field are reproduced in Fig. 7.10. These data allow comparison of the data of normal and anomalous trichromats. The functions show that the protanomalous and deuteranomalous trichromats have minima near 490 and 500 nm, respectively, at the positions of the neutral points of the corresponding dichromat. The sensitivity at these minima are reduced compared with data for normal trichromats. Above 500 nm colorimetric purity discrimination improves and at 565 nm reaches a level similar to that of a normal trichromat. There is a suggestion of a broad secondary minimum in the yellow-green region. The Nelson (1938) and McKeon and Wright (1940) data showed trends similar to the Chapanis (1944) data and further demonstrated considerable interobserver variability characteristic of anomalous trichromats.

STILES-CRAWFORD EFFECT OF THE SECOND KIND (SCE 2)

The Stiles-Crawford effect of the second kind (SCE 2) is a color phenomenon described in Chapter 6 for the normal trichromat. The SCE 2 wavelength shifts in anomalous trichromats (Walraven & Leebeck, 1962; Voke, 1974; Walraven, 1976) were much larger than in normal trichromats; the greatest shifts occurred for the deuteranomalous trichromat. Further, for wavelengths above 560 nm the direction of wavelength shift with decentration was to shorter wavelengths. In comparison, in normal trichromats the shift is to longer wavelengths; i.e., in a normal trichromat the apparent hues of yellows, oranges, and reds shift to more reddish hues. Walraven (1976) has interpreted the data as reflecting self-screening (Chapter 3).

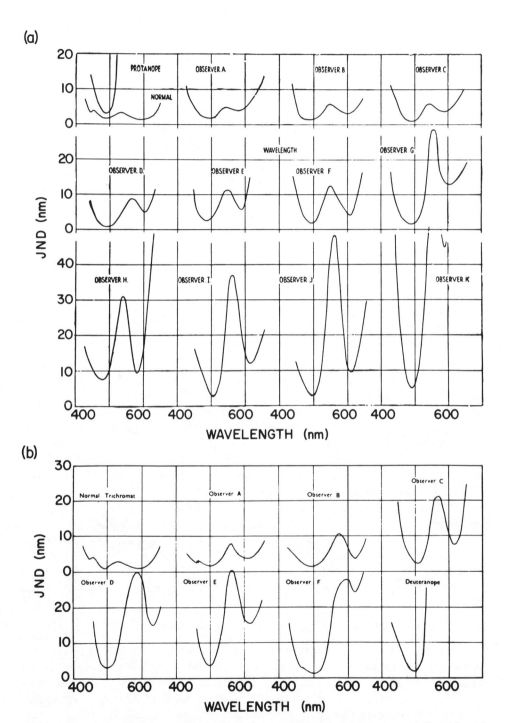

Fig. 7.9. Wavelength discrimination curves for anomalous trichromats. (a) Data for 11 protanomals arranged in order of severity of defect. The first diagram shows the curves for a normal and for a protanope. (b) Hue discrimination curves for 6 deuteranomals, 1 normal, and 1 deuteranope. [From Wright, W. D. *Researches on normal and defective color vision*. London, Kimpton, 1946 (reproduced with permission of Kimpton).]

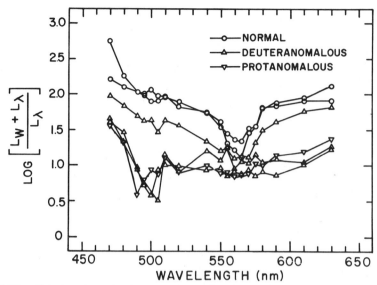

Fig. 7.10. Colorimetric purity discrimination thresholds for anomalous trichromats. Data for a normal trichromat are shown for comparison. [Data redrawn from Chapanis, 1944.]

PSYCHOPHYSICAL CORRELATES OF
THE VISUAL PHOTOPIGMENTS

Anomalous trichromats make a unique Rayleigh match and therefore have two visual photopigments active at wavelengths above 500 nm. Attempts to derive the spectral sensitivities of the corresponding two receptor mechanisms using partial bleaching techniques were made by de Vries (1948b), Wald (1966), Walraven, Van Hout, and Leebeck (1966), Watkins (1969a, b), Piantanida and Sperling (1973a, b), Sperling and Piantanida (1974), and Walraven (1976) but with variable success. The technique of reflection densitometry is not suitable for detection of two photopigments sensitive above 500 nm in the anomalous trichromat (Rushton, 1970).

Estimates of the absorption spectra of the anomalous pigments derived from techniques other than partial bleaching were reported by Lobanova and Speranskaya (1961), Wald (1966), Alpern and Torii (1968a, b), Pokorny, Smith, and Katz (1973), Rushton, Powell, and White (1973), Pokorny, Moreland, and Smith (1975), and Piantanida, Bruch, Latch, and Varner (1976). Figure 7.11 shows some estimates of the anomalous photopigments in deuteranomalous and protanomalous trichromats.

Color Perceptions of Protan and Deutan Observers

The color vision characteristics of a color-defective observer can be specified by color-matching performance, spectral sensitivity, and wavelength and colorimetric purity discrimination. These characteristics allow insights into the types of discriminations made by color defectives but do not address the problems of their color experiences. Experimental studies that aim to investigate color experience include hue estimation and hue cancellation.

Color defectives are a minority in a society that has developed a color vocabulary too rich for their needs; nevertheless, color terms are used with skill by many color defectives. Dichromats may be comfortable using the term "orange" in daily life although they may

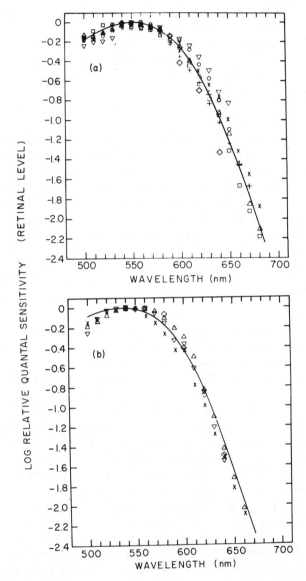

Fig. 7.11. Estimates of the absorption spectrum of the anomalous visual photopigment of deuteranomalous (a) and protanomalous (b) trichromats. Data are expressed as log relative quantal sensitivity at the retina. The solid lines are proposed visual photopigment absorption coefficients using the single-pigment hypothesis and based on analysis of red–green matches. ◇, Rushton, Powell, and White (1973a, b, c); ○, de Vries (1948b); □, Wald (1966); +, Walraven, Van Hout, and Leebeck (1966); Δ, Alpern and Torii (1968a, b); ▽, Piantanida and Sperling (1973a,b); ×, Piantanida, Bruch, Latch, and Varner (1976). [From Pokorny, J., & Smith, V. C. *Journal of the Optical Society of America,* 1977, *67,* 1196–1209 (reproduced with permission of the Optical Society of America).]

not be able to differentiate long-wavelength spectral lights reliably in a laboratory situation. Laboratory tests use small fields and spectrally pure colors, putting color defectives at a disadvantage in comparison with their experiences in daily life, where they may make few errors. Of course, two stimuli, although of the same chromaticity for a dichromat (being located on the same isochromatic line of the chromaticity diagram), can be differentiated if they arouse different sensations of brightness or lightness. Many congenital dichromatic observers reach maturity without realizing that there is anything abnormal about their color vision.

A feature characteristic of abnormal red–green vision is heightened chromatic contrast, described by Nagel (1904) and reviewed by Chapanis (1949). The feature is easy to demonstrate when a 670 nm (red) light and a 589 nm light are presented side-by-side. The color defective says the 589 nm field appears "green," although when the 670 nm field is extinguished the test field is said to be yellow (the hue remains relatively constant for normals). Heightened chromatic contrast occurs not only when different spectral radiations are present side by side but also when different luminances of the same spectral radiation are present. A protanope, for example, is likely to call the less radiant of two long-wavelength spectral fields "red."

COLOR PERCEPTIONS OF DICHROMATS

Some understanding of dichromatic color perception comes from a consideration of the confusion lines in the CIE diagram. By associating the coordinates in the x, y chromaticity diagram with their usual unique color appearance to normal trichromats, colors confused by the two types of dichromats can be estimated. For both protanopes and deuteranopes one isochromatic line lies on the spectrum locus from 540 to 700 nm; red–green dichromats confuse greens, yellows, and reds. It is customary to say that protanopes confuse reds with dark browns, pale blues with purples and magentas, blue-greens, whites, and red-purples, and light greens with light browns (fawns); deuteranopes confuse reds, oranges, and light browns, blues, violets, and blue purples, blue-greens, whites, and purples, and light greens, magentas, and purple reds.

The confusion line passing through equal-energy white is called the *minor neutral axis;* it indicates precisely which colors and in particular which monochromatic radiation (neutral point) can be completely matched with the equal-energy white. An axis orthogonal to the minor axis is called the *major axis,* and the remaining chromatic sensations can be plotted on it—at the intersection with the minor axis there is an achromatic hue; above, there is "yellow" with increasing saturation; and, below, there is "blue," also with increasing saturation. Accordingly, the visible spectrum to the observer having either protanopia or deuteranopia is said to appear in these three hues.

There is a type of observer for whom this prediction can be verified—namely, the unilateral color defective. Although rare, such observers do exist. Judd (1948) reviewed the early literature on unilateral color defects. One experiment of interest is to compare the color percepts of the two eyes. Sloan and Wollach (1948) performed this experiment. Their observer, a high school student, had a deuteranopic right eye. The left eye was also not normal: using the left eye the subject failed screening plates and showed a deutan error accumulation on the FM 100-hue test. His color match measured on the anomaloscope was normal; thus he was not a true deuteranomalous trichromat, as is often quoted in literature. Color names for spectral colors presented to the deuteranopic eye included blue for wavelengths below 500 nm, white at 500–505 nm, and yellow above 505 nm; the color names for lights presented to the fellow eye were normal. When comparison lights were presented simultaneously to the two eyes, spectral wavelengths at two spectral regions, 451–453 and 584 nm, appeared the same to the two eyes.

A related experiment consists of asking the unilateral dichromat to match the colors seen by the dichromatic eye to colors seen in the normal eye. Such data have been reported by Graham and Hsia (1961) for an observer with a color-defective eye and a normal eye. The color-defective eye was classified as deuteranopic although there were subtle differences in color matching compared with classical deuteranopes. An experiment was arranged to allow the observer to compare the appearance of spectral colors between the two eyes. The results showed that the color-defective eye appreciated only two chromatic hues. White was seen at the neutral point (502 nm). Wavelengths below the neutral point could be matched to 470 nm in the normal eye, i.e., appeared blue. Wavelengths above the neutral point could be matched to 570 nm in the normal eye, i.e., appeared yellow.

MacLeod and Lennie (1974) compared color perceptions in the eyes of an observer who was deuteranopic in one eye and deuteranomalous in the other. This observer could match all wavelengths below the neutral point in the deuteranopic eye to a wavelength of about 474 nm in the deuteranomalous eye. All wavelengths above the neutral point could be matched to a wavelength of about 610 nm. The observer was asked to set unique hues for his deuteranomalous eye; unique blue occurred at 466 nm and unique yellow at 589 nm. It is of interest that the colors seen in the dichromatic eye do not correspond to the wavelengths set as unique hues by the trichromatic eye. MacLeod and Lennie interpret these data as throwing doubt on the opponent process interpretation of color.

As previously noted, although many dichromats are surprisingly good at naming color fields correctly in the everyday world, these skills are less apparent in the laboratory, where small spectral fields are used. There have been at least four recent studies of the color naming of the dichromat. The studies indicated that the dichromat, like the normal trichromat, will use the response categories blue, green, yellow, and red to describe the spectrum (Luria, 1967; Weitzman & Kinney, 1967; Boynton & Scheibner, 1967; Scheibner & Boynton, 1968). However, it should not be inferred that dichromats have four unique sensory percepts corresponding to these names. The response category blue is used as by the normal observer. The response green shows a peak between 490 and 510 nm. Above 500 nm, the use of response categories green, yellow, and red depends on luminance: with a dark surround and low luminance stimuli, deuteranopes are likely to call spectral stimuli above 510 nm red; at high luminance, they may call such stimuli yellow. Although typically the response category red is not well differentiated from the categories green and yellow for wavelengths above 510 nm, some deuteranopes reliably differentiate these response categories even when luminance is controlled (Scheibner & Boynton, 1968). For the protanope the category red is used for dark stimuli and yellow is used for higher-luminance stimuli. Again, a few protanopes will differentiate the response categories green, yellow, and red in a consistent wavelength-dependent fashion for equiluminant stimuli (Scheibner & Boynton, 1968).

Another approach to understanding dichromatic color perception is the derivation of chromatic opponent-response functions. The classical experiments of Hurvich and Jameson showed that the normal trichromat has two chromatic opponent response functions, one a three-component function r-g-r for red-green called V_2 and one a two-component function b-y for blue-yellow called V_3 (Chapter 3). The functions were measured using four fixed cancellation stimuli chosen to be the observer's unique hues: a long-wavelength stimulus cancelled "greenness," a unique yellow stimulus cancelled "blueness," a unique green stimulus cancelled "redness," and a unique blue stimulus cancelled "yellowness" of spectral lights. Romeskie and Yager (1978) found that only two cancellation stimuli were necessary for dichromats, one below and one above the neutral point. Romeskie and Yager (1978) thus obtained only one chromatic response function from either a protanope or a deuteranope; both resembled the V_3 function of normal trichromats, although there were differences in the shape of the y component between protanope, deuteranope, and normal trichromat.

These studies confirm that for small fields, dichromatic observers have color perceptions that extend on a blue–yellow discrimination axis separated by a neutral area. For the reported cases of unilateral dichromacy the color perceptions of the dichromatic eye were a reduction form of the normal or anomalous eye. With larger fields many dichromatic observers have an added dimension of color discrimination mediated by their two cone photopigments and a rhodopsin receptor (see above). The perceptual correlates for large fields are unknown.

COLOR PERCEPTIONS OF ANOMALOUS TRICHROMATS

In the case of anomalous trichromats, the possibility exists of a truly different color vision. A unilateral deuteranomalous observer, a self-observation of Reichert (1916), was studied by von Kries (1919) and later by Trendelenburg (1941b). Von Kries (1919) compared the color names for the normal eye with those for the deuteranomalous eye. "Violet" was not perceived in the deuteranomalous eye. Short wavelengths were reported as "blue" shading to "grayish-blue" at 480 nm; 488 and 496 nm appeared almost colorless to the deuteranomalous eye. Above 535 nm the spectrum was predominantly seen as "yellow," "pure yellow" being reported from 559 to 591 nm. The hue at 680 nm was described as "yellow with a trace of red." These data suggest a reduction in apparent saturation for many spectral hues in addition to a reduction in the chromatic content of the spectrum above 520 nm. Trendelenburg (1941b) noted that although anomaloscope examination of the fellow eye was normal, there were errors on pigment tests *(Pigmentfarbenanomalie)*. The defect was transmitted to a daughter who was deuteranomalous.

Hue estimation of brief foveal flashes was reported by Smith, Pokorny, and Swartley (1973). A 12' diameter spectral light was flashed for 12 msec. Deuteranomalous observers were asked to report the chromatic content by percentage using the response categories blue, green, yellow, and red. Typical data for two deuteranomalous trichromats are shown in Fig. 7.12. All deuteranomalous observers who were tested used all four colors in describing the spectrum. Blue was used for wavelengths below 500 nm, peaking at about 450 nm. The category blue was used similarly by deuteranomalous and normal trichromats. The categories green, yellow, and red were not as well differentiated by the deuteranomalous trichromats, with overlapping use of the red and green categories. The category green peaked at 500–520 nm, yellow showed a broad peak from 540 to 610 nm, and red peaked at long wavelengths. The observers showed considerable interobserver variability in their choices of the response categories at a given luminance level. However, for all observers an increase in luminance allowed the response category yellow to dominate the red and green categories.

The wavelength locations associated with the perception of the unique hues for anomalous trichromats differ from those of normals. Rubin (1961) asked normal and anomalous trichromats to find the wavelengths corresponding to a set of color percepts. The percepts included three unique hues, "blue," "green," and "yellow." In addition, settings for "cyan" (a perfect balance of blue and green) and "orange" (a balance of red

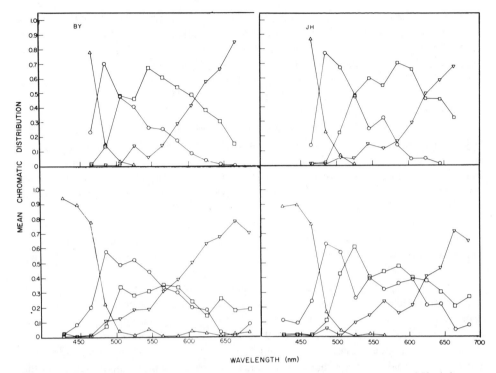

Fig. 7.12. Hue estimation curves for two deuteranomalous trichromats. Upper: 250 td; lower: 25 td. [From Smith, V. C., Pokorny, J., & Swartley, R. *American Journal of Psychology*, 1973, 86, 115–131 (reproduced by permission of the University of Illinois Press).]

and yellow) were requested, although on the basis of the von Kries (1919) data, the percepts blue-green and orange are not appreciated by the deuteranomalous eye. Table 7.3 shows the results. The wavelengths associated with unique hues were shifted to shorter wavelengths for protanomalous trichromats and to longer wavelengths for deuteranomalous trichromats than the wavelength locations used by normal trichromats. The deuteranomalous trichromats were unable to find a setting for unique blue. At short wavelengths they did not perceive "violet" (or a reddish component to blues). The percept of "blue" simply increased in apparent saturation as wavelength decreased. Hurvich and Jameson (1964) have confirmed that the spectral locus of unique yellow is shifted to

Table 7.3*

Mean Wavelengths at Which the Three Classes of
Trichromats Located the Five Hues and the Corresponding
Standard Deviations (nm)

	278 Normals	12 Protanomals	32 Deuteranomals
Orange	601.1 ± 2.4	590.4 ± 3.1	611.7 ± 3.4
Yellow	576.6 ± 2.0	563.1 ± 3.0	583.4 ± 2.9
Green	517.5 ± 5.7	501.7 ± 3.3	519.6 ± 3.5
Cyan	494.3 ± 1.7	488.3 ± 2.3	497.6 ± 2.1
Blue	468.3 ± 3.1	467.7 ± 4.0	none

*From Rubin, M. L. *American Journal of Ophthalmology*, 1961, *52*, 166–172, (reproduced with permission of the Ophthalmic Publishing Company).

shorter wavelengths (569–576 nm) for protanomalous trichromats and to longer wavelengths (590–600 nm) for deuteranomalous trichromats compared to its locus (575–590 nm) for normal trichromats. The data of Rubin (1961) and Hurvich and Jameson (1964) were based on the self-adjustment technique. Smith, Pokorny, and Swartley (1973) found that for small, brief flashes the color-naming data were too variable to allow determination of unique hue loci of deuteranomalous trichromats for yellow and that blue did not have a unique locus.

Romeskie (1978) used a color-naming technique with a 1° field presented for 1 sec with four protanomals and two deuteranomals. Romeskie could not obtain a locus for unique yellow in three anomalous trichromats (two protanomals and one deuteranomal) but did obtain unique blue for the two deuteranomalous trichromats. There is therefore considerable variance in whether or not the percepts of "unique" blue and yellow exist for all anomalous trichromats.

Romeskie (1978) measured chromatic opponent response functions in six anomalous trichromats. Four cancellation stimuli were necessary for the anomalous trichromats as for normal trichromats. The V_3 response (b-y) was approximately normal, but the V_2 (r-g) response was much reduced.

Finally, color discriminations of anomalous trichromats also give insight into perceptual aspects of anomalous color vision. The chromatic discrimination losses are specific to the R-G axis of discrimination and extend along the confusion lines of the corresponding dichromat (Farnsworth, 1947; Birch, 1973). This fact forms the basis for the successful pigment plate tests, which depend on discrimination loss for detecting red–green anomalous trichromacy. The saturation discrimination function suggests that the spectrum above 500 nm is relatively desaturated. Pokorny and Smith (1977) suggested that the long-wave part of the spectrum has reduced chromatic content for anomalous trichromats. The colors of their spectrum might be conceived as including saturated blues fading into a grayish region, extremely desaturated greens, then yellows, and, finally, relatively desaturated oranges.

The Anomaloscope

DIAGNOSIS OF RED–GREEN DEFECTS

The anomaloscope (Chapter 5) is principally used to diagnose the red–green color defects; three subtypes of protan and three subtypes of deutan observers have been recognized (Franceschetti, 1928). Anomaloscope matching ranges measured by Pickford (1958a) on the Pickford-Nicolson anomaloscope are depicted in Fig. 7.13. Typical Rayleigh matching data are summarized in Table 7.4. In the protan series, the simple protanomalous trichromat (abbreviated PA) makes a unique match that contains a higher proportion of red primary compared with the normal match. To a normal trichromat the mixture fields at the protanomalous match appear orange in comparison with the yellow test field. On average, the matching range is somewhat wider than that of a normal trichromat. The extreme protanomalous trichromat (abbreviated EPA) has a wide matching range that includes the simple protanomalous match and the normal match and may extend to one of the primaries. The protanope (abbreviated P) as a dichromat matches the test light to the green primary, the red primary, and all possible mixtures of the primaries. The protanopic luminosity loss for long wavelengths is expressed on the Nagel

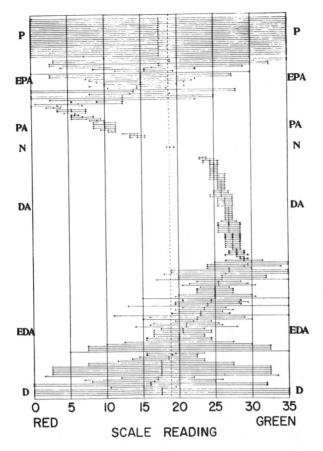

Fig. 7.13. Matching ranges and midpoints for 191 major red–green defectives on the Pickford anomaloscope. One normal subject is shown in the middle for comparison. P, protanopes; EPA, extreme protanomals; PA, protanomals; D. deuteranopes; EDA, extreme deuteranomals; DA, deuteranomals; N, normal. [From Pickford, R. W. *Advancement of Science,* 1958, *15,* 104–117 (reproduced with permission of the British Association for the Advancement of Science).]

model I anomaloscope in the different luminance settings of 589 nm light used in the matches (Fig. 7.14)—the 589 nm light is set at a relatively dim level in the match to 670 nm and at a relatively high level in the match to 545 nm. In the deutan series the simple deuteranomalous trichromat (abbreviated DA) makes a unique match that contains a higher proportion of green primary than the normal match. To a normal trichromat the mixture fields at the deuteranomalous match appear greenish in comparison with the yellow test field. On the average the matching range is somewhat wider than that of the average normal trichromat. The extreme deuteranomalous trichromat (abbreviated EDA) has a wide matching range that includes the simple deuteranomalous match and the normal match and that may extend to one of the primaries. The deuteranope (abbreviated D), as a dichromat, matches the yellow test light to the green primary, the red primary, and all possible mixtures of the primaries. The approximately normal deuteranopic luminosity is represented on the Nagel model I anomaloscope by approximately equal luminance settings of the 589 nm test light to either primary and all mixtures (Fig. 7.14).

Table 7.4
Summary of Anomaloscope Behavior

Description	Abbreviation	Rayleigh Matching Behavior	AQ*
Normal trichromat	N	Unique narrow match	1.0 (0.72–1.33)
Protan defects			
Simple protanomalous trichromat	PA	Narrow match displaced to red Luminosity loss for red primary	< 0.25 (0.15–0.50)
Extreme protanomalous trichromat	EPA	Wide match including PA and N matches and sometimes one of the primaries Luminosity loss for red primary	—
Protanope	P	Matches full range Luminosity loss for red primary	—
Deutan defects			
Simple deuteranomalous trichromat	DA	Narrow match displaced to green Normal luminosity	4.0 (2.0–5.6)
Extreme deuteranomalous trichromat	EDA	Wide match including DA and N matches and sometimes one of the primaries Normal luminosity	—
Deuteranope	D	Matches full range, normal luminosity	—

*Quotients given only for normal and simple anomalous trichromats.

208

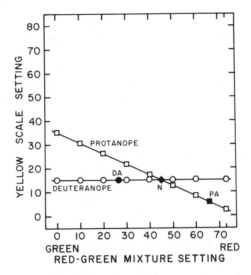

Fig. 7.14. Small-field brightness matches made by a protanope and a deuteranope on the Nagel model I anomaloscope.

MIDMATCHING POINT AND MATCHING RANGE

According to the principle of the alteration system, the anomalous trichromat's match reflects the fact that one or more of his or her visual photopigments differ from those of normal trichromats. Thus the midmatch point has theoretical significance: when a trichromat accepts a narrow match, the midmatching point is determined by the absorption spectra of the visual photopigments and the lens transmission function.

In contrast, the matching range is an indication of the observer's chromatic discriminative ability. The matching range is a measurement of importance in the practical situation. On average, the matching range of the simple anomalous trichromat is wider than that of the normal trichromat. The distribution of match widths of anomalous trichromats is variable, with occasional anomalous trichromats having narrow matching ranges.

For the Nagel anomaloscope the matching range is independent of the midmatching point for normal and deuteranomalous trichromats. This statement is true in practice (Waaler, 1927; Willis & Farnsworth, 1952) and reflects the design of the instrument (Pokorny & Smith, 1977). Rayleigh equations for protanomalous trichromats measured on the Nagel anomaloscope theoretically may show dependence of matching width on midmatch position (Pokorny & Smith, 1977), but too few protanomalous trichromats have been investigated for a statistical demonstration of this fact. Since for the most frequent type of anomalous trichromacy, deuteranomalous trichromacy, the midmatching point and matching range are independent, it follows that the midmatching point does not indicate the practical severity of the color defect (Verriest, 1960b; see also Hurvich, 1972).

EXTREME ANOMALOUS TRICHROMACY

Extreme anomalous trichromacy is defined only by performance at the anomaloscope. The studies discussed above (Anomalous Trichromacy) did not differentiate simple and extreme anomalous trichromacy. According to the Franceschetti classification the extreme anomalous trichromat is an observer with a wide matching range that includes the normal match, the match of the corresponding simple anomalous trichromat, and perhaps one of the primaries (Franceschetti, 1928). Not all researchers accept the Franceschetti classification of extreme anomalous trichromacy as a unique entity. A different classification was proposed by Trendelenburg and Schmidt (1935): they defined as extreme anomalous trichromats those anomalous trichromats who showed "tuning," a widened matching range only after staring at their match (the equation under *Umstimmung;* see Chapter 5). In this view, the extreme anomalous trichromat is an anomalous trichromat with poor chromatic discriminative ability.

MINIMALLY AFFECTED ANOMALOUS TRICHROMACY
(Minmalanomale Trichromaten)

A few anomalous trichromats have excellent chromatic discrimination. Their Rayleigh midmatch point is typical of anomalous trichromatic vision, but they pass screening tests. In the German literature such observers are sometimes called *minimale Protanomalen* or *minimale Deuteranomalen* (Vierling, 1935). The majority of screening plates that have been validated with an anomaloscope detect 95–99 percent of all anomalous trichromats. Thus "minimally affected" protanomaly and deuteranomaly comprise perhaps 1–5 percent of the anomalous trichromatic population.

ANOMALOUS QUOTIENT

The anomalous quotient (Trendelenburg, 1929) is a common method of presenting the midmatching point of a trichromat's Rayleigh equation (Chapter 5). Anomalous quotients may be used to compare data from different laboratories if the identical set of primaries is used in both laboratories. A word of caution is in order: The anomalous quotient is independent of the luminance ratio of the primaries but not of the spectral distribution of the primaries. Different versions of the same model anomaloscope with nominally identical primaries may give slightly different ranges of anomalous quotients for anomalous trichromats (e.g., Waaler, 1927; Trendelenburg & Schmidt, 1935; Willis & Farnsworth, 1952). The most probable explanation of such discrepancy among these studies is in differences between the actual transmission spectra of the primaries, which were nominally identical.

Schmidt (1955b) noted that when the anomalous quotients of normal and anomalous trichromats are replotted as percentiles as a function of log(AQ) they have similar variance. The data of Waaler (1927) and Willis and Farnsworth (1952) show a similar result. Schmidt (1955b) suggested the source of variability to be common in the three groups. Variance of the anomalous quotient must be attributed to variation in inert ocular pigments and/or to variation in the shape or spectral location of the visual photopigments. Moreland (1972) suggested that the major source of variation was in the inert pigments. Pokorny and Smith (1976) determined that the normal range of variability of inert ocular pigment of the lens accounts for two-thirds of the variation of green–red ratios in normal trichromats. The remaining one-third was due to receptoral variation—for example, variation of effective optical density of photopigment absorption spectra in the population (Smith, Pokorny, & Starr, 1976) or in the characteristic photopigment spectra (Smith, Pokorny, & Starr, 1976; Alpern & Pugh, 1977; Alpern & Moeller, 1977).

INTERPRETATION OF ANOMALOSCOPE MATCHES

According to the reduction theory for dichromacy, the dichromat should accept the Rayleigh match of the normal trichromat. Further, if dichromacy occurs by "loss" of a class of photopigment (e.g., MWS for deuteranopes) and assuming alteration of only that class of photopigment in the corresponding anomalous trichromat (M'WS for deuteranomalous trichromats), the dichromat will also accept the color match of the corresponding anomalous trichromat. In comparison, hypotheses of reduction by collapse for dichromacy or alteration of two or more classes of visual photopigment in anomalous trichromacy give the prediction that dichromats will not accept matches of the corresponding anomalous trichromat. The anomaloscope behavior is therefore important in differentiating these theoretical interpretations of red–green color defect.

In general, the dichromat does accept the matches of both the normal trichromat and the corresponding anomalous trichromat. Quantitative data were given by Mitchell and Rushton (1971b). Rushton, Powell, and White (1973) and Hurvich and Jameson (1978) showed that protanopes accept protanomalous and normal trichromatic matches. Although these experimental data are true in a population comparison, a given individual dichromat, e.g., a protanope, may or may not accept the color matches made by a given individual protanomalous trichromat or a given individual normal trichromat.

Procedures in which an individual is asked to accept or reject a different person's color match are called confrontation experiments. Acceptance of another's match in confrontation may fail because of individual differences in inert ocular pigments combined with receptoral variation (Alpern & Pugh, 1977; Alpern & Moeller, 1977; Alpern & Wake, 1977; Pokorny & Smith, 1977). On the other hand, acceptance may occur because of poor chromatic discrimination (Hurvich, 1972; Hurvich & Jameson, 1978). The confrontation experiment therefore provides only weak evidence for or against a given theoretical interpretation.

Transmission and Frequency of Red–Green Color Defects

Horner (1876) and others established by means of the study of extensive pedigrees that the mode of transmission of the protan and deutan defects is identical to that of hemophilia; the disease occurs chiefly in males and is transmitted through females who generally are not affected themselves (Fig. 7.15). Following Morgan's (1910) studies of sex-limited transmission in Drosophila, Wilson (1911) and others suggested that these color defects depend on pathologic genes carried by the X chromosome. Various pedigrees are reviewed by François and Verriest (1961a) and Franceschetti, François, and Babel (1974).

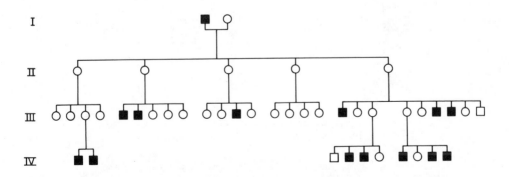

Fig. 7.15. Horner's (1876) pedigree showing that red–green color vision defects occur in males in each generation. ○, female; □, male; solid symbols indicate affected members.

TERMINOLOGY FOR X-CHROMOSOME–LINKED INHERITANCE

X-chromosome–linked (or sex-linked) inheritance refers to traits carried on the sex chromosomes. The female has two X chromosomes, one inherited from the mother and one from the father, with matching genetic loci (homologues). The male has one X chromosome inherited from the mother and a Y chromosome inherited from the father. X and Y chromosomes have some matching genetic loci (homologous portion) and some nonmatching loci (nonhomologous portion). If a gene occurs on the X chromosome at a locus for which no matching gene occurs on the Y chromosome, X-chromosome–linked inheritance results. In X-chromosome–linked recessive inheritance the affected female must inherit a defective gene on both X chromosomes, that is, from each parent. The male inheriting the defective gene from his mother will always show the defect, since he has no normal gene to oppose expression of the defect. Females who have one defective gene are called carriers. The affected males (who give an X chromosome to daughters and a Y chromosome to sons) pass the defective gene to all their daughters, who will be carriers, and to none of their sons.

Genes that occupy matching positions on a pair of chromosomes are called alleles. When more than one trait can be determined at a given gene position (locus), there are multiple alleles. Some traits—for example, color vision—are determined by sets of multiple alleles active at more than one gene locus. In X-chromosomal inheritance, the male is called a *hemizygote*—a *simple hemizygote* when he has a defective allele at one gene locus, a *compound hemizygote* if he has defective alleles at each of two gene loci. There are a number of terms that are used to describe the deduced genotype of the female. The *homozygote* has matched pairs of alleles; the *heterozygote* has nonmatched pairs of alleles. The *simple heterozygote* has unmatched alleles at only one gene locus; the *mixed, compound,* or *double heterozygote* has unmatched alleles at more than one locus. There are two subtypes of compound heterozygote illustrated in Fig. 7.16 for a woman with two

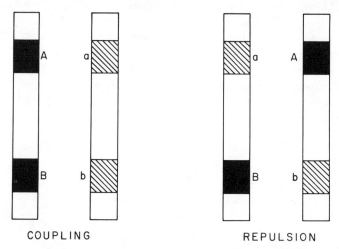

COUPLING   REPULSION

Fig. 7.16. Diagram of the two types of compound heterozygote. (left) Abnormal genes a, b are on the same chromosome and are said to be coupled. (right) Abnormal genes a, b are on opposing chromosomes and are said to be in repulsion. Genes that tend to be transmitted together from generation to generation are said to be linked either in coupling or in repulsion.

normal alleles (A, B) and two abnormal alleles (a, b). If the abnormal alleles (a, b) occur on the same chromosome, the compound heterozygosity is said to be coupled; if abnormal alleles (a, b) occur on homologous chromosomes, the compound heterozygosity is said to be in repulsion. An alternative terminology is used by Jaeger (1972), who differentiates two types of compound heterozygote. The allelic compound heterozygote has unmatched abnormal alleles at one locus (e.g., a_1, a_2, BB). Such a female will be color defective. The nonallelic compound heterozygote has unmatched alleles at more than one locus (e.g., Aa_1, Bb_1).

TRANSMISSION OF RED–GREEN COLOR DEFECTS

It was established by means of the study of families affected by different defects that in a woman the simultaneous presence of a gene for protan defect and a gene for deutan defect generally gives a primarily normal phenotype (Fig. 7.17a), while the simultaneous presence of a gene for dichromatism and a gene for the corresponding anomalous trichromatism results in anomalous trichromatism (Fig. 7.17b). By analogy with the multiple allelic systems governing eye color in Drosophila, Just (1925) propounded the now generally accepted theory of multiple alleles for red–green color defects, one set for the protan and one for the deutan defects.

A further point to be clarified was whether the protan and deutan allelic series occur at the same locus of the X chromosome (one-locus hypothesis) or at two different loci (two-loci hypothesis). Genealogies consistent with the two-loci hypothesis are shown in Figure 7.17c. In Vanderdonck and Verriest's (1960) pedigree a woman proven to be a repulsion compound heterozygote had two normal sons, both proven X, Y males; the data can be explained only by crossing over between the two loci. A more recent (Fig. 7.17c) pedigree showing a similar finding is that of Went and de Vries–de Mol (1976). Recent work shows that the loci are close to each other (Siniscalco, Filippi, & Latte, 1964; Fraser, 1969; Arias & Rodriquez, 1972) on the short arm of the X chromosome (Lindsten, Fraccaro, Polani, Hamerton, Sanger, & Race, 1963). Kalmus (1962) and Siniscalco, Filippi and Latte (1964) suggest that the deutan and protan loci are situated on either side of the gene for glucose-6-phosphate dehydrogenase deficiency.

Today, we attribute the X-chromosome–linked color defects to the activity of two sets of genes, one governing a protan series of defects and one governing a deutan series of defects. At the protan locus the alleles are genes for normal color vision, simple protanomaly, extreme protanomaly, and protanopia. A similar set exists for the deutan locus. Color matching using the Rayleigh equation allows differentiation of the various defects. The presumed genotype for the protan series of alleles is designated by the letter A in upper or lower case and for the deutan series by the letter B in upper or lower case. Table 7.5 gives the terminology for allele series and the genotype and the phenotype for the simple hemizygote.

In the simple heterozygous female a dominance pattern among the alleles has been found. In the definition of recessive X-chromosome–linked inheritance, if the female has a normal gene on one X chromosome she has a primarily normal phenotype. What happens, though, when she has abnormal alleles on both X chromosomes? For color vision the rule is that the phenotype will resemble that of the least serious defect (Fig. 7.17b). With one allele for simple protanomalous trichromacy and the other for simple (genotype a_1B, a_1B) or extreme protanomalous (a_1B, a_2B) trichromacy or protanopia (genotype a_1B, a_3B), the color vision is that of simple protanomalous trichromacy. With one allele for extreme protanomalous trichromacy and the other for extreme

Table 7.5

Genotypes and Phenotypes for Males (Simple Hemizygotes) With Congenital Red–Green Color Vision Defects

Protan Alleles				Deutan Alleles			
Symbol for Protan Allele Sequence	Genotype for Hemizygote	Phenotype		Symbol for Deutan Allele Sequence	Genotype for Simple Hemizygote	Phenotype	
A	AB	N	Normal	B	AB	N	Normal
a_1	a_1B	PA	Simple protanomalous trichromat	b_1	Ab_1	DA	Simple deuteranomalous trichromat
a_2	a_2B	EPA	Extreme protanomalous trichromat	b_2	Ab_2	EDA	Extreme deuteranomalous trichromat
a_3	a_3B	P	Protanope	b_3	Ab_3	D	Deuteranope

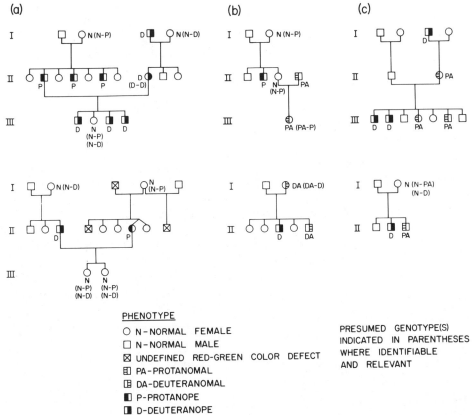

Fig. 7.17. Examples of the hereditary transmission of the X-chromosome—linked color vision defects. (a) A female inheriting two defective genes, one for a protan defect and one for a deutan defect, usually has normal color vision. The upper pedigree is redrawn from Franceschetti (1949); the lower pedigree is redrawn from Franceschetti and Klein (1957) as expanded by Franceschetti, François, and Babel (1974). (b) A female inheriting two defective genes from the same series (either protan or deutan) usually shows the color defect, and it will be the "least serious." The upper pedigree is redrawn from Waaler (1927); the lower pedigree is redrawn from Brunner (1930), abbreviated pedigree 18. (c) A female who is a carrier for two defective genes, one for a protan defect and one for a deutan defect, may have sons with normal color vision, protan defect, or deutan defect. These are examples of crossing over according to the two-loci hypothesis. Upper pedigree is redrawn from Vanderdonck and Verriest (1960); lower pedigree is redrawn from Went and de Vries—de Mol (1976).

protanomalous trichromacy (a_2B, a_2B) or protanopia (a_2B, a_3B), the color vision is extreme protanomalous trichromacy. Protanopia occurs only with two alleles for protanopia (a_3B, a_3B). The dominance sequence for both protan and deutan genes is shown in Table 7.6.

The evidence for the multiple-allele hypothesis was that dichromacy and anomalous trichromacy appeared to represent independent alleles. For example, a simple heterozygote for protanopia should not have sons with protanomalous trichromacy. This expectation is realized in the great majority of cases. Nevertheless, there are rare pedigrees showing variable manifestation in which a simple heterozygote has sons including normal and anomalous trichromats and dichromats (Göthlin, 1924; Brunner,

Table 7.6
Dominance Sequence for Heterozygous Females

Normal trichromacy dominant to:	simple anomalous trichromacy
	extreme anomalous trichromacy
	dichromacy
Simple anomalous trichromacy dominant to:	extreme anomalous trichromacy
	dichromacy
Extreme anomalous trichromacy dominant to:	dichromacy

1930). Intrafamily variability has been reported to be less than interfamily variability (Pickford, 1967; Went and de Vries–de Mol, 1976). Variable manifestation also occurs rarely between eyes of a color-defective observer (reviewed by Waardenburg, 1963b). Some of these cases, the so-called unilateral observers, were discussed above.

The separate existence of an allele for extreme anomalous trichromacy was postulated by Franceschetti (1928). A pedigree showing extreme anomalous trichromacy as an uniquely inherited entity that obeys the dominance sequence in the simple heterozygous female (Ab₁, Ab₂) was published by Grützner and Schrapp (1974). Nevertheless, some researchers do not think that EPA and EDA should have separate recognition, since some pedigrees show alternation of simple and extreme anomalous trichromacy (Jaeger, 1972). Extreme anomalous trichromacy also has been considered to represent action of a separate modifying gene (Trendelenburg & Schmidt, 1935).

FREQUENCY OF THE PROTAN AND DEUTAN DEFECTS

The frequency in males is practically identical to the gene frequency because males are homozygous for the X chromosome and the phenotype corresponds almost always to the genotype. The overall frequency is approximately 8 percent in European whites if one considers only statistics established by valid diagnostic methods (data compiled by Hsia & Graham, 1965 are listed in Table 7.7). The frequency is higher (10 percent) for whites in the U.S. (Willis & Farnsworth, 1952). As for non-Europeans (Kherumian & Pickford, 1959), Mongols are less frequently affected (4–5 percent), and the frequency is still lower in blacks (1.5–4 percent), Australian aborigines (1–2 percent), and some of the red peoples (native Americans or Amerinds) (1–2 percent). Post (1962) suggested that these different frequencies are real; he hypothesized that selection relaxation has allowed an increase in frequency of defective alleles in European populations.

The frequency in women is approximately 0.42 percent according to a combined sample of 24,666 from four studies of European white females (Table 7.7). This observed value is in good agreement with the theoretical value, which can be calculated from the frequency in males (taken as 8 percent), taking into account that compound heterozygous women (Jaeger's nonallelic compound heterozygotes) are normal. On the basis of the percentages of phenotypes observed by Waaler (1927) in males, one can predict that 0.36 percent of women should be deuteranomalous, 0.03 percent protanomalous, and less than 0.01 percent deuteranopic and 0.01 percent protanopic, giving a total of 0.41 percent. In practice there may appear to be a greater proportion of protanopic women than predicted, since occasional heterozygous females exhibit the full color defect (see below, The Heterozygote Female). By contrast, according to the hypothesis that no segregation of protan and deutan defects occurs, the expected frequency is 0.64 percent.

The frequency in "intersexes" obeys the expectation of X-chromosome–linked

Table 7.7

Percentages of Protans and Deutans in Various Populations as
Reported by Different Investigators

Population	Waaler (1927)	von Planta (1928)	Schmidt (1936)	François, Verriest, Mortier, & Vanderdonck (1957)	Kherumian & Pickford (1959)
	Norwegians	Swiss	Germans	Belgians	French
Males	9049	2000	6863	1243	6635
Females	9072	3000	5604	None	6990
Protanope	0.88	1.60	1.09	0.97	2.62
Protanomalous	1.04	0.60	0.68	1.05	
Deuteranope	1.03	1.50	1.97	1.37	6.33
Deuteranomalous	5.06	4.25	4.01	4.91	
Male total (observed)	8.01	7.95	7.75	8.30	8.95
Female total (observed)	0.40	0.43	0.36	—	0.50
Female total (calculated on male total)	0.64	0.63	0.60	—	0.80
Female total (calculated on basis of male protans and deutans)	0.41	0.38	0.39	—	0.47

From Hsia, Y., & Graham, C. H. Graham (Ed.). *Color blindness in vision and visual perception.*
New York, John Wiley & Sons, 1965 (reproduced with permission of John Wiley and Sons, Inc.).

recessive inheritance (Walls, 1959b; Franceschetti, 1960). In Turner syndrome (with genotype X0) the frequency of the protan and deutan defects resembles that in males. In Klinefelter syndrome (with genotype XXY) the frequency is similar to that in females although about 3 percent higher, since nondisjunction can occur at different miotic stages.

COMPOUND HEMIZYGOTES

Compound hemizygotes are males who inherit genes for defective color vision for both protan and deutan defects. These observers are rare but of great importance, since they provide test cases of the various theories of color defect. Cases of presumed compound hemizygotes include those of Walls and Mathews (1952), Pickford (1962), Siniscalco, Filippi, and Latte (1964), Latte, Filippi and Siniscalco (1965), and Arias and Rodriguez (1973a, b). In both the Pickford (1962) and the Walls and Mathews (1952) reports there was no independent confirmation of genes for both protan and deutan defects in the family. In the Siniscalco, Fillippi, and Latte (1964) pedigree the mother was known to carry genes for both protanopia and deuteranopia and had three sons; one was a protanope, one was a detueranope, and one was presumed to be a compound hemizygote for protanopia and deuteranopia (a₃b₃). This last observer was color defective; he made errors on clinical color tests typical for both protanopia and deuteranopia. Long-wavelength spectral sensitivity measured by absolute threshold (and by brightness matching on an anomaloscope) showed values intermediate between protan and deutan observers. The Arias and Rodriguez (1973a, b) pedigrees are from a genetic isolate with documentation of extreme protanomaly paired with various deutan defects. One observer with EPA and DA (Arias, 1976) (presumed genotype a₂b₁) made a narrow Rayleigh match shifted to green in the deuteranomalous range. The yellow brightness match was not normal but indicative of long-wavelength luminosity loss. Measured increment thresholds on chromatic backgrounds appeared the same as for protan observers. On screening plates he behaved as a protan. Arias (1976) comments that the subject's chromatic discrimination, as that of his cousins, also compound hemizygotes, was far superior to that observed in EPA (genotype a₂B); for example, the subject passed the Farnsworth Panel D-15 test, which is failed by the EPA. Arias (1976) noted this mixed defect, i.e., green-shifted Rayleigh equation with reduced luminosity, in all compound hemizygotes of EPA with a gene from the deutan series. Arias and Rodriguez (1973a, b), for example, describe a compound hemizygote for deuteranopia and extreme protanomaly whose anomaloscope matching was deuteranomalous with a wide matching range that did not include the normal match.

THE HETEROZYGOUS FEMALE

The mother or female child of a male with X-chromosome–linked color defect is a heterozygous carrier for the defective gene. The color vision in simple and compound heterozygotes is often said to be normal; however, carrier females do show color vision abnormalities.

Simple heterozygotes. There are many instances of simple heterozygous women who show a complete classical defect of color vision despite the presumed presence of a normal gene. The cases have been summarized by Franceschetti (1960) and François and Verriest (1961a). This finding is particularly frequent in carriers of protanopia. Many authors have shown that the majority of simple heterozygotes exhibit some signs of subnormal color vision. These findings may be significant only in a comparison of a group of heterozygous women with a control group. A research interest in recent years has been accurate identification of the carrier state in individual cases.

The most obvious abnormality is the so-called *Schmidt sign,* discovered by Schmidt (1934, 1955a) in protan carriers. The defect consists of a reduction in the relative luminous efficiency curve to a position halfway between the normal curve and the curve of the corresponding male hemizygote. The existence of the *Schmidt sign* has been confirmed by a large number of other authors using different psychophysical methods (reviewed by Verriest, 1972a). A number of these authors also noted an abnormality in the relative spectral luminous efficiency function of deutan carriers consisting of a reduced sensitivity at short wavelengths (Verriest, 1972a). Adam (1969) termed this finding the *de Vries sign* because it was described first by de Vries (1948).

Increment thresholds measured on chromatic backgrounds also show abnormalities. Ikeda and Urakubo (1968) and Ikeda, Hukami, and Urakubo (1972) used the Boynton (1961) HTRF test to evaluate heterozygotes and discovered abnormalities in heterozygotes for protan defects. De Vries– de Mol (1977) and de Vries– de Mol, Went, van Norren, and Pols (1978) found that protan and deutan heterozygous females can be reliably distinguished from each other and from homozygotes by their increment threshold spectral sensitivities on red and green chromatic backgrounds.

Other minor abnormalities are indicative of a loss in chromatic discriminative ability.

Some of these abnormalities are not significant on an individual basis. They include the following:

1. Difficulties in reading correctly some pseudoisochromatic tests (reviewed by Verriest, 1972).
2. Abnormalities at the anomaloscope. There may be a small displacement of the mean Rayleigh match toward red in the protan carriers and toward green in the deutan carriers (reviewed by Verriest, 1972a), brightness matching may be abnormal (Piantanida, 1971), there may be an increased scatter in the Rayleigh match (reviewed by Verriest, 1972a), or there may be exaggerated simultaneous color contrast similar to that observed in the cases of anomalous trichromatism (Walls & Mathews, 1952).
3. Abnormalities in hue and saturation discrimination. These findings include elevated $\Delta\lambda$ on measure of the wavelength discrimination curve (Möller-Ladekarl, 1934), increased errors on the FM 100-hue test (Krill & Schneiderman, 1964; Verriest, 1972a), abnormalities of hue discrimination and colorimetric purity discrimination using pigment tests (reviewed by Verriest, 1972a), and abnormalities of color identification of a 1' target presented along the horizontal meridian between 0° and 10° (Grutzner, Born, & Hemminger, 1976).

The explanation of the color defects observed in carrier females is the Lyon inactivation hypothesis (1961), sometimes called Lyonization. Lyon proposed that early in embryonic life one of the X chromosomes in each cell becomes inactive. Descendents of a given cell have the same active chromosome as the parent cell. Inactivation is random, with equal probability for either maternal or paternal chromosome. The cells of the carriers are thus a mosaic representing an admixture of paternally derived and maternally derived cells. A number of authors have attempted to demonstrate mosaicism in the female carrier of X-chromosome–linked color defect (Krill & Beutler, 1964; 1965; Grützner, Born, & Hemminger, 1976).

Compound heterozygotes.   François and Verriest (1961a) summarized the pedigrees with known compound heterozygotes. To these pedigrees, those of Went and de Vries–de Mol (1976), Jaeger and Lauer (1976), and Arias (1976) have been added. The color vision of the compound heterozygote is as diverse as for the simple heterozygote: some appear normal (Franceschetti, 1949; Franceschetti & Klein, 1957; Pickford, 1950; Ichikawa & Majima, 1974; Arias, 1976; Jaeger & Lauer, 1976) and some show color defects (Walls & Mathews, 1952; Jaeger, 1951; François & Verriest, 1961a). Unfortunately, the genotype is always inferred, and there are often multiple possibilities to explain the phenotype, as discussed by François and Verriest (1961a) and Ichikawa and Majima (1974). Finally, it is noteworthy, although unexplained, that females with complete achromatopsia with normal visual acuity (see below) are usually compound heterozygotes (François, Verriest, & DeRouck, 1955).

UNILATERAL COLOR DEFECT

The origin of unilateral color disturbance remains obscure (de Vries–de Mol & Went, 1971). For the male cases possibilities include somatic backmutation. For female cases the possibility of Lyonization can be added. Lyonization could be a factor in males only if they demonstrated two X chromosomes (i.e., XXY). In the de Vries–de Mol and Went study (1971) of the unilateral color defective described by Bender, Ruddock, de

Vries–de Mol, and Went (1972), this possibility was ruled out by a buccal smear. To these genetic possibilities trauma or environmental factors must be added, as should the possibility that the defect is of cortical origin (see Chapter 8). At this time, there is no satisfactory explanation for asymmetry of color vision, and probably no single explanation will describe all cases. Some cases definitely reflect assymmetric manifestation (Trendelenburg, 1941b; Waardenburg, 1963b); others may reflect cortical defects (see Chapter 8).

Theoretical Issues

Theoretical accounts of congenital red–green defects have been a major interest since the initial recognition of the defects. The greatest interest in theoretical approaches has concerned the number and spectral position of the cone visual photopigments of color defectives. Few researchers have produced explicit analysis concerning the interobserver variability of anomalous trichromats or of presumed chromatic opponent processing in anomalous trichromats and dichromats. One exception is the theoretical analysis of Jameson and Hurvich (Jameson & Hurvich, 1956; Hurvich & Jameson, 1962), reviewed in depth by Hurvich (1972). As a general comment, the transformation from the visual photopigments to the opponent channels is not yet worked out for normal trichromats. It is therefore not surprising that there are yet few accounts of abnormal color vision that include the chromatic opponent channels.

CONE VISUAL PHOTOPIGMENTS

Modern theory reflects two basic approaches—theories whose starting point is the anomaloscope behavior, including the hypothesis of two multiple-allele series, and theories whose origin is some other aspect of defective color vision.

Theories based on anomaloscope behavior. Analysis of color-matching data led von Kries (1899; see also 1924) to conclude that anomalous trichromacy is an alteration system in which one or more of the visual photopigments differ from normal in their spectral position. Alpern and Torii (1968a) examined this notion for protanomalous trichromacy and concluded that protanomaly was indeed an alteration system. The von Kries (1899) hypothesis leads to the generally accepted view that the protan and deutan gene sequences govern the formation of normal and abnormal cone visual photopigments. Table 7.8 shows for each allele series a likely λ_{max} for the visual photopigment. The uncertainty concerning extreme anomalous trichromacy is reflected in the fact that no visual photopigment can be assigned to the a_2, b_2 alleles. These photopigment maxima were based on the work of Pokorny and Smith (1977). Modern theorists associated with this type of approach include Wald (1966), Vos and Walraven (1971), and Ruddock and Naghshineh (1974). In terms of the description of congenital color defects as reduction, alteration, and collapse systems, Wald (1966), Vos and Walraven (1971), and Ruddock and Naghshineh (1974) combine a reduction system for dichromacy with an alteration system for anomalous trichromacy.

It is usually assumed that the alleles A, a_1, a_2, B, b_1, and b_2 determine individual structures with unique absorption characteristics (Wald, 1966). The gene frequency reflects genetic drift and population and mutation frequencies for each allele. However, Ruddock and Naghshineh (1974) have proposed that the abnormal absorption spectra associated with the a_1, a_2, b_1, and b_2 alleles occur as a result of admixture of two

Table 7.8
Theoretical Predictions for Multiple-Allele Hypothesis

	Protan Alleles				Deutan Alleles		
Allele	λ_{max} of Photopigment*	Phenotype With Normal Allele at Deutan Locus	Photopigments Corresponding to Phenotype	Allele	λ_{max} of Photopigment*	Phenotype With Normal Allele at Protan Locus	Photopigments Corresponding to Phenotype
A	560	Normal	534 560	B	534	Normal	560 534
a_1	541	Simple PA	534 541	b_1	553	Simple DA	560 553
a_2	?	Extreme PA	534 ?	b_2	?	Extreme DA	560 ?
a_3	Missing†§ or 534‡	Protanope	534	b_3	Missing† or 560‡§	Deuteranope	560

*λ_{max} of visual photopigments are for quantal sensitivity at the receptor (Smith & Pokorny, 1972; Pokorny, Smith, & Katz, 1973; Pokorny & Smith, 1977).
†Theory of Wald (1966).
‡Theory of Ruddock and Naghshineh (1974) and Piantanida (1974).
§Theory of Walls and Mathews (1952).

normal visual photopigments in a single cone; i.e., the allele structure is governing the proportions of two normal photopigments mixed within the cone outer segment. It is hypothesized that anomalous trichromacy occurs because one of the photopigments serves as a screening pigment for the other. Ruddock and Naghshineh (1974) suggest that gene frequencies are identical for protans and deutans but that the phenotype of simple deuteranomalous trichromacy is more frequent because small admixtures of the photopigments have more effect on the Rayleigh match for deuteranomalous than for protanomalous trichromats. Verriest (1960b) had previously noted that photopigment admixture could serve as a possible explanation for anomalous trichromacy.

Another hypothesis involves the concept that protanomalous trichromacy may represent normal photopigment or photopigments in an abnormally low effective optical density (Baker, 1966; Alpern & Torii, 1968a, b). Alpern and Torii (1968b) showed that this proposal is incorrect.

The Schouten hypothesis (de Vries, 1948) is a special case in which the shifted visual photopigment of protanomalous trichromats is hypothesized to be identical to the shifted visual photopigment of deuteranomalous trichromats. Pokorny, Smith, and Katz (1973) and Pokorny, Moreland, and Smith (1975) suggested that Schmidt's (1955) Rayleigh equation data were not compatible with the Schouten hypothesis. However, MacLeod and Hayhoe (1974) and Hayhoe and MacLeod (1976) suggested that anomalous color-matching data from Wright's laboratory (McKeon & Wright, 1940) may be consistent with the Schouten hypothesis.

The various theories disagree on the action of the a_3 and b_3 alleles. Some authors (Wald, 1966; Vos & Walraven, 1971) postulate that no viable photopigment is formed under dominance of the a_3, b_3 allele. Wald (1966) assumes that a normal cone mosaic occurs, i.e., that the remaining two photopigments occupy a full complement of cones. It is also possible to postulate that the photoreceptor as well as the photopigment is nonviable and that protanopes and deuteranopes have a reduced cone mosaic (Vos & Walraven, 1971). These possibilities have not been differentiated and represent a weakness of this type of theory.

In an alternate approach, Piantanida (1974) and Ruddock and Naghshineh (1974) postulated that the a_3 and b_3 alleles do govern formation of a visual photopigment. The protan allele, a_3, governs a photopigment identical (Ruddock & Naghshineh, 1974) or virtually identical (Piantanida, 1974) to the normal photopigment formed at the B allele. Similarly, the deutan allele, b_3, governs a photopigment identical (Ruddock & Naghshineh, 1974) or virtually identical (Piantanida, 1974) to the normal photopigment formed at the A allele.

Finally, it is possible to suggest that at the a_3 allele no viable visual photopigment is formed, while at the b_3 allele a visual photopigment identical to that governed by the A allele is formed (Walls & Mathews, 1952).

Compound hemizygotes (see above) are important because they may help to distinguish the various possibilities. Presumed compound hemizygotes for deuteranopia and an allele for protanomaly (possible genotypes a_1b_3, a_2b_3) were anomalous trichromats with a unique Rayleigh match (Arias & Rodriguez, 1973a, b), suggesting that the b_3 allele governs a photopigment. The presumed compound hemizygote for protanopia and deuteranopia (a_3b_3), as suggested by Sinascalco, Filippi, and Latte (1964) and Latte, Filippi, and Sinascalco (1965), was color defective, not normal, as predicted by the theories of Ruddock and Naghshineh (1974) or Piantanida (1974), or monochromatic, as predicted by the theory of Vos and Walraven (1971).

Theories based on other considerations.   Jameson-Hurvich theory: Jameson and Hurvich (1956) postulated that the deutan gene regulates a spectral shift of all three cone photopigments to longer wavelengths and the protan gene regulates a spectral shift of all three photopigments to shorter wavelengths; in addition, the amount of the shift may vary from individual to individual. The Jameson-Hurvich theory postulates an alteration system for both dichromacy and anomalous trichromacy. An additional neural factor (discussed below) differentiates dichromatic and trichromatic observers, giving an alteration system with a further modification by a collapse system.

Applied to dichromacy, the theory states that the protanope will have three classes of visual photopigment. All classes demonstrate a (yoked) spectral shift to shorter wavelengths in comparison with the normal visual photopigments. The deuteranope also has three classes of visual photopigments, and all demonstrate a yoked spectral shift to longer wavelengths. A third class of observer is the "neuteranope," a term suggested by Hurvich (1972) to describe the Aitken-Leber-Fick (Graham, 1965b) fusion deuteranope, a dichromat with three classes of visual photopigments identical to those of normal trichromats. According to the Jameson-Hurvich theory, dichromacy is said to result from "neural loss." The theory was derived from color perception data and does not address the findings of the pedigree studies. There is no explanation of the evidence that produced the multiple-allele hypothesis or of the observed allele frequencies, nor is there prediction for the compound hemizygote. Psychophysical studies of increment thresholds (reviewed above) and color matching do not support the hypothesis that all three visual photopigments are shifted in red–green color defect. Recently, Hurvich and Jameson (1978) reported Rayleigh matches of normal and anomalous trichromats and dichromats and concluded that the von Kries hypotheses are correct for a population study.

Alpern theory: A novel approach was recently proposed by Alpern and his co-workers (Alpern & Moeller, 1977; Alpern & Pugh, 1977; Alpern & Wake, 1977); they suggest that there is a natural variation in the in the absorption spectra of the visual photopigments and that the λ_{max} may vary over a 7–8 nm range. A color defect occurs with a defective allele at the P or D locus. With an allele for color defect at the P locus, the observer has two photopigments from the D set and therefore has two active visual photopigments in the long-wavelength range, but since there is variability in the photopigment spectra, the two photopigments need not be identical. If these are well separated in λ_{max} the phenotype is anomalous trichromacy. If they are very close, the phenotype is dichromacy. The Alpern hypothesis is a replacement theory and could be considered a receptoral collapse system.

The Alpern hypothesis was derived from psychophysical studies of spectral sensitivity. According to the Alpern hypothesis, there is no need for multiple alleles. A weakness of the theory is that the variance (given the total range of 7–8 nm) is too small to give correct predictions of the expected distribution of anomaly and anopia. If each class of photopigments shows normal variation and color defect occurs when two visual photopigments are chosen from the same class, the usual outcome would be a 0–1 nm difference between the pair of absorption spectra. Such observers would probably be dichromats. Thus for both protan and deutan defect there should be many more dichromats than extreme anomalous trichromats or simple anomalous trichromats. Even if a rectangular rather than normal distribution were assumed, there would still be more dichromats than simple anomalous trichromats. Further, the relative frequencies of anomaly and anopia should be identical for both protan and deutan genes. The Alpern hypothesis also predicts that all compound hemizygotes should have trichromatic color vision within normal limits. This expectation is not realized in observers presumed to be compound hemizygotes (reviewed above).

Another issue, now principally of historical interest, concerned the finding that occasional deuteranopes do not show relative luminous efficiency loss at short wavelengths. Willmer (1949) proposed the existence of two forms of deuteranopia; one, type I, was characterized by a normal luminosity function and represented a fusion or Aitken-Leber-Fick observer; the other, type II, characterized by reduced sensitivity at short wavelengths, represented a loss or König type of observer. Alpern, Mindel, and Torii (1968) suggested that although previous studies of partial bleaching in deuteranopes had not revealed two photopigments active above 520 nm, the type I deuteranope, being relatively rare, may simply not have been included in the sample of deuteranopes under study. Alpern, Mindel, and Torii (1968) therefore specifically studied a deuteranope who fulfilled Willmer's (1949) criteria for a type I (fusion) deuteranope. Their study revealed no evidence for two photopigments active above 520 nm. They concluded that deuteranopia is always a reduction system by loss and suggested that varation in the luminosity function of deuteranopes reflects variation in the density of the macular pigment.

CHROMATIC DISCRIMINATIVE ABILITY

A major feature of individuals having anomalous color vision is interobserver variability in studies of colorimetry, wavelength and colorimetric purity discrimination, and hue naming. Wavelength and saturation discrimination functions of different individual anomalous trichromats vary from those appearing close to normal to those appearing close to dichromatic. Interobserver variability occurs also in the large and variable matching ranges measured on the anomaloscope (Fig. 7.12). Anomaloscope matching ranges, the total errors on the Farnsworth-Munsell 100-hue test, and the shape of the wavelength discrimination function are correlated (Lakowski, 1971a), suggesting that all reflect a common source of discrimination loss in each individual. Mitchell and Rushton (1971) and Rushton, Powell, and White (1973) stated that the precision of brightness discrimination made by normal and anomalous trichromats is similar. Helve's (1972a) analysis of FM 100-hue data shows that the discrimination loss experienced by dichromats and anomalous trichromats is primarily in judgments of the redness–greenness component of color fields.

Researchers have questioned whether or not the appearance of a continuous range of variability in judgments of redness–greenness might not represent a continuous variation in a biologic substrate—for example, either in the absorption spectra of the visual photopigment (Ruddock & Naghshineh, 1974; Alpern & Moeller, 1977; Alpern & Pugh, 1977; Alpern & Wake, 1977) or in a "neural" weighting constant on an opponent channel (Hurvich & Jameson, 1962; 1978).

The concept of a continuous gradation in visual photopigment spectra has appeared in two rather different forms, that of Ruddock and Naghshineh (1974) and that of Alpern and his co-workers, both described above. Although the prediction of the photopigment is quite different, both hypotheses share as a natural consequence the prediction of a continuous gradation of chromatic discriminative ability. A weakness, however, is the concomitant prediction common to both theories that Rayleigh midmatch point is correlated with the matching range, a prediction not borne out by data (Verriest, 1960b; see also Hurvich, 1972).

Hurvich and Jameson (1962; 1978) postulated that variation in Rayleigh equation match widths for normals and anomalous trichromats may reflect variation of a weighting constant on an r-g opponent channel. Their most recent model thus includes two postulates, (1) an alteration system for anomalous trichromacy and (2) an independent reduction of neural activity in opponent channels. The adoption of two postulates allows prediction of match widths both of those occasional anomalous trichromats who show superior discrimination and of those who show reduced discriminatory ability.

Attempts to relate variability in anomalous trichromats to a biologic substrate ignore the natural statistical variability of normal observers. Normal trichromats also show interobserver variablility in the FM 100-hue test scores and in Rayleigh match widths on the Nagel anomaloscope. Pokorny and Smith (1977), using for a theoretical base visual photopigments as in Fig. 7.11, compared the statistical distribution of chromatic discriminations in normal and anomalous trichromats, allowing for similar statistical variation in both groups. They concluded that the close overlap of the visual photopigments of anomalous trichromats adequately explained both the poorer than normal (average) discrimination as well as the larger variability of this class of observer typified by the acceptable match range on the anomaloscope. Within the population, some anomalous trichromats may show discrimination as sensitive as some normal trichromats. Factors that contribute to variability in discrimination may be similar in both anomalous and normal trichromats, without the necessity of postulating an independent source of biologic variation.

THE BLUE–YELLOW DEFECTS

Congenital blue–yellow defects are much rarer than red–green defects. Often, their existence as true stationary, inherited defects has been questioned, since the acquired nature of blue–yellow defects can be easily overlooked. Nevertheless, both dichromatic and anomalous trichromatic tritan defects are classically described.

Autosomal Dominant Tritan Defect

The tritan defect is characterized by a lack of function of the mechanism that allows normals to discriminate colors that differ by the amount of short-wavelength light they contain. This is a relatively rare (incidence 1 in 10,000 to 1 in 60,000) defect with autosomal dominant inheritance (Kalmus, 1955). In autosomal dominant inheritance the individual inheriting a defective gene will show the defect, and the family pedigree will have affected members in each generation. Two concepts have been applied to autosomal dominant inheritance—penetrance and manifestation. Penetrance refers to the observed frequency of the genotype. The expected proportions of affected descendents in generation x is 0.5^{x-1}. If the observed frequency is less than this, the gene is said to show incomplete penetrance. Manifestation (also called expressivity) refers to the symptoms of the defect expressed in the phenotype. Autosomal dominant defects are characerized by wider inter- and intrafamilial variation in the symptoms and are said to show variable manifestation (or expressivity). Incomplete penetrance is difficult to establish in human pedigrees, and difficulties are further complicated by the variable manifestation. The large, four-generation family of autosomal dominant tritan defect reported by Henry, Cole, and Nathan (1964) and updated by Smith, Cole, and Isaacs (1973) included 66 descendents of the presumed generation I tritan. Table 7.9 compares the observed with the

Table 7.9

Proportion of Tritans in a Family With Autosomal Dominant Tritan Defect*

Generation	Descendents	Affected Descendents	Observed Proportion	Expected Proportion
I	1	1	1	1
II	5	2	0.4	0.5
III	16	4	0.25	0.25
IV	34	4	0.118	0.125

*Pedigree of Henry, Cole, and Nathan (1964), updated by Smith, Cole, and Isaacs (1973).

expected proportion of affected descendents, assuming complete penetrance. The observed frequencies are close to expected and are consistent with complete penetrance at least in this family. The severity of manifestation of the tritan defect is variable from one family member to another (Henry, Cole, & Nathan, 1964); there are many cases of "incomplete tritanopia" consistent with this typical variability—one member may be a dichromat, another may be a trichromat. Since an alteration system cannot be demonstrated in these observers, Cole, Henry, and Nathan (1964) suggested that such observers be termed incomplete tritanopes rather than tritanomals (a terminology that has been used frequently in the past). Since incomplete tritanope is a contradictory term, some researchers may prefer to use the all-inclusive term tritan.

COLOR MATCHING

Color matching for tritanopes has been reported by Fischer, Bouman, and ten Doesschate (1951), Wright (1952), Sperling (1960), and Cole, Henry, and Nathan (1966). Judd, Plaza, and Farnsworth (1950) used Munsell colors to evaluate chromaticity confusions. The tritanope can match all spectral colors to a mixture of two primaries. Usually one is chosen above 565 nm and one is chosen below 565 nm. The incomplete tritanope refuses many of the dichromatic matches. The unit coefficients shown in Fig. 7.18 represent an average of seven tritanopes from Wright's study (1952) with data normalized at 582.5 nm. The tritanopic color-matching data show the existence of pairs of wavelengths that have identical tritanopic coefficients. Such pairs of wavelengths must themselves be identical and are called confusion colors. Confusion colors may be directly plotted on a chromaticity chart (Wright, 1952) and are shown on the 1931 x, y CIE chromaticity diagram (Fig. 7.19). The confusion colors of the tritanope converge toward the short-wavelength region of the diagram. Thomson and Wright (1953) calculated the convergence point in the Judd (1951a) revised x, y diagram to be $x = 0.1748, y = 0.0044$. Thomson and Wright (1953) and Vos and Walraven (1971) used these values to derive receptor fundamentals. Other recent theoretical estimates are $x = 0.1748, y = 0.0006$ (Walraven, 1974) and $x = 0.1748, y = 0$ (Smith & Pokorny, 1975). The line passing from the convergence point through the equal-energy white intersects the spectrum locus at 569 nm. Cole, Henry, and Nathan (1966) measured the neutral points for two tritanopes to a 6500 K white and obtained values of 568 and 570 nm.

SPECTRAL SENSITIVITY

When determined by heterochromatic flicker photometry, the relative luminous efficiency curve is normal or nearly so (Wright, 1952; Sperling, 1960), possible slight defects in the short-wavelength section being hard to separate from the normal variation caused by prereceptoral absorption (Wright, 1952). Increment thresholds measured on a

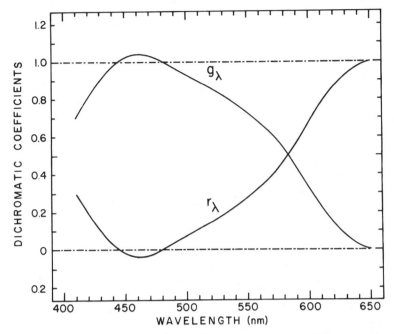

Fig. 7.18. Average WDW dichromatic coefficient curves for seven tritanopes. The primaries were 650 and 460 nm, with normalization at 582.5 nm. [Redrawn from Wright, 1952.]

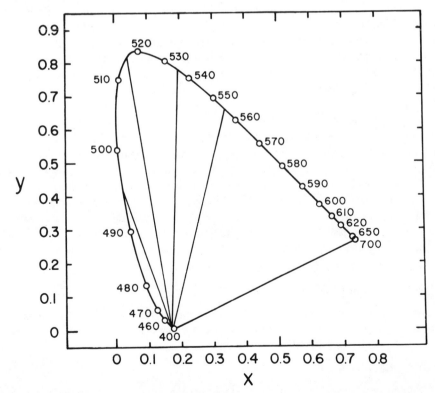

Fig. 7.19. The average confusion loci for tritanopes on the CIE chromaticity diagram calculated from average tritanopic coefficients of Fig. 7.18.

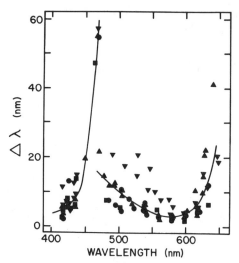

Fig. 7.20. Wavelength discrimination curves for four tritanopes. (Redrawn from Wright, 1952).

white background demonstrate reduction in sensitivity at short wavelengths, since the normally obtained peak at 451 nm is absent (Verriest & Uvijls, 1977a, b).

WAVELENGTH AND COLORIMETRIC PURITY DISCRIMINATION

Wavelength discrimination was reported by Fischer, Bouman, and ten Doesschate (1951) and Wright (1952). Wavelength discrimination data measured by Wright (1952) for four tritanopes are shown in Fig. 7.20. The $\Delta\lambda$ steps are large in the wavelength range 400–480 nm and may be unobtainable in the spectral region near 460 nm. Below 440 and above 520 nm the wavelength discrimination is as good as that of normal trichromats. The incomplete tritanope shows elevated $\Delta\lambda$ thresholds at 460 nm but otherwise normal discrimination.

Colorimetric purity discrimination was reported by Cole, Henry, and Nathan (1966) for the spectral region 480–650 nm. No colorimetric purity discrimination is obtained at the neutral point (about 570 nm for an equal-energy white). At other wavelengths, purity discrimination was similar to that of normal observers. Reduced purity discrimination would be expected for wavelengths below 480 nm, a range not investigated by Henry, Cole, and Nathan (1964). Since to the tritanope wavelengths below 460 nm have confusion wavelengths in the green, the purity discrimination of short-wavelength lights will be equivalent to that for the matching confusion color (Smith & Pokorny, 1973b). The purity discrimination of tritanopes would thus show a second minimum just below 400 nm.

INCREMENT THRESHOLDS

Increment thresholds were measured by Cole and Watkins (1967) and Padmos, van Noren, & Faijer (1978). They found that the Stiles $\pi_1 - \pi_3$ (i.e., blue) mechanisms were either absent or severely depressed.

THEORETICAL ISSUES

Although autosomal dominant tritan defect has often been considered a photopigment defect by analogy with the X-chromosome–linked defects (Smith, Cole, & Isaacs, 1973), there is no evidence for this view. A recent electroretinographic study demonstrated that the a-wave spectral sensitivity of tritans to a short-wavelength test stimulus of 45° visual angle determined under a bleaching-level "yellow" adaptation stimulus of 70° visual angle did indeed have the form of the SWS photopigment (Padmos, van Norren, & Faijer, 1978) although considerably reduced in sensitivity compared with normal trichromats. The psychophysical thresholds obtained under identical test conditions were virtually unobtainable in the tritans. These findings suggest a retinal origin for the autosomal dominant tritan defect.

Alpern (1976) has emphasized the variability of the published color-matching data for tritanopes, questioning the merit of using an average tritanopic copunctual point in deriving König fundamental response curves. Smith and Pokorny (1975) also noted difficulties, since the majority of published König fundamentals do not predict tritanopic color-matching data. The discrepancies may be attributed to macular pigment variation, as emphasized by Judd, Plaza, and Farnsworth (1950), to variation in effective optical density of the photoreceptors (Pokorny, Smith, & Starr, 1976), and/or to variation in visual photopigment absorption spectra (Alpern, 1976).

Anomalous Trichromacy

An anomalous trichromacy has been recognized since Hartung's self-observation (Engelking, 1925; Hartung, 1926; Engelking & Hartung, 1927) and called tritanomaly. It is characterized by some chromaticity confusions. In the Engelking-Trendelenburg equation the tritanomalous observer uses more blue primary than the average normal trichromat. The inheritance is unknown, and the defect must be a rare one, Hartung's case being one of the few well-documented ones. Schmidt (1942; 1970) described a case interpreted as tritanomaly in a woman. Moreland and Young (1974) describe a man diagnosed as "marginally tritanomalous."

Color Perceptions of Tritan Observers

Based on the direction of the minor axis, we may infer some properties of color perception in tritan observers. Chromatic perceptions would be predicted as "green" with increasing saturation between the neutral point (570 nm) and 460 nm and "green" with decreasing saturation below 460 nm. Chromatic perceptions would be predicted as "red" with increasing saturation for wavelengths above the neutral point. This expectation was not confirmed in a color-naming procedure used by Walls (1964) or in the hue estimation data reported by Smith (1973) using a technique similar to that of Boynton and Gordon (1965). In the Smith (1973) study the tritanope used "blue" and "green" interchangeably at short wavelengths. Above 500 nm the color-naming behavior was approximately normal.

Diagnosis of Tritan Defects

On measurement of the Rayleigh equation the tritanope makes a unique match that falls within the distribution of matches made by normal trichromats. To diagnose tritanopia it is necessary to design a special color match; for example, an observer who matches a violet light to a green light is classified as a tritanope. Screening tests that indicate an abnormal accumulation of errors may also be an indication of a tritan defect. However, many acquired defects mimic tritan defect (see, e.g., Jaeger, 1956; Cox, 1960; 1961a, b; Verriest, 1963; Krill, Smith, & Pokorny, 1970). Thus it is always imperative to rule out eye disease.

Several researchers have questioned the identity of congenital tritanopia as a unique genetic entity. Krill, Smith, and Pokorny (1970; 1971) drew attention in particular possible confusion of congenital tritan defect with autosomal dominant optic atrophy (ADOA), a disease of identical inheritance. Some patients with ADOA have only mildly reduced visual acuities (5/6– 6/9) but a pronounced color defect. Such patients have color vision identical to that for congenital tritan defect. Implicit in the suggestion of Krill, Smith, and Pokorny (1971) is the hypothesis that tritanopia is an inherited disorder associated with ADOA and resulting from the same genetic defect. Krill, Smith, and Pokorny (1970) suggested these diagnostic criteria for tritanopia: (1) visual acuity must be normal in all family members; (2) the central visual fields must be normal; and (3) the optic nerves must appear normal in all family members. These criteria have been applied in recent studies (Smith, Cole, & Isaacs, 1973; Went, Volker-Dieben, & de Vries– de Mol, 1974). Further, many of the tritans tested by Wright were reexamined and found to fulfill the criteria for a unique genetic entity (Neuhan, Kalmus, & Jaeger, 1976).

Diagnosis of tritanomalous vision hinges on establishing that color matches with WDW normalization differ from those of normal trichromats. The Moreland equation (Moreland & Kerr, 1978) may prove helpful in locating a "suspected" tritanomal.

MINOR COLOR ABNORMALITIES

Minor abnormalities of color vision occur among normal trichromats (Verriest, 1968). They have been studied in Germany and Scotland, and two different terminologies have developed. For the most part, these abnormalities are subtle and recognized primarily statistically; this fact is reflected in the classifications, which are neither widely used nor understood. Nevertheless, an individual case may prove a difficult and puzzling problem to the unwary examiner.

German Classification

In the German classification (reviewed by Heinsius, 1959; Trendelenburg, 1961) three major classes of minor color abnormality are recognized. An observer is considered a "completely normal" trichromat (*unbedingt normale Trichromate*) if the absolute matching range is less than 5 scale units on the Nagel anomaloscope in neutral adaptation (*Neutralstimmung*) and less than 10 scale units with continued observation (tuning or *Umstimmung*) and the midmatching point falls near the average normal match (Engelking, 1933; Hartung, 1935; Schmidt, 1935; Heinsius, 1961). Data on the time course of *Umstimmung* in normal subjects were reported by Verriest and Popescu (1974).

The first class of minor color abnormality is the *bedingt normale* (Vierling, 1935) or *noch normale* (Trendelenburg, 1964) *Trichromate*, i.e., "almost normal." The midmatching point of the Rayleigh equation falls at the extremes of the normal range. There is no evident abnormality of chromatic discriminative ability. These minor deviations of the Rayleigh equation have been ascribed to abnormally high (*starker Makulatingierung*) or abnormally low (*schwacher Makulatingierung*) levels of macular pigment (Grützner, 1971). In modern versions of the Nagel anomaloscope the green primary is at 545 nm, and macular pigment effects should be minimal. Other possible explanations include abnormality of lens, variation in photopigment absorption spectra, early retinal degenerations, or abnormality in a female heterozygous for congenital red– green color defect.

The second class of minor color abnormality, defined by Trendelenburg (1929) and also by Hartung (1935), is the *farbenschwache Trichromaten* (color-weak trichromats). The classification was subdivided into *Farbenasthenopie,* which is characterized by an enlarged matching range for the Rayleigh equation only under conditions of fatigue, i.e., after staring at the match for several seconds, and *Farbenamblyopie,* in which the matching range for the Rayleigh equation is wide for all conditions of measurement (Rosmanit, 1914; Engelking, 1933; Hartung, 1935; Schmidt, 1935; Hensius, 1959; 1961). Grützner (1971) showed that these observers do have an enlarged $\Delta\lambda$ in a wavelength discrimination test.

A third class of minor color abnormality is described by Vierling (1935) as the *minimalanomale Trichromaten* (minimally affected anomalies). Of these, the minimally affected protanomalous and deuteranomalous trichromats were described above.

Another term, *Pigmentfarbenanomalie* (pigment color defect), was used to describe observers with normal Rayleigh matches who make errors on pigment tests. The term "anomaly" is misleading, since with a normal Rayleigh match there is no evidence of an alteration system; *Pigmentfarbenamblyopie* might be a better term. Grützner (1971) disputed the classification, and it may be possible to explain the commission of a few errors on pigment tests as the result of prereceptoral absorption, and/or poor chromatic discrimination. However, there are occasional observers who have a normal and narrow Rayleigh equation but fail screening plates (Vierling, 1935; Engelbrecht, 1944; Heinsius & Grevsmuht, 1951; Stams, 1965; Verriest, 1968).

Scottish Classification

The Scottish classification of minor color abnormality was developed by Pickford (1951; 1958a) and Lakowski (1965). The classification is a statistical one. Pickford (1951; 1958a) and Lakowski (1965a; 1971a) recognize two classes of minor color abnormality—the weak color-normal observer and the deviant color-normal observer.

The weak color normal is the observer whose Rayleigh equation midpoint is within normal range but whose acceptance range exceeds twice the modal value for the population. By this definition, color-weak observers comprise 20 percent of the normal population (Pickford, 1957; Pickford & Lakowski, 1960; Lakowski, 1965a; 1971a). Such observers show poor spectral wavelength discrimination (Lakowski, 1971a).

The deviant color normal is the normal trichromat whose Rayleigh equation lies within the normal distribution and has a normal matching range but whose midpoint is displaced greater than two standard deviations from the mean. By this definition, the deviant color-normal observers comprise 4 percent of the normal population (Pickford, 1963; Lakowski, 1965a). These types of deviations may be ascribed to extreme values (high or low) of lens pigmentation and/or to variation in the width or spectral maxima of the visual photopigment absorption spectra (Smith, Pokorny, & Starr, 1976; Pokorny, Smith, & Starr, 1976; Alpern & Moeller, 1977; Alpern & Pugh, 1977; Alpern & Wake, 1977).

Lakowski (1965a) extended the classification to the blue–yellow match. He noted that these minor color abnormalities occur most frequently in older age groups. This finding again emphasizes the fact that minor color abnormalities described in unselected populations may occur in observers with lens or retinal changes due to aging, in observers with incipient eye disease, or in females who are heterozygous for a congenital red–green defect.

THE ACHROMATOPSIAS

The achromatopsias comprise a group of disorders in which color perception is either entirely absent (complete achromatopsia) or severely defective (incomplete achromatopsia). Achromatopsia as a stationary inherited congenital disorder was recognized as early as the 17th century (Waardenburg, 1963a, b). These defects have proved fascinating to researchers since that time, and a vast and confusing terminology has developed. Table 7.1 gives a classification of the achromatopsias. Excellent reviews of individual cases are given by Waardenburg (1963a, b) and François, Verriest, and DeRouck (1955). It is usually assumed that the rod system is normal in achromatopsia with reduced visual acuity. However, Pinckers (1972a) and Krill (1977) have noted decreased scotopic ERGs in some cases of complete achromatopsia with reduced visual acuity, and it is possible that some individuals may show a progressive disorder involving rods as well as cones. At this point it is not known whether such individuals represent a separate form of progressive cone–rod degeneration or whether they reflect individual variation in the defective gene for achromatopsia with reduced visual acuity. Such individuals require careful followup and study. It is always important to establish the diagnosis carefully. Achromatopsia with reduced visual acuity can be confused with cone and cone–rod degenerations.

Complete Achromatopsia With Reduced Visual Acuity

Complete achromatopsia shows autosomal recessive inheritance. Usually, the defect occurs in one or more male and female children in a family with no history of previous defect. In a high proportion of cases there is a history of consanguinity. The incidence of complete achromatopsia is about 0.003 percent (Waardenburg, 1963). The visual acuity is and 0.1. In infancy and childhood there is often an obvious pendular nystagmus. By adolescence the nystagmus is usually suppressed to a great extent. The near vision may be better than distance vision, possibly because change in eye position on convergence helps to arrest the nystagmus (Krill, 1977). There may be concomitant strabismus or exotropia and some minor degree of direct corneal astigmatism. Many achromats show aversion to high light levels and will avoid bright, sunny environments. The fundus generally appears disease-free on ophthalmoscopic examination and fluorescein angiography. Subtle fundal abnormalities include absence of foveal reflex and irregular distribution of the macular pigment. The latter finding is most evident in blue-light photography of the fundus. There is temporal pallor of the optic discs in 20 percent of the cases (François & Verriest, 1961a). The ERG shows absent photopic and normal scotopic components (Krill, 1968). The EOG is normal.

Because of their visual complaints, the majority of achromats are referred to an eye clinic, where the terminology achromatopsia or total color blindness is used. The term monochromacy (monochromatism) is more frequently used in the vision research literature with respect to psychophysical evaluation of color matching and chromatic discrimination.

COLOR VISION CHARACTERISTICS—COLOR MIXTURE

The complete achromat can match any two wavelengths by adjusting the radiance of one, i.e., only one primary (monochromat) is required for color mixture. The data expressed as the relative energy of the matching stimulus for a spectral primary light of fixed energy will resemble the scotopic relative luminous efficiency curve of normal observers $(V'\lambda)$.

SPECTRAL SENSITIVITY

The spectral sensitivity function at all luminances and for all techniques of measurement corresponds to the scotopic relative luminous efficiency curve of normal trichromats. When the curve is measured with central fixation, it may be necessary to correct the $V'\lambda$ curve for macular pigment absorption (Alpern, Falls, & Lee, 1960; Verriest, 1971a).

CHROMATIC DISCRIMINATION

The achromat is unable to make discriminations on the basis of purely chromatic changes.

OTHER PSYCHOPHYSICAL FUNCTIONS

The normal trichromat shows a duplex function for dark adaptation, flicker fusion frequency, and visual acuity that has been attributed to independent function of rods and cones. The complete achromat does not show normal duplex function and furthermore does not show a Purkinjé shift; his or her vision appears to be mediated by the rod mechanism.

EVIDENCE FOR CONE FUNCTION

The visual findings indicate a primary absence of cone function in complete achromatopsia. There have been reports of duplex function in dark adaptation (Sloan & Newhall, 1942; Lewis & Mandelbaum, 1943; Walls & Heath, 1954; François, Verriest, & DeRouck, 1955; Sloan, 1958; Auerbach & Kripke, 1974), visual acuity, FFF, and increment thresholds (Hecht, Shlaer, Smith, Haig, & Peskin, 1938; 1948; Verriest & Uvijls, 1977a, b). A recent study of electroretinograms (Auerbach & Merin, 1974) from 39 achromats indicates that residual photopic function may occur in the majority of complete achromats, although photopic function is not generally evident under conventional electroretinographic techniques. Such duplex function might be considered as indicative of cone as well as rod function, although in measurements of visual acuity, FFF, and increment thresholds the presumed "cone" branch of achromats does not show the range of the cone branch observed in normal trichromats. Further, the spectral sensitivity of the presumed "cone" branch is that of the scotopic curve. Lewis and Mandelbaum (1943), Hecht, Shlaer, Smith, Haig, and Peskin (1948), and Sloan (1958) interpreted these duplex data as indicating the presence of "day rods," an idea first attributed to von Kries. Walls and Heath (1954) have suggested that duplex function might be attributed to the presence of short-wavelength-sensitive cones. There is a form of incomplete achromatopsia in which the short-wavelength-sensitive cones are found; however, in complete achromatopsia of autosomal recessive inheritance there is no evidence for a short-wavelength-sensitive photopigment. The Stiles-Crawford effect of the rapidly adapting branch is that of cone photoreceptors, not that of rod photoreceptors (Alpern, Falls, & Lee, 1960). This finding of a Stiles-Crawford effect typical of cones in a receptor with the spectral response of rhodopsin has led to the concept of the "rhodopsin cone." Complete achromats presumably have some residual cone photoreceptors that contain a visual photopigment of spectral characteristics similar to those of rhodopsin. To complicate this discussion further, Conner and MacLeod (1977) reported that duplex FFF can be measured in rod photoreceptors of normal trichromats. Their finding leaves open the possibility that duplex function in achromatopsia may under some conditions be mediated by rods.

PATHOLOGY OF COMPLETE ACHROMACY

There have been four histologic studies of the eye in complete achromatopsia. All four studies agreed in the finding of normal-appearing rods in normal quantities. There are major differences between the four studies in the findings of cone photoreceptors. In the earliest study (Larsen, 1921) there were normal peripheral cones, but foveal cones showed abnormal morphology. In the second study (Harrison, Hoefnagel, & Hayward, 1960) the eye was not obtained until 40 hours after death; despite considerable autolysis of the photoreceptor layer, cones in reduced numbers could be identified in the periphery. There were few receptors of any kind in the macula. The third study (Falls, Wolter, & Alpern, 1965) revealed normal and abnormal cones throughout the retina. An outstanding feature was the low proportion of cone photoreceptors outside the fovea. Foveal cones, although of abnormal morphology, were normal in number. The researchers also suggested that there was no foveola. A ganglion cell layer was observed in all sections of the foveal region. In the most recent study (Glickstein & Heath, 1975), there were no photoreceptors in the fovea and a reduced number of normal and abnormal cones throughout the retina. There was a genuine fovea with interruption of the ganglion cell and inner nuclear layers. As in the Falls, Wolter, and Alpern (1965) study, the proportion of extrafoveal cone photoreceptors was low, about 5–10 percent of that observed in the normal eye. It is impossible to reconcile these studies beyond the statement that severe cone abnormality always occurred. Cones that are abnormal in morphology and/or few in number are present in the retina. Presumably, these cones contain a visual photopigment with the spectral response of rhodopsin.

X-Chromosome–linked Incomplete Achromatopsia

An X-chromosome–linked recessive form of incomplete achromacy was first described by Spivey, Pearlman, and Burian (1964) and Spivey (1965). This form is now recognized as a unique genetic entity and has been identified with an entity termed blue monocone monochromacy, first described by Blackwell and Blackwell (1957; 1961). An alternative term is π_1 cone monochromacy (Alpern, Lee, & Spivey, 1965). These terms, blue monocone monochromacy and π_1 cone monochromacy, are misnomers—the clinical description is that of the incomplete achromat but with a residual dichromatic color vision. Unfortunately, this terminology is also somewhat contradictory!

X-chromosome–linked incomplete achromatopsia with reduced visual acuity is similar in most respects to complete achromatopsia. There is reduced visual acuity, pendular nystagmus, aversion to bright lights, and the minimal ocular signs, including abnormal distribution of macular pigment, described for the complete form. François, Verriest, Matton–Von Leuven, DeRouck, and Manavian (1966) have noted concomitant myopia. There is a Purkinjé shift at a moderate photopic illumination and residual color perception. The visual acuity is quite variable, ranging from 0.33 to 0.1. Such variability may occur within a family, or a given observer may have a difference of two lines on the acuity chart between eyes. This finding is unusual in congenital X-chromosome–linked recessive hereditary diseases, which usually show symmetric visual results.

COLOR MATCHING

Clinical color vision has been studied extensively in X-chromosome–linked incomplete achromacy (François, Verriest, Matton-Von Leuven, DeRouck, & Manavian, 1966; Daw & Enoch, 1973). Alpern, Lee, Maaseidvaag, and Miller (1971) studied color mixture in two observers. At mesopic and low photopic levels the observers were dichromatic, requiring two primaries for color mixture. Their data revealed the activity of two visual photopigments, one with the spectral characteristics of rhodopsin and one with the spectral characteristics of short-wavelength–sensitive cones. At low mesopic and scotopic levels the observers became monochromatic, behaving as complete achromats. At high photopic levels the observers again became monochromatic, using only the short-wavelength–sensitive photopigment.

SPECTRAL SENSITIVITY

Studies of brightness matching (Blackwell & Blackwell, 1961; Alpern, Lee, & Spivey, 1965) and flicker photometry (Verriest, 1971a) demonstrated a spectral response similar to that of the SWS cone photopigment of the normal trichromat at high photopic levels and a spectral response similar to that of rods (CIE $V'\lambda$) at low photopic levels. At an intermediate luminance Blackwell and Blackwell (1961) were able to demonstrate a mixed function in which the blue cones and the $V'\lambda$ mechanism showed linear summation. Alpern, Lee, and Spivey (1965) were not able to obtain a mixed function on their X-chromosome–linked incomplete achromats. Pokorny, Smith, and Swartley (1970) also found a mixed SWS and $V'\lambda$ function using an increment detection task (Fig. 7.21). When measured with central fixation, the relative luminous efficiency function must be corrected for macular pigment in order to fit the $V'\lambda$ (Blackwell & Blackwell, 1961; Alpern, Lee, & Spivey, 1965; Pokorny, Smith, & Swartley, 1970; Verriest, 1971a).

CHROMATIC DISCRIMINATION

The Alpern, Lee, Maaseidvaag, and Miller (1971) study shows that X-chromosome–linked incomplete achromats have dichromatic color vision. The majority of these observers do make reliable color discriminations. This behavior is evidenced by correct identification of "blues" and "yellows" (Daw & Enoch, 1973) and a consistent red–green axis on the FM 100-hue and Panel D-15 tests.

OTHER PSYCHOPHYSICAL TESTS

Green (1972) and Daw and Enoch (1973) measured contrast sensitivity, and Daw and Enoch (1973) reported on the Westheimer function for the SWS cones in X-chromosome–linked incomplete achromatopsia. The contrast sensitivity peaks at 1 cycle/deg, and the Westheimer function shows a minimum at 1°.

EVIDENCE FOR CONES CONTAINING RHODOPSIN

Alpern, Lee, Maaseidvaag, and Miller (1971) were able to demonstrate a Stiles-Crawford effect typical of cone photoreceptors in their observer. Daw and Enoch (1973) were unable to replicate the finding. This discrepancy probably reflects variability in the populations of "rhodopsin cones." Further, there is considerable variability of fixation among incomplete achromats. Incomplete achromats do not always use foveal fixation (Siegel, Graham, Ripps, & Hsia, 1966), and their choice of fixation changes with luminance (Siegel & Bruno, 1964). The Pokorny, Smith, and Swartley (1970) observer

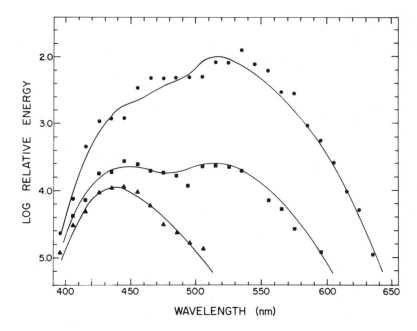

Fig. 7.21. Increment threshold spectral sensitivity functions for an X-chromosome–linked recessive incomplete achromat. The log relative energy at threshold is shown as a function of wavelength. Upper curve (●), dark adapted; middle curve (■), background of 0.4 td; lower curve (▲), background of 6.2 td. The solid line fitted to the dark-adapted data is the CIE (1951) $V'\lambda$ function modified by macular pigment screening. The solid line fitted to the 6.2 td background is the Stiles π_1 function, representative of the SWS sensitive cones. The solid line fitted to the 0.4 td background is a mixed function representing linear summation of the $V'\lambda$ and π_1 functions. [From Pokorny, J., Smith, V. C., & Swartley, R. *Investigative Ophthalmology*, 1970, *9*, 807–813 (reproduced with permission of the Association for Research in Vision and Ophthalmology).]

used foveal fixation at high luminances but when dark-adapted used an area 1° or 2° to the superior retina (unpublished communication). Other incomplete achromats may fixate at 4° or more in the parafovea (Siegel & Bruno, 1964; Siegel, Graham, Ripps, & Hsia, 1966).

THE HETEROZYGOUS FEMALE

Female carriers of X-chromosome–linked achromatopsia often show minor abnormalities (Spivey, Pearlman, & Burian, 1964; Goodman, Ripps, & Siegel, 1965; Krill, 1977). Abnormalities of color vision include excessive errors with a deutan axis on the FM 100-hue test and matches displaced toward the green primary on the Nagel anomaloscope. The spectral sensitivity function may be depressed for wavelengths below 550 nm. There may be delayed dark adaptation, and the fusion frequency may be reduced on the electroretinogram.

EXPLANATION OF X-CHROMOSOME–LINKED INCOMPLETE
ACHROMATOPSIA

It has been postulated that X-chromosome–linked incomplete achromatopsia results from a combination of two alleles for dichromacy (a_3, b_3) at the protan and deutan loci (Alpern, 1974). According to this hypothesis, which implies a reduction theory for red–green dichromacies, the X-linked incomplete achromat is a compound hemizygote for protanopia and deuteranopia. A compound hemizygote for protanopia and deuteranopia was found in the Siniscalco, Filippi, and Latte (1964) pedigree. The observer had color vision "intermediate between protanopia and deuteranopia." He was not an incomplete achromat. The alternative possibility is that X-chromosome–linked incomplete achromatopsia is a unique genetic entity.

Autosomal Recessive Incomplete Achromatopsia

In contrast to the many reports concerning complete and X-chromosome–linked incomplete achromatopsia, there have been few psychophysical studies of the autosomal recessive incomplete achromat. In a review of 230 cases of achromatopsia, François, Verriest, and De Rouck (1955) documented diverse residual color perception in 15 cases of incomplete achromatopsia. In their 1959 review, François and Verriest (1959a) added little further information. The paucity of documented cases may reflect the fact that an autosomal recessive incomplete achromat is likely to receive a diagnosis of cone dysfunction or cone degeneration.

Franceschetti, Jaeger, Klein, Ohrt, and Rickli (1958) suggested that both incomplete and complete achromatopsia occurred in the same pedigree, indicating that they were phenotypic variations of the same genotype. This result, however, may have reflected their choice of test, the Nagel anomaloscope, compounded by the typical variation in chromatic discrimination occurring among incomplete achromats. For example, residual color perception is more obvious when large stimulus fields are used (Jaeger, 1950; Baumgardt & Magis, 1954).

Inasmuch as different types of residual color vision occur in incomplete achromatopsia, the condition appears to comprise multiple genotypes. Jaeger (1950; 1953), for example, studied three incomplete achromats, two with neutral points in the blue-green and one with a neutral point in the yellow-green. Sloan (1954) and Goodman, Ripps, and Siegel (1965) also noted diverse findings when screening color vision of incomplete achromats. Even allowing for the cases with presumed X-chromosome–linked inheritance, there is still a diversity of color vision findings indicative of multiple genotypes.

Smith, Pokorny, and Newell (1978, 1979) reported two distinguishable forms of incomplete achromatopsia of apparent autosomal recessive inheritance. In one form (protan type) (Smith, Pokorny, & Newell, 1978) there was a unique type of dichromatic color vision and protanopic photopic luminosity function. In this family of a consanguineous marriage 4 of 15 children were affected, showing the usual signs of achromatopsia, with visual acuities of 6/60 to 6/180, pendular nystagmus, and aversion to bright lights. The ERG showed minimal photopic responses. No abnormality of rod function was present. In the other form (deutan) (Smith, Pokorny, & Newell, 1979) there was trichromatic color vision and deuteranopic photopic luminosity function. There were four affected members in three families. The visual acuities ranged from 6/18 to 6/60, and pendular nystagmus occurred only in those with most severely affected visual acuity. The ERG showed minimal photopic response and a reduced high radiance scotopic response.

COLOR MATCHING

Color tests included extended Rayleigh matches and dichromatic coefficients. For the protan type, Rayleigh matches were displaced to red. One of the affected children was studied using an 8° field. The patient showed dichromatic color mixture at low and moderate photopic luminances using primaries of 450 and 650 nm. Analysis of the matches indicated dichromatic color matches mediated by two visual photopigments—the normal MWS cone photopigment and a photopigment with the spectral characteristics of rhodopsin. For the deutan type the Rayleigh matches were again shifted to red but showed normal luminance. Analysis of the extended Rayleigh series showed that red–green color matches were mediated by the normal LWS cone photopigment and a photopigment with spectral characteristics of rhodopsin. Dichromatic matches using primaries of 450 and 650 nm were not accepted, indicating the presence of a SWS photopigment.

SPECTRAL SENSITIVITY

Spectral sensitivity was measured using heterochromatic flicker photometry at 140 td. In the protan type the relative luminous efficiency function resembled the spectral sensitivity of the isolated MWS visual photopigment (observed in protanopes), confirming the presence of the MWS cones. In the deutan type the relative luminous efficiency function resembled the spectral sensitivity of the isolated LWS visual photopigment (observed in deuteranopes), confirming the presence of the LWS cones.

These types of color vision in autosomal recessive incomplete achromatopsia were not previously fully documented. The studies emphasize that adequate recognition of different forms of autosomal recessive incomplete achromatopsia requires evaluation of color matching and spectral sensitivity rather than clinical screening techniques.

Achromatopsia With Normal Visual Acuity

Achromatopsia with normal visual acuity is an extremely rare disorder (1 in 10^8 of the population). The individuals are usually termed cone monochromats (Pitt, 1944). In their exhaustive survey of the literature François, Verriest, and De Rouck (1955) confirmed only 15 cases, including the cases of Pitt (1944) and Weale (1953). Some of these individuals showed residual color perception. There have been three or four additional reports (Sloan, 1946; Adachi-Usami, Gavriysky, Hecht, Schenkel, & Scheibner, 1974; Alpern, 1974). A difficulty in reviewing the literature is that achromatopsia with normal visual acuity is often called "atypical achromatopsia," a term also used for incomplete achromatopsia with reduced visual acuity.

No inheritance pattern is recognized. In several of the cases, family pedigrees reveal coexisting red–green color defects. Female cases are nearly always compound heterozygotes for red–green color defects (François, Verriest, & De Rouck, 1955). There is no evidence of cone abnormality. Visual acuity is normal; the ophthalmoscopic examination is normal; the electroretinogram shows no evidence of a cone dysfunction syndrome.

COLOR MATCHING

The complete achromat with normal visual acuity can match any two wavelengths by adjusting the radiance of one—i.e., only one primary is required for color mixture (monochromat).

SPECTRAL SENSITIVITY

The spectral sensitivity function takes one of two forms. It may show sensitivity loss at long wavelengths and appear similar to that of the protanope. These observers have been termed the protan or "protanoid" type of cone monochromat. An observer of this type was studied by Weale (1953; 1959), Fincham (1953), Gibson (1962), and Ikeda and Ripps (1966). Another of Weale's (1953) observers was studied by Baumgardt (1955). Alternatively, the luminous efficiency function may appear similar to the normal photopic (or deuteranopic) function. In this case the observer has been termed the deutan or "deuteranoid" type of cone monochromat; an observer of this type was studied by Alpern (1974).

CHROMATIC DISCRIMINATION

In theory, the achromat is unable to make discriminations on the basis of purely chromatic changes; however, in several cases of achromatopsia with normal visual acuity there are reports that some observers do show residual color perception if the field of view is sufficiently large (Crone, 1956; Krill & Schneiderman, 1966).

INTERPRETATION

It has been generally agreed that achromatopsia with normal visual acuity is a postreceptoral defect; a review of the studies, however, suggests that this view is over simplified.

The protan type. A female observer of the protan type was fully studied by Weale (1953; 1959), Fincham (1953), Gibson (1962), and Ikeda and Ripps (1966). The observer was a monochromat with a protanopic luminous efficiency function. Chromatic fringes served as a cue for accomodation (Fincham, 1953). Normal Stiles π mechanisms could be demonstrated in her fovea (Gibson, 1962). By densitometry Weale (1959) was able to measure two visual photopigments active in the red–green range. These findings are suggestive of a postreceptoral defect occurring in higher visual pathways. However, Ikeda and Ripps (1966) noted that the electroretinographic spectral sensitivity agreed with the psychophysical spectral sensitivity in demonstrating long-wavelength luminous efficiency loss. Ikeda and Ripps suggest that the defect of the LWS cone occurs distal to the site of b-wave generation, similar to the defect observed in congenital night blindness (Ripps, 1976), placing the defect in the outer synaptic layer.

The deutan type. Alpern (1974) studied a male achromat with approximately normal (or deuteranopic) luminous efficiency. The observer could match exactly every spectral light to a single standard light by appropriate adjustment of radiance. From retinal densitometry there was evidence for only one cone visual photopigment, in the red–green range. The observer's data were similar to those of deuteranopes. Alpern (1974) showed a Stiles π_1 function indicating the presence of the SWS cone, and he concluded that his achromat combined a photopigment defect with a postreceptoral defect.

INCOMPLETE FORMS AND INTERMEDIATE CASES

There are reports of incomplete forms of achromatopsia with normal visual acuity. These cases have been termed atypical (Krill & Schneiderman, 1966) or pseudomonochromats (Jaeger, 1950). Some cases are reviewed by Waardenberg (1963) and François and Verriest (1959a). There is not sufficient information to allow analysis of their color vision.

There are also reports of observers with mildly reduced acuity (6/9 to 6/15) and severe unclassified color defects. As an example, there are the three exceptional cases of Sloan (1954). Such observers do not show nystagmus or photophobia. They are classed sometimes as incomplete achromats with normal visual acuity and sometimes as incomplete achromats with reduced visual acuity. An understanding of the color vision defects of these exceptional observers would require both spectral sensitivity and color-matching analysis. In addition, careful ophthalmoscopic examination and long-term follow-up is required to rule out subtle progressive macular disease.

Diagnosis of Achromatopsia

COMPLETE ACHROMATOPSIA WITH REDUCED VISUAL
ACUITY

Reduced visual acuity, pendular nystagmus, extinguished photopic ERG, and normal-appearing retina are clinical findings that make diagnosis of complete achromatopsia relatively easy in the infant or young child. Today, with routine medical care and early visual screening the majority of patients are seen in their first decade. Occasional patients do escape detection and are first seen at an age when the pendular nystagmus is suppressed. Fluorescein angiography and electroretinography may be necessary to differentiate these patients from those with central cone degenerations.

The complete achromat makes a characteristic set of matches on examination of the Rayleigh equation. Since the achromat is a monochromat, a color match can be made to any red–green mixture for which the test radiance can be adjusted appropriately. To the achromat, on the Nagel model I anomaloscope the green primary appears much brighter than the red primary. The yellow scale is therefore turned near the top of its range in matching greenish mixtures and near zero when matching red. The result is a characteristic slope when the yellow scale value is plotted for the various red–green mixtures (Fig. 7.22). On arrangement tests the patient makes a characteristic "scotopic" pattern on an axis that lies between the classic deutan and tritan axes (Sloan, 1954; Verriest, Buyssens, & Vanderdonck, 1963). There are large error accumulations (400–800 errors) on the FM 100-hue test.

X-CHROMOSOME–LINKED INCOMPLETE ACHROMATOPSIA

X-chromosome–linked incomplete achromatopsia shows clinical findings similar to those of complete achromatopsia although with better visual acuity. The X-chromosome–linked form of incomplete achromatopsia is suggested when the affected patient gives a family history of affected brothers, maternal male cousins, or maternal grandfather. The anomaloscope examination give results identical to those for complete achromatopsia (Fig. 7.22).

On clinical screening the patient shows a deutan axis on arrangement tests, making 400 or more errors on the FM 100-hue test. On specialized psychophysical testing of

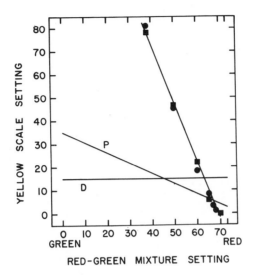

Fig. 7.22. Typical brightness matches made by complete achromat (solid square) and X-chromosome-linked recessive incomplete achromat (solid circle).

spectral sensitivity, the patient shows an inverse Purkinjé shift (Chapter 6). At scotopic, mesopic, and low photopic levels peak sensitivity occurs near 500 nm (or, if foveal fixation is used, it may be shifted to 530 nm by macular pigment screening). At higher photopic levels peak sensitivity shifts to shorter wavelengths, around 440–450 nm (Fig. 7.21).

AUTOSOMAL RECESSIVE INCOMPLETE ACHROMATOPSIA

The autosomal recessive incomplete achromatopsias have been poorly recognized in the past, and clinical screening is not definitive. The diagnosis is suggested in any patient who has unexplained reduced visual acuity with normal ophthalmoscopic examination and fluorescein angiogram accompanied by characteristic ERG and color vision findings. Photopic components of the ERG are recordable but reduced in amplitude. The results of clinical color vision screening show a scotopic pattern on arrangement tests. The Rayleigh equation may be displaced to red in the protanomalous range, showing either protan or deutan brightness matching. These patients have residual color vision that differs from the type I color defect seen in central cone degeneration (Smith, Pokorny, & Newell, 1978, 1979). The diagnosis is established by psychophysical studies of spectral sensitivity and color matching

ACHROMATOPSIA WITH NORMAL VISUAL ACUITY

Observers with achromatopsia and normal visual acuity are very rare and are usually "found" by chance. Since the visual acuity is normal, this type of patient is unlikely to be referred to an eye clinic. On R-G screening plate tests the observers behave either as protans or deutans depending on their luminous efficiency function. They also miss the B-Y screening plates. There may be a 200–300-error accumulation on the FM 100-hue test with a predominant tritan axis (Krill & Schneiderman, 1966). Diagnosis of complete achromatopsia requires psychophysical evelution of color matching of various spectral wavelengths to a single primary wavelength.

Jennifer Birch, M. Phil.

I. A. Chisholm, M.D.

Paul Kinnear, Ph.D.

Marion Marré, M.D.

A. J. L. G. Pinckers, M.D.

Joel Pokorny, Ph.D.

Vivianne C. Smith, Ph.D.

Guy Verriest, M.D.

8

Acquired Color Vision Defects

AGING*

Visual acuity, the extent of the visual field, the absolute and differential sensitivity, flicker fusion frequency, amplitude of the electroretinogram, and color discrimination improve during childhood and adolescence, achieve their maximum values in the third decade, and thereafter deteriorate progressively with chronologic age.

Although the evolution before puberty and in the very old is obscured by psychological factors, the gradual improvement during youth and the gradual deterioration during senescence of chromaticity discrimination has been demonstrated by subject performance with the Color Aptitude Test (Gilbert, 1957), the FM 100-hue test (Verriest, Vandevyvere, and Vanderdonck, 1962), and the assessment of the matching range at the Pickford-Nicolson anomaloscope (Lakowski, 1958; Ohta & Kato, 1976). In addition, these studies showed that in senescence, chromatic discrimination for the blue–yellow axis was much more affected than for the red–green axis (Figs. 8.1 and 8.2). During senescence the Rayleigh equation is shifted progressively towards green (Boles-Carenini, 1954; Lakowski, 1962), while the relative luminous efficiency at short wavelengths is decreased in both scotopic vision (Crawford, 1948) and photopic vision (Ruddock, 1965a, b; Verriest, 1970a) (Fig. 8.3). The degradation of color vision in the elderly is a most important phenomenon. As with other aspects of visual performance, color vision can be improved only by using higher illuminances and by taking care to avoid glare, to which older subjects are more sensitive (Weale, 1963; Verriest, 1971b).

---

*Contributed by Guy Verriest, M.D.

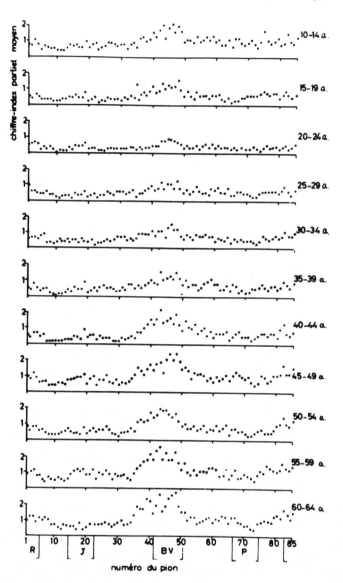

Fig. 8.1. Mean FM 100-hue scores in different age groups (illuminant C, illuminance of 100 lux). [From Verriest, G., Vandevyvere, R., & Vanderdonck, R. *Revue d'optique théorique et instrumentale* (Paris), 1962, *41*, 499–509 (reproduced with permission of Masson, Editeur).]

Lakowski (1962) and Verriest, Van de Velde, and Vanderdonck (1962), by simulating the effects of old age with neutral-density filters in front of young eyes, showed that the senile changes in foveal color vision were due mainly to the progressive yellowing of the nucleus of the crystalline lens (Chapter 3). Weale (1961) showed that this effect is exaggerated by senile miosis, since the central part of the lens is thicker than its peripheral parts. There is no evidence that the amount of the inert yellow macular pigment, which shows individual variation, should be a factor in age-dependent color vision changes (Chapter 3).

Verriest and Uvijls (1977a) concluded that receptoral factors account for the changes

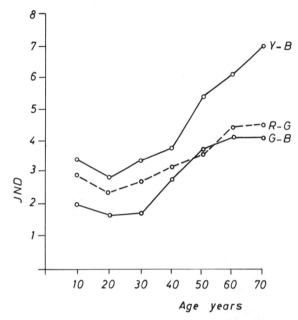

Fig. 8.2. Mean matching ranges in jnd units on the Pickford-Nicolson anomaloscope in different age groups. [From Ohta, Y. & Kato, H. *Modern Problems in Ophthalmology,* 1976, *17*, 345– 352 (reproduced with permission of S. Karger AG).]

in color vision during adolescence. They compared central and peripheral achromatic increment thresholds for equal-energy monochromatic objects on a white background of 10 cd m⁻² in three age groups of normal subjects (10– 15, 16– 41, and 60– 76 years). When compared with the median group, the youngest group was more sensitive peripherally, as expected from the changes in lens transmittance, but was less sensitive foveally, especially for the shortest and longest wavelengths, which can be explained only by retinal changes (Fig. 8.4).

REFRACTIVE MEDIA*

When the spectral curve of transmission for one or more of the prereceptoral ocular structures is altered in such a way that a portion of the visible spectrum is preferentially more absorbed than normal, the deviant color match is attributed to an absorption system (Chapter 4). The most common variety of an absorption system occurs in brownish senile nuclear cataract. Such affected lenses absorb short-wavelength light (Bucklers, 1930), with the result that the spectral curve of relative luminous efficiency shifts toward longer wavelengths (Verriest, 1970b) (Fig. 8.5). The Rayleigh equation shifts toward green (Lakowski, 1962), but the anomalous quotient does not depend on the wavelength of the comparison light, as predicted in an absorption system (François & Verriest, 1957a). There is a type III acquired blue– yellow defect (described in the 19th century; Karantinos, 1971; Pinckers, 1972b), especially when visual acuity has dropped below 0.2 (François & Verriest, 1968).

Young normal crystalline lenses absorb more light of short than long wavelengths. The absence of the lens in the light pathway either by its surgical removal (aphakia) or by

---

*Contributed by Guy Verriest, M.D.

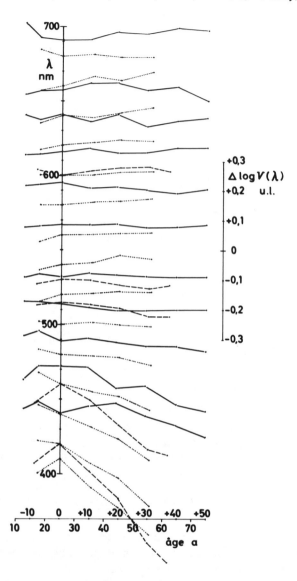

Fig. 8.3. Mean variation with age of the relative luminous efficiencies of several wavelengths of the visible spectrum for photopic vision (dashed lines: Ruddock, 1965; continuous lines: Verriest, 1970) and for scotopic vision (point lines: Crawford, 1949). [From Verriest, G. *Nouvelle Revue d'Optique Appliquée,* 1970, *1,* 107–126 (reproduced by permission of Masson, Editeur).]

its displacement (lens luxation) produces a sensory condition that is opposite to that of brownish senile nuclear cataract. The shorter wavelengths are less absorbed than in a normal eye. The spectral curve of relative luminous efficiency shows an improvement of sensitivity at short wavelengths, with no significant difference between young and elderly aphakic subjects (Verriest, 1972b; 1974b) (Fig. 8.6). Under conditions of scotopic vision, an ultraviolet radiation at 365 nm should be as luminous as a radiation at 546 nm to the aphakic subject (Goodeve, Lythgoe, & Schneider, 1941). In aphakia, the Rayleigh equation is slightly shifted to red (Lakowski, 1962), but color discrimination is clinically

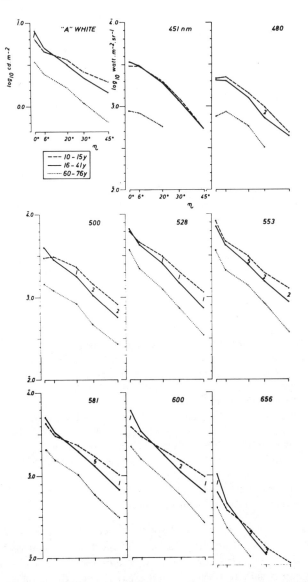

Fig. 8.4. Mean retinal profiles for white and monochromatic circular objects of 116′ diameter against a 10 cd m² white background in three age groups. [From Verriest, G. & Uvijls, A., *Documenta Ophthalmologica*, 1977, *43*, 217–248 (reproduced with permission of W. Junk BV).]

normal or even superior for the discrimination of blue hues (de Mattiello & Gonella, 1976). During the first days after the removal of the lens, the subject can experience cyanopsia because of the sudden increase in the blue end of the spectrum; in the following days the subject can experience erythropsia as a result of glare, especially when exposed to bright lights with a dilated pupil. The differences in color vision between a unilateral aphakic eye and a normal fellow eye can be corrected by wearing a yellowish spectacle or contact lens before the aphakic eye.

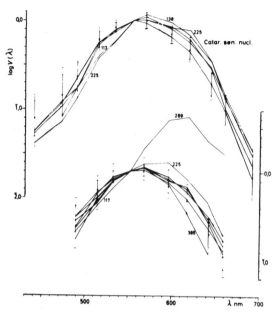

Fig. 8.5. Individual spectral curves of luminous efficiency relative to that of λ = 552 nm obtained by heterochromatic flicker photometry at 55 td (upper panel) and 415 td (lower panel) in eight cases of nuclear senile cataract. Normal range spread is indicated by the vertical bars. In five cases the efficiencies of the longer wavelengths are increased while those of shorter wavelengths are reduced. In no. 289, a case with dichromatic type III color defect and 0.2 visual acuity, only the higher level of retinal illumination could be used. The shift of the curve toward the right is so pronounced that the maximum of the function is at about 610 nm instead of about 555 nm. [From Verriest, G. *Color 69*. Göttingen: Musterschmidt Verlag, 1970, pp. 115–130 (reproduced with permission of Musterschmidt Verlag).]

Pathologic discoloration of the refractive media also causes absorption system defects. The characteristic xanthopsia of jaundice has been recognized from antiquity. At short wavelengths, the spectral curve of relative luminous efficiency is depressed, and the Rayleigh equation is shifted toward the red (Seki, 1954). Helmbold (1932) wondered if there was not also a neural component to this color defect. Hemorrhages in the refractive media cause erythropsia, which changes to chloropsia as the blood is resorbed (Helmbold, 1932). Alpern, Bastian, Pugh, and Gras (1976) studied extensively a case of hypercupremia with brown deposits on Descemet's membrane and on the anterior and posterior lens capsules. The Rayleigh equation was shifted toward the green. The mathematical treatment of the color-matching functions showed that the mechanism of the defect was an absorption system, not an alteration system, and that the spectral absorption was maximal at 430 nm. A similar absorption curve was given by the comparison of the CIE V'_λ curve with the subject's peripheral absolute threshold curve of scotopic relative luminous efficiency.

Corneal scars, white cataracts, and vitreous opacities do not disturb color vision. Colored halos are observed when the transparency of the optic media is altered by

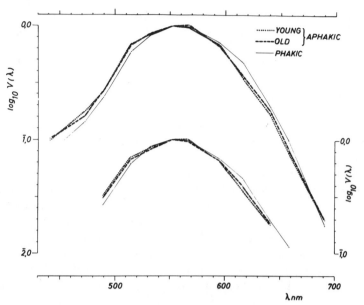

Fig. 8.6. Mean spectral curves of luminous efficiency relative to λ = 552 nm obtained by heterochromatic flicker photometry at 55 td (upper panel) and 415 td (lower panel) in 28 young aphakic eyes, in 27 old aphakic eyes, and in 126 control phakic eyes. All differences between the means of the young and old aphakic eyes are nonsignificant. Nearly all differences between the means of the aphakic and phakic eyes are significant at the 0.01 level; the aphakic and phakic eyes are significant at the 0.01 level; the aphakic means are greater than the phakic ones from 441 to 514 nm and smaller from 595 to 658, but they are again greater for λ = 691 nm. [From Verriest, G. *Modern Problems in Ophthalmology*, 1973, *13*, 314–317 (reproduced with permission of S. Karger AG).]

numerous homogeneous particles that are of a different refractive index than those of the surrounding media, e.g., the presence of blood cells in the precorneal film, in the corneal stroma, or in the anterior chamber, corneal edema of acute glaucoma, and incipient cataract. Such halos are best seen in a dark room when looking at a bright light source. The inner ring is blue, the outer red. The halo diameter varies as the reciprocal of the particle size, being smaller when the particle size is large.

An eccentric pupil exaggerates chromatic aberration. Besides the effects of reduced visual acuity on the performance for given color vision tests, uncorrected ametropia is said to shift the Rayleigh equation to red in hypermetropia and to green in myopia (Wienke, 1960; Cernea & Constantin, 1977). Malignant myopia can give rise to an obvious type III acquired blue–yellow defect, but this is then due to the concomitant chorioretinal degeneration.

ALBINISM AND CONGENITAL NIGHTBLINDNESS*

Congenital deficiencies of color vision are discussed in Chapter 7; here, we consider albinism (in which the lack of pigment in the uvea is associated with a foveal hypoplasia) and congenital night blindness.

Albinism, either generalized or confined to the eyes, is accompanied by a shift of the Rayleigh equation toward red and often by a certain degree of enlargement of the

---

*Contributed by Guy Verriest, M.D.

matching range at the anomaloscope (Pickford, 1958b; Pickford & Taylor, 1968; Krill & Fishman, 1971; Taylor, 1976). Electroretinographic spectral sensitivity is shifted toward long wavelengths, especially at the higher levels of illuminance, because of the reflection of light from the blood of the choroidal vessels (Dodt, Copenhaver, & Gunkel, 1959; Krill & Lee, 1963); the psychophysical spectral curve of relative luminous efficiency does not show this feature (Verriest, 1964). Color discrimination can become severely defective when albinism is associated with chorioretinal degeneration.

In *essential night blindness* (dominant autosomal, recessive autosomal, or sex-linked recessive inheritance) color discrimination is usually normal. Rarely, there may be a type III acquired blue–yellow defect (Armington & Schwab, 1954; Ohta, 1969; Verriest, 1970b). The spectral curve of relative luminous efficiency is photopic (Dieter, 1929). Verriest (1970b) showed relative long-wavelength–sensitivity loss in a case of sex-linked recessive night blindness with myopia and type III blue–yellow acquired color defect. In Oguchi disease color discrimination can be either normal or slightly defective with a blue–yellow axis (François & Verriest, 1968). This result corresponds to the narrowing of the blue isopter often described in the older literature. The blue–yellow defects in congenital and acquired night blindness have been used as a proof that the cone pigment prosthetic groups should be linked in some way with vitamin A (Le Grand, 1972).

FUNDUS DETACHMENT*

Choroidal Detachment

The choroid is loosely in contact with the sclera for most of its area, being adherent only at the optic foramen, at the periphery, and at the points of emergence of the vortex veins. The physical conditions therefore exist that might favor collection of fluid between choroid and sclera in the suprachoroidal space.

Uveochoroidal detachment is commonly seen following intraocular surgery or ocular injury. These detachments, single or multiple, are to be found in the peripheral portion of the fundus. They are usually of short duration, and in general visual sequelae are not prominent. Records of color analysis are not available in the literature.

Choroidal detachments unassociated with injury are uncommon. They are multiple or annular in form, have an inflammatory basis, and are true choroidal effusions. They are usually long standing and affect central visual function due to an accompanying maculopathy. On resolution of the choroidal detachment, a pigmentary disturbance remains marking the area of the detachment. The disturbance of central visual function can be demonstrated by use of the FM 100-hue test even after successful resolution of the effusion by antiinflammatory drugs (Fig. 8.7).

Retinal Detachment

Retinal detachment by virtue of the physical separation of the photoreceptors from the pigment epithelium and their consequent degeneration is accompanied by severe visual dysfunction in the area of the detachment. Reports on color vison defect in retinal detachment have been available from the turn of this century. Köllner (1907a) reported data obtained from his examination of 36 patients, 32 of whom presented a blue–yellow defect. François and Verriest (1957a) questioned whether the blue–yellow defect they found was due to the detachment per se or to the predisposing myopia, since they were

---

*Contributed by I. A. Chisholm, M.D., and A. J. L. G. Pinckers, M.D.

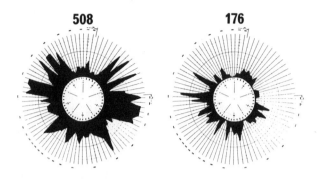

Fig. 8.7. FM 100-hue test pattern obtained from a patient showing uveochoroidal effusion (left) before therapy and (right) after 4 months of therapy with corticosteroids.

unable to demonstrate blue–yellow defects in nonmyopic eyes with retinal detachment. This disparity was amplified in the further study by François, Verriest, DeRouck, and DeVos (1962), who demonstrated that both type I acquired red–green and type III acquired blue–yellow defects could be identified in patients with retinal detachment. Recent reports have shown that a blue–yellow defect can be aroused by the detachment itself (Koliopoulos & Theodosiadis, 1972; Martin, Menezo & Lopez, 1972; Chisholm, McClure, & Foulds, 1975). Marré (1973), while agreeing that a blue–yellow defect exists, maintains that the blue mechanism is the most severely affected. The various color defects noted by François and Verriest (1957a), Gaillard (1962), and Koliopoulous and Theodosiadis (1972) in retinal detachment are summarized in Table 8.1, where it can be seen that type III acquired blue–yellow defect is the most common.

Functional visual recovery following successful retinal detachment surgery by means other than visual acuity was explored by Chisholm, McClure, and Foulds (1975). The patients studied fell into two groups, depending on whether the macula was involved in the area of detachment or not. Examination by the FM 100-hue test of patients with an intact macula showed a predominant type III acquired blue–yellow defect preoperatively, whereas a generalized depression of chromatic discrimination accompanied by a higher error score was found when the macula was detached (Fig. 8.8). Recovery of function was gauged by observing the changing FM 100-hue test plot (Fig. 8.9) or error score (Foulds, Reid, & Chisholm, 1972). When the error score of the recovering eye was related to the score of the fellow nondetached eye, an exponential pattern of recovery was identified in each group; by this means it was possible to demonstrate a gradual and continuing functional improvement in the macula-detached group over an extended period (Fig. 8.10) (Chisholm, McClure, & Foulds, 1975).

Table 8.1
Retinal Detachment: 95 Eyes

Color Vision	Eyes
Normal	20
Congenital defect	2
Type I acquired red–green defect	8
Type III acquired blue–yellow defect	45
Unclassified acquired defect	20

From François and Verriest, 1957a; Gaillard, 1962; Koliopoulos and Theodosiadis, 1972.

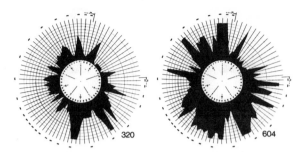

Fig. 8.8. FM 100-hue test pattern in retinal detachment (left) with macula intact and (right) accompanied by a detachment of the macula. [From Chisholm, I.A., McClure, E., & Foulds, W.S. *Transactions of the Opthalmological Society of the United Kingdom* 1975, *95,* 167–172 (reproduced with permission of the Ophthalmological Society of the United Kingdom).]

Pigment Epithelial Detachment

A pathologic process in the choroid resulting in exudation from the choriocapillaris may lead to a localized collection of serous fluid under the pigment epithelium and detachment from Bruch's membrane: Such collections of fluid may be single or multiple and may remain localized or extend through into the subretinal space, causing an additional localized serous retinal detachment (Gass, 1967). The posterior pole of the eye

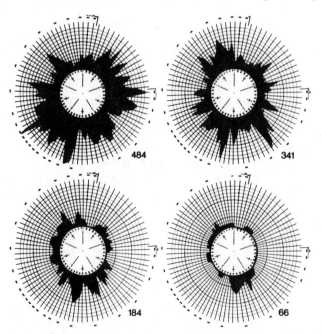

Fig. 8.9. Changing FM 100-hue test pattern after successful retinal detachment surgery. [From Foulds, W. D., Reid, H. R. C. & Chisholm, I. A. *Modern Problems in Ophthalmology,* 1972, *12,* 49–57 (reproduced with permission of S. Karger AG).]

COLOUR DISCRIMINATION RECOVERY following successful Retinal Detachment Surgery

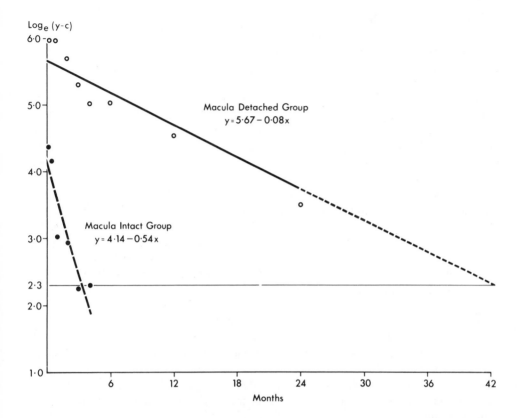

Fig. 8.10. Change in FM 100-hue test error score illustrating the rate of functional recovery after successful retinal detachment surgery. The rate of recovery when the macula is intact is rapid. When the macula is detached, recovery is slow and extends over 3 years. [From Chisholm, I. A., McClure, E., & Foulds, W. S. *Transactions of the Ophthalmological Society of the United Kingdom,* 1975, *95,* 167–172 (reproduced with permission of the Ophthalmological Society of the United Kingdom).]

seems to be more prone to such changes than other areas of the retina. As pertinent to this section, only central serous retinopathy and central serous detachment accompanying congenital optic pit will be discussed. Localized pigment epithelial detachment at the macula will be discussed under Macular Degenerations and acute posterior multifocal placoid pigment epitheliopathy under Chorioretinitis.

CENTRAL SEROUS RETINOPATHY

This is the term given to an apparently spontaneous serous detachment developing in the macular area, frequently of obscure etiology, usually self-limiting, but possibly recurrent. Clinically, the condition consists of a circumscribed area of serous detachment at the macula that causes a variable reduction in macular function. In their study of the color vision defect, Jaeger and Nover (1951) observed two phenomena: (1) a type III acquired blue–yellow color defect that persisted after resorption of the serous fluid and (2) a Rayleigh equation that was displaced toward red and that was reversible. The extent of the color vision defect was correlated with the decline in visual acuity (Fonta, 1972), the depth of the lesion, and the activity of the leaking area but not with the diameter of the serous lesion (Metge, Jayle, Vola, Fonta, & Aurran, 1972). Dorne (1971) observed that when acuity dropped below 0.50 the type III acquired blue–yellow defect developed into achromatopsia, and further observed that the color vision deficiency was one of the earliest signs of this condition. A type III blue–yellow defect has been detected by the FM 100-hue test by Coscas and Legras (1970) and Pinckers (1975a). Abnormal test performance on the Roth 28-hue test was detected by Dorne (1971). The use of Umazume-Ohta test plates has been advocated by Ohta (1972) and Pinckers (1976a) for the early diagnosis of this condition. Other methods of color vision analysis, including the F2 plate, the Farnsworth Panel D-15, and the AO HRR plates, have been found of varying sensitivity by Legras and Coscas (1972). The authors felt that this lack of test corroboration was dependent on the degree of edema present.

A characteristic change in the increment spectral sensitivity curves is frequently encountered in central serous retinopathy. Using white backgrounds, there is a selective lowering in the sensitivity to the short and middle-range wavelengths, so that the 600 nm peak becomes prominent as the normal peak at 451 nm declines (Verriest & Uvijls, 1977a). This curious change of the spectral curve of relative luminous efficiency was earlier reported by Zanen and Meunier (1965). Smith, Pokorny, and Diddie (1978) showed that the displaced Rayleigh equation was caused by receptor disorientation.

SEROUS DETACHMENT SECONDARY TO OPTIC PIT

Congenital pit of the optic disc is often complicated by macular abnormalities, which include secondary serous detachment or pigmentary changes at the macula. In 16 of 24 cases (Kranenburg, 1959) central color recognition was found to be disturbed, principally for blue and yellow. Farpour and Babel (1968) described either "protan" or "tritan" defects, while Mustonen and Varonen (1972) found normal color vision or poor color discrimination.

Hereditary Vitreo Retinal Disorders

SEX-LINKED RECESSIVE VITREO RETINAL DEGENERATION
(JUVENILE HEREDITARY RETINOSCHISIS)

In its fully expressed form, this hereditary ocular disease is characterized by maculopathy, which evolves through a series of stages, vitreous degenerations with the formation of veillike membranes and peripherally placed retinal cysts. Color vision has been reported normal by Ricci (1960), Carr and Siegel (1970), and Denden (1975). Verriest (1964) observed a color vision defect without predominant axis. A red–green discrimination loss with a reduction in red sensitivity (type I defect) was reported by Geiser and Falls (1961) and Deutman (1971). Blue–yellow defects, however, are frequently observed (Verriest, 1964; Vainio-Mattila, Eriksson, & Forsius, 1969; Krill & Deutman, 1972a). Helve (1972b) demonstrated a blue–yellow defect in 81 eyes using the FM 100-hue test and concluded that the color vision abnormality resulted from a deep lesion of the macular sensory retina. Some subjects have been reported as passing the Farnsworth Panel D-15. Patients investigated by Pinckers, Nabbe, and Bogaard (1976) showed a red–green confusion with Lanthony's Desaturated Panel or showed a type I red–green arrangement on the FM 100-hue test (Table 8.2). Harris and Yeung (1976)

Table 8.2
Color Vision in Peripheral Chorioretinal Dystrophies

	Eyes Examined	Normal	Slight Defect	Type I Acquired r-g Defect	Type III Acquired b-y Defect	Achromatopsia
I: Peripheral chorioretinal dystrophies (François & Verriest, 1968)	157	35	19	15	75	—
II: Retinitis pigmentosa and central involvement (Pinckers, 1971a)	43	4	8	13	1	17
III: Peripheral chorioretinal dystrophy (Pinckers, 1971a)	54	24	21	—	9	—
1. Typical retinitis pigmentosa	15	6	6	—	3	—
2. Atypical retinitis pigmentosa	34	17	11	—	6	—
3. Unilateral retinitis pigmentosa	1	1	—	—	—	—
4. Bardet-Biedl syndrome	4	—	4	—	—	—

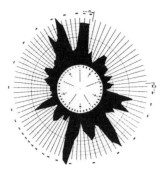

Fig. 8.11. FM 100-hue test pattern in juvenile hereditary retinoschisis. [From Harris, G.S. & Yeung, J. *Canadian Journal of Ophthalmology*, 1976, *11*, 1–10 (reproduced with permission of the Canadian Journal of Ophthalmology).]

demonstrated blue–yellow defects on the FM 100-hue test in affected subjects (Fig. 8.11), and by examining both male and female blood relations they were able to show that nonaffected relatives of either sex had poorer color discrimination than the population in general (Fig. 8.12).

There is a form of foveal retinoschisis with autosomal recessive inheritance. Lewis, Lee, Martonyi, Barnett, and Falls (1977) described bilateral foveal dystrophy in three young women; the disorder resembled the macular involvement in juvenile sex-linked retinoschisis, although it was less severe. In all three cases, the Nagel anomaloscope revealed a Rayleigh equation shifted to red, while other tests (AO HRR, Ishihara, Farnsworth Panel D-15, FM 100-hue) gave normal results. When such a foveal retinoschisis accompanies a rod–cone dystrophy, there is a mild to moderate type I red–green defect (Noble, Carr, & Siegel, 1978).

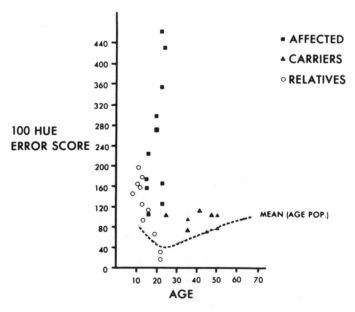

Fig. 8.12. Distribution of FM 100-hue test error scores for the normal population and juvenile hereditary retinoschisis. [From Harris, G. S. & Yeung, J. *Canadian Journal of Ophthalmology*, 1976, *11*, 1–10 (reproduced with permission of the Canadian Journal of Ophthalmology).]

AUTOSOMAL DOMINANT HYALOID RETINAL DEGENERATION
(WAGNER SYNDROME)

A blue–yellow defect in subjects suffering from Wagner syndrome was observed by
Guillaumat, Rouchy, and Arrata (1970) and confirmed by Verriest (1974). Half of the 16
subjects diagnosed as suffering from Wagner syndrome examined by Pinckers (1970a)
had an elevation of the FM 100-hue test score. In those patients whose retina was intact, a
blue–yellow defect was found but was considered to be due to the simultaneous presence
of nuclear cataract (Pinckers & Jansen, 1974). In an attempt to evaluate how far myopic
(and thus the fundus) changes resembling malignant myopia are part of Wagner
syndrome, Pinckers (1970a) examined 14 myopic eyes with a refractive error greater than
6 diopters. In only one subject was an abnormality of the FM 100-hue test detected.

RECESSIVE HYALOID TAPETORETINAL DEGENERATION
OF GOLDMANN FAVRE

In this disease, electrophysiologic examination reveals a severe disturbance. Color
vision examined by means of the AO HRR plates was reported as normal by Carr and
Siegel (1970). A deficiency without predominant confusion was reported by Blanck,
Polliot, and Bernard (1973). François, DeRouck and Cambie (1974) examined three
patients, two of whom had a red–green defect and one a combined red–green and
blue–yellow defect.

Senile Retinoschisis

This uncommon condition, found as a rule in the sixth or seventh decade, occurs as
an extension of a peripheral microcystoid degenerative process affecting the middle layer
of the retina. The surface of the schisis shows a snowflake appearance, and may be found
in association with pavingstone or cobblestone degeneration of the retina. No color vision
analysis has been reported in this condition.

DIFFUSE AND CENTRAL CHORIORETINAL DYSTROPHIES

In this section the chorioretinal dystrophies are arbitrarily subdivided into diffuse or
preferentially extramacular diseases and the macular diseases. In peripheral dystrophies
the macular area is often also affected; in such cases routine color vision examination by
means of plate tests, arrangement tests, and anomaloscope reflects the macular
involvement.

Diffuse Chorioretinal Dystrophies

These dystrophies have in common that their localization is primarily extramacular
and so mostly affect the rod function, although a diffuse cone dysfunction with relatively
intact macular area is not excluded. A combined rod–cone dystrophy is common.

ROD DYSTROPHIES

According to François and Verriest (1968), a type III blue–yellow defect is a characteristic feature of peripheral retinal involvement. The results of color vision examination in rod dystrophies are often not very clear, and this is certainly due in many cases to simultaneous macular involvement. Table 8.2 shows the results of color vision examination in cases of peripheral retinal dystrophies with and without macular involvement (François & Verriest, 1968; Pinckers, 1971a). A type I red–green defect was not found in eyes with exclusive peripheral involvement.

Typical retinitis pigmentosa. In typical retinitis pigmentosa, the results of color vision examination are reported variously as normal (Cox, 1960; 1961a, b; Verriest, 1964; Pinckers, 1971a) type III blue–yellow defect (Köllner, 1906; François & Verriest, 1956a; 1957a; Ohta, 1957; Cox, 1960; 1961a, b; Verriest, 1964; Kurata, 1967b; Aspinall, Adams, & Hayreh, 1973), type I red–green defect due to macular involvement or a congenital deficiency or concomitant Stargardt disease (François & Verriest, 1956a; 1957a; Grützner, 1961; Pinckers, 1971a), total achromatopsia (Goodman & Ripps, 1960; Verriest, 1964). A blue–yellow defect in retinitis pigmentosa *sine pigmento* was observed by Leber (1871b). Color vision was reported to be normal in some cases of dominantly inherited retinitis pigmentosa (Berson, Gouras, & Gunkel, 1968) and sex-linked retinitis pigmentosa (Berson, Gouras, Gunkel, & Myrianthopoulos, 1969).

According to Ohta (1957) there are three stages. In the first stage there is a normal Rayleigh match; the FM 100-hue test is disturbed only if the illumination is diminished. In the second stage there is a pseudoprotanomaly, and the FM 100-hue test shows a type III acquired blue–yellow defect even in normal illumination. In the third stage the anomaloscope match widens to the green, while the FM 100-hue test shows a chaotic cap arrangement. The pattern of cap arrangement with the Farnsworth Panel D-15 and FM 100-hue test is variable (François & Verriest, 1956b; Bozzoni, 1959; Verriest, 1964; Pinckers, 1975a); there is occasionally a slight concomitant red–green defect (Verriest, 1964). In cases with normal visual acuity, a mild type III blue–yellow defect may occur. If visual acuity has dropped to 0.7 or less, there is a moderate blue–yellow defect; if visual acuity has dropped to 0.1 or less, there is a severe color vision disturbance (Verriest, 1964).

Massof, Finkelstein, Starr, Kenyon, Fleischman, and Maumenee (1979) reported bilateral symmetry in FM 100-hue test error scores. Further, they observed a negative correlation (-0.73) between the logarithm of the error score and the percentage of normal visual field preserved. The disturbance of color vision is not correlated, however, with the ERG and EOG changes (Imaizumi, 1967). The spectral luminosity curve remains generally normal, although blue darkening or scotopization is sometimes observed (Larsen, 1923; Verriest, 1970b).

Massof and Finkelstein (1979) suggested that different subclasses with retinitis pigmentosa may be identified by means of color adaptometry. Color perimetry reveals reduced blue sensitivity (François, Verriest, & Israel, 1966). Even if foveal color discrimination is still normal, a blue–yellow defect is found at 7° and 10° eccentricity (François, Verriest, & Metsälä, 1964). François and Verriest (1962) evaluated color vision in 50 patients using the Farnsworth Panel D-15. Color vision was considered normal if the Farnsworth Panel D-15 result was normal or showed a few minor errors (12 patients), mildly defective if there were a few type III errors (12 patients), and severely defective if there were major type III errors (26 patients).

Sandberg and Berson (1977) measured the tvr curves in retinitis pigmentosa and showed abnormalities in both blue (π_1 or π_3) and longer-wavelength cone mechanisms (either π_4 or π_5) at 10° from the fovea.

Atypical forms of retinitis pigmentosa. In inverse retinitis pigmentosa, Verriest (1964) observed either a type III blue–yellow defect as observed in retinitis pigmentosa or a type I red–green defect as observed in juvenile macular degeneration. In central retinitis pigmentosa Hommer and Thaler (1977) noted a color vision defect resembling "protanomaly" in a younger patient and "protanopia" in an elder one. In our opinion this color vision defect is an acquired type I red–green defect. It is likely that other retinal specialists would have classified these patients as dominant progressive cone or foveal dystrophy (see below, Cone Dystrophies). In a unilateral case Pearlman, Saxton, and Hoffman (1976) obtained normal plate results.

In sector retinitis pigmentosa color vision can be either normal or characterized blue–yellow, red–green, or completely defective, just as in typical retinitis pigmentosa (Bisantis, 1971; Dralands, Evrard, Pouchon, Rommel, & Stanescu, 1971; Thaler, Heilig, & Slezak, 1972; Ivandic, 1972; Pinckers, 1975a; Abraham, Ivry, & Tsvieli, 1976).

In pericentral retinitis pigmentosa the reports are the same as for typical retinitis pigmentosa and sector retinitis pigmentosa. Further, the spectral luminosity curve is depressed at long wavelengths (Miglior, Spinelli, & Castellani, 1969; Hommer, 1969; François, De Rouck, Cambie and De Laey, 1972a; Pinckers, 1975a).

Myotonic dystrophy. In myotonic dystrophy the color vision defect can be the only ophthalmic symptom of the disease (Remky, 1972). Color vision, however, may be normal (Burian & Burns, 1967), defective without predominant confusions (Babel & Tsacopoulos, 1970), or show a blue–yellow defect. Babel (1975) examined 11 subjects with the Ishihara, anomaloscope and one (unspecified) Farnsworth test—he observed normal color vision in two cases, "deuteranomaly" in two cases, and a disturbed color vision without prominent confusions in seven cases.

Retinitis punctata albescens. Color vision is usually reported to be normal. Although there may be no errors on the Ishihara test, the Farnsworth Panel D-15 and FM 100-hue test often reveal a type III acquired blue–yellow defect (Franceschetti, François, & Babel, 1963).

Verriest (1964) observed a type III blue–yellow defect as in retinitis pigmentosa. Color vision can be affected early in the disease—he found in one case a severe defect when visual acuity was 0.9. Other reports note various defects of color vision in retinitis punctata albescens: normal or slightly disturbed (Meyer, 1941; Vannas & Setala, 1958; Smith, Ripps, & Goodman, 1959), red–green defect (Bietti, 1937), a type III blue–yellow defect (François & Verriest, 1956a), or total color blindness (Atkinson, 1932; Tamai, Setogawa, & Kandori, 1966).

Choroideremia. In choroideremia color vision may be normal (Saebo, 1948; Cox, 1960; 1961a, b; Takki, 1974). A low-discrimination type is described by MacCulloch (1969) and Fouanon, Ardouin, Perdriel, and Dary (1971). Pameyer, Waardenburg, and Henkes (1960) reported a case with normal anomaloscope performance and red–green

Farnsworth Panel D-15 defect; red–green defects were described by Verriest (1964) and Kurstjens (1965), blue–yellow defects by Jaeger and Grützner (1962), Verriest (1964) and Kurstjens (1965), and an acquired blue–yellow defect by Blackwell and Blackwell (1970). Kurstjens (1965) examined color vision in 19 cases and reported 9 cases with normal color vision, 5 with a blue–yellow defect (AO HRR, Farnsworth Panel D-15), 2 with a moderate type I defect (Ishihara, AO HRR), and 3 with a severe type I defect (Ishihara, Farnsworth Panel D-15, Nagel anomaloscope).

Carriers have normal color vision (Pameyer, Waardenburg, & Henkes, 1960; Verriest, 1964) but elevated thresholds in the blue–green part of the spectrum (Jaeger & Grützner, 1962).

Gyrate atrophy of choroid and retina. In gyrate atrophy of choroid and retina, Kurstjens (1965) found normal color vision in six cases (AO HRR, Farnsworth Panel D-15) and a type III defect in one case. Verriest (1964) observed a type I defect similar to that found in juvenile macular degeneration. Takki (1974a), in an examination of 15 cases, was the first to demonstrate hyperornithinemia in gyrate atrophy. In testing color vision with the Farnsworth Panel D-15 she found normal color vision (6 youngest cases), a blue–yellow defect (5 cases), indefinite defects due to poor visual acuity (3 cases), or unrecordable color vision (1 case). Hyperornithinemia was also found by McCullogh and Marliss (1975, 1 case), who observed color vision and reduced visual acuity of 0.2. Recently, a marked deficiency of ornithine aminotransferase in transformed lymphocytes of a patient with gyrate atrophy was reported (Kaiser-Kupfer, Valle, & Del Valle, 1978) In cultured fibroblasts an L-ornithine-ketoacid transaminase deficiency was established (Deutman, Sengers, & Trijbels, 1978).

Neuronal ceroid lipofuscinosis. The late infantile or Jansky-Bielschowsky type and the juvenile or Spielmeyer-Vogt type of amaurotic familial idiocy are characterized by the accumulation of lipofuscin material; hence these types are called neuronal ceroid lipofuscinosis (NCL).

In contrast to typical retinitis pigmentosa, the early *b*-wave alterations in NCL suggest that the process starts in the bipolar Müller cell layer. The cones are involved earlier than the rods. The clinical course of the disease suggests a progression from the bipolar Müller cell layer toward the receptors and at the same time a progression from the posterior pole toward the retinal periphery (Pinckers & Hoppe, 1978). Ultrastructural studies (Goebel, Fix, & Zeman, 1974; Goebel, Zeman, & Damaske, 1977) are consistent with the clinical progression. The data suggest an early deterioration of color vision. However, the patients are very young, and hence a reliable evaluation of color vision is difficult. Verriest (1964) examined two cases—one had normal color vision and one an acquired red–green defect.

Pinckers and Bolmers (1974) observed 18 cases, of which they could carry out a reliable color vision examination of only 4; 3 patients displayed a dichromatic red–green defect and 1 subject could perform a correct naming only of large colored surfaces. Beckerman and Rapin (1975) observed a "protan" red–green color defect.

Niemann-Pick lipoidosis. Sebestyén and Gálfi (1969) observed a 12-year-old boy with Niemann-Pick disease and reported normal central color vision.

Hypobetalipoproteinemia. Yee, Herbert, and Bergsma (1976) examined three subjects with atypical retinitis pigmentosa in familial hypobetalipoproteinemia (Bassen-Kornzweig) with the AO HRR and Farnsworth Panel D-15; color vision was normal.

Pigmented paravenous retinal atrophy. In pigmented paravenous retinochoroidal atrophy, Saraux, Béchetoille, Offret, and Nou (1974) and Pearlman, Kamin, Kopelow and Saxton (1975) found normal color vision. François and Verriest (1976) examined five cases (ten eyes) and found normal color vision in five eyes but a blue–yellow defect in three eyes.

CONE DYSTROPHY

The term cone dystrophy refers to the cone disturbance detected by elec-troretinography (François, de Rouck, Verriest, de Laey, & Cambie, 1974). The type I color vision defect refers to a color vision defect associated with cone disturbance. Both terms represent symptoms of central cone disease that need not be present at the same time. The cone dysfunction syndrome (Goodman, Ripps, & Siegel, 1963) includes stationary or progressive congenital and acquired conditions that show reduced visual acuity, color defect, and abnormal cone ERG.

In this section syndromes are described that are characterized either by cone dystrophy and a type I acquired red–green defect or by just one of these symptoms. For differential diagnostic purposes the macular dystrophies have to be taken into account. It has to be emphasized that a transition between different forms of cone dystrophy is not excluded. Since the cone dystrophies are basically diagnosed by means of the ERG, there is a risk that some entities or their stages do not differ essentially from macular diseases (described below).

There are three possible combinations of cone dystrophy and type I acquired red–green defect: (1) the combination of a cone dystrophy and a type I defect, (2) the presence of a cone dystrophy without a type I defect, and (3) a type I defect without cone dystrophy. Abraham and Sandberg (1977) reported four cases with foveal atrophy, central scotoma, and mild to moderate acquired red–green defect with either a normal ERG or an ERG with diminished cone and rod activity; this is an example of the transition of central cone involvement (third type) to diffuse cone involvement (first type or cone dystrophy).

Cone dysfunction and type I acquired red–green defect. Goodman, Ripps, and Siegel (1963) describe under the name progressive cone degenerations patients who manifest a progressive loss of visual acuity and color vision associated with cone dysfunction but little or no scotopic ERG defect. Color vision varies from normal to a total acquired achromatopsia (Berson, Gouras, & Gunkel, 1968). In the early stages, type III acquired blue–yellow defect can be found along with type I acquired red–green defect (Steinmetz, Ogle, & Rucker, 1956). This disease has also been called progressive cone dystrophy (Deutman, 1971) and diffuse cone disease (Krill, Deutman, & Fishman, 1973). The macular alterations resemble those found in chloroquine retinopathy.

Krill and Deutman (1972a) state that severe color vision defects are present when visual acuity drops to 0.5 or 0.3, which is relatively early compared to other macular diseases. These authors divide their patients into two groups on the basis of performance on the Nagel anomaloscope. In the first group the results of the anomaloscope display a severe disturbance, even with a relatively good visual acuity—the Rayleigh match is wider than normal and is spread to both the red and green ends. In the second group the Rayleigh equation is wider than normal but displaced only to the red end. In both groups the FM 100-hue test shows a red–green defect initially. The FM 100-hue test progresses to a scotopic pattern, while the anomaloscope matches widen eventually to achromatopsia. These symptoms are characteristic of a type I acquired red–green defect and have been described for acquired cone dysfunction by many authors. There is a severe color vision defect when vision drops to 0.5 or less; color vision sometimes is lost completely (François, 1974).

In progressive generalized cone dysfunction (François, de Rouck, Verriest, de Laey, & Cambie, 1974) all cases show a marked disturbance of color vision, usually a type I acquired red–green defect. The ophthalmoscopic and fluoroangiographic pictures are variable. When the disease is progressive, a rod dysfunction sooner or later becomes evident, resulting in the clinical picture of a generalized cone–rod disease with predominating cone dysfunction symptoms (Goodman, Ripps, & Siegel, 1963).

Pearlman, Owen, Brounley, and Sheppard (1974) described a dominant inherited cone dystrophy in nine members of one family (AO HRR, Ishihara, FM 100-hue test); the onset occurs some years after birth and the disease is progressive, leading eventually toward achromatopsia. In one case color vision was normal when first tested but 4 years later was red–green defective. Patients who showed gross disturbance of color discrimination appeared to have normal thresholds for π_4 and π_5 functions, suggesting a postreceptoral site for the red–green discrimination defect.

Hansen, Larsen, and Berg (1976) reported a familial syndrome (seven patients) of progressive cone dystrophy, degenerative liver disease, endocrine dysfunction, and hearing defect. The results of color vision examination were as follows: Farnsworth Panel D-15, one case normal, three cases showing a scotopic pattern; F_2 plate, either the green symbol seen or no symbols seen; Ishihara, all cases defective; AO HRR, all cases red–green and blue–yellow defective. The FM 100-hue test error score in the case with normal Farnsworth Panel D-15 was 282 without predominant axis.

In two siblings with electroretinographically diagnosed cone–rod dystrophy, Stanescu and Michiels (1976) observed a color vision defect of the "protanope" (i.e., type I) type (Ishihara, Farnsworth Panel D-15, Nagel anomaloscope). Auerbach and Kripke (1976) reported a family (five cases) with progressive cone dystrophy. They observed myopia, photophobia, scotopic pattern on color vision tests, and absent cone ERG. These "achromats" claimed to have had good color vision when they were young. The inheritance of the disease was autosomal dominant. Verriest and Uvijls (1977a) demonstrate in cone dysfunctions a characteristic scotopization of the spectral sensitivity curves of the affected retinal areas, with reduced sensitivity for long wavelengths. Color perimetry shows the retinal areas for which cone function is impaired. An interesting fact for diagnostic, prognostic, and followup purposes is that these authors find in generalized cone dysfunction a perimetric deficit extending to eccentricities of 20° and beyond. In comparison, in Stargardt disease scotopization is generally restricted to 6° (or, in a few cases, to 20°).

Cone dysfunction without type I acquired red–green defect. There are several reports of an electroretinographic cone dysfunction without a significant impairment of color vision (Goodman, Ripps, & Siegel, 1963). Pinckers and Thijssen (1974) observed myopia and normal color vision (AO HRR, Farnsworth Panel D-15, FM 100-hue test, anomaloscope) or a blue–yellow defect. The combination of cone dysfunction without color vision disturbance is called oligocone trichromatopsia (Van Lith, 1973) or peripheral cone disease (Krill, Deutman, & Fishman, 1973). At least some cases of peripheral cone disease are due to myopic chorioretinal degeneration (in French, *choroidose myopique*), as noted by Pinckers and Deutman (1977).

Type I acquired red–green defect without cone dysfunction. In central cone involvement (Krill, Deutman, & Fishman, 1973) there is a severe type I color vision defect but a normal ERG. There are indications that the ERG after some years will reveal a definite cone abnormality; in such cases "central cone involvement" is perhaps an early stage of progressive cone dystrophy.

Dominant progressive foveal dystrophy (Deutman, 1971) closely resembles Stargardt disease but differs from it because of its dominant mode of transmission. It generally occurs somewhat later in life, and its progression is less rapid than in Stargardt disease. The different mode of inheritance proves that for Stargardt disease and dominant progressive foveal dystrophy two different genes are responsible (François, 1974). Color vision examination reveals the same stages as for Stargardt patients (see below). In a recent study Pinckers, Deutman, and Notting (1976) suggest that some cases listed as dominant Stargardt disease in fact are really dominant cystoid macular dystrophy (below).

Macular Dystrophies

While the diseases described above are selected mainly on the basis of the electroretinographic findings, this section enumerates macular dystrophies on the basis of the clinical picture. Of course this division is arbitrary, but this is not the moment to propose a new classification of chorioretinal dystrophies.

STARGARDT DISEASE

Stargardt (1909) originally described a disease with autosomal recessive inheritance and the clinical picture of a macular lesion developing to an oval-shaped (often sharply delineated) atrophic area surrounded by yellowish dots. Perhaps Behr's (1920) unitarism is the cause of confusion that still exists concerning the nomenclature of macular disease. Stargardt disease was first identified as "juvenile macular degeneration with selective photopic involvement" by François, Verriest, de Rouck, and Humblet (1956) and fully described by François, Verriest, and de Rouck (1962). Stargardt disease is a slowly progressive macular degeneration ultimately resulting in an acquired (central) achromatopsia. According to Pinckers (1971b) the more classic symptoms of Stargardt disease do not appear until visual acuity has dropped to 0.2 or less, although individual variations are possible; if visual acuity is 0.1 or less, the EOG and the color vision are always disturbed. Photophobia is present but seldom a predominant feature. Visual acuity improves in mesopic circumstances. The ERG is normal in most cases (23 of 32 patients) (Pinckers, 1971b), but a cone dysfunction may occur. The EOG initially is normal (11/32), but becomes subnormal (18/32) and occasionally flat (3/32) (Pinckers, 1971b). In subjects with an affected macular ERG (MERG) an altered visual evoked cortical potential (VECP) pattern will be present; the VECP can be affected even if the amplitudes of the ERG are still normal (Fiore, Korol, & Babel, 1975).

Because Stargardt disease is the classical example of a type I acquired red–green defect, a detailed description of the results of color vision examination is given below.

Ishihara (12th edition).   A normal reading is an exception.

AO HRR (2nd edition).   The initial response is normal. As a first sign, the red–green plates, P_7 and D_7, are missed, later followed by other misreadings. Once the transition toward achromatopsia starts, the blue–yellow plates, T_{18} and T_{+17} are missed. The most insensitive blue–yellow plates are T_{19} and T_{+19}.

F_2 plate.   In early stages the green symbol is seen; later neither symbol is seen.

Farnsworth Panel D-15.   The sequence of deterioration is as follows: normal to minor error to red–green confusions to a scotopic arrangement. A blue–yellow confusion is exceptional (Fig. 8.13).

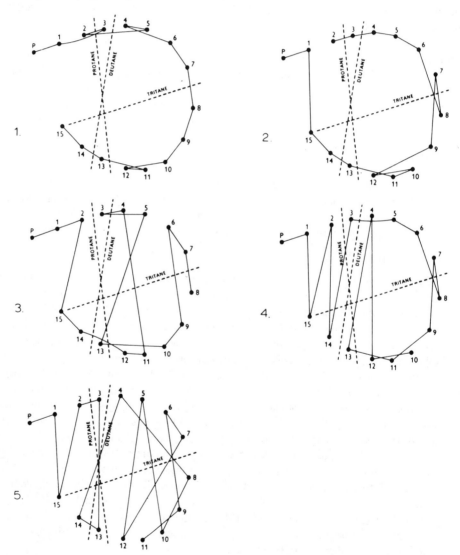

Fig. 8.13.   Sequence of Farnsworth Panel D-15 performance in Stargardt disease in members of one family.

FM 100-hue test. In individual cases the FM 100-hue test plots can show a curious axis rotation. Starting with a normal pattern the total error score may increase without a prominent error accumulation or a smooth monopolar accumulation of the purple caps. A marked accumulation at yellow and purple caps is frequently found; this shifts to the scotopic pattern and finally to a chaotic cap arrangement (Fig. 8.14).

Anomaloscope (Nagel model II). One of the first things to be noted is diminished long-wavelength sensitivity; the Rayleigh match is displaced and broadened toward the extreme end of the red scale; later the equation zone is broadened toward the green end; ultimately, the setting is that of (central) achromatopsia (Fig. 8.15).

Pinckers (1970b; 1971b) observed that the FM 100-hue test is very useful for observing progression in followup examinations. The FM 100-hue test results are often more pathologic than the anomalous quotient, which is of course very altered when the Farnsworth test patterns are scotopic. The stage preceeding color vision deficiency can be recognized by means of a retinal profile or by the determination of a luminance–visual acuity curve (Bessière, Vérin, Rougier-Houssin, & LeRebeller, 1969). Zanen and

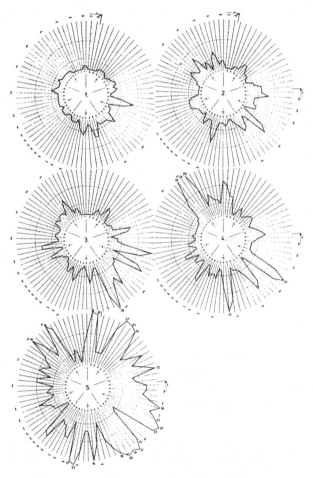

Fig. 8.14. FM 100-hue test results in Stargardt disease in the same family as represented in Fig. 8.13.

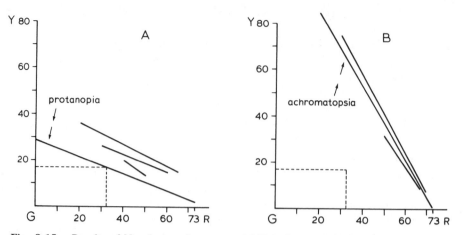

Fig. 8.15. Results of Nagel anomaloscope model II performance in Stargardt disease in the same family as represented in Figs. 8.13 and 8.14. (a) Includes a case of congenital protanopia; (b) includes a case of congenital achromatopsia. The dotted lines indicate the normal Rayleigh match (17 Y and a red–green mixture of 32.5 units).

Meunier (1969) confirm that in Stargardt disease there is a receptoral lesion; they found that the relative spectral luminosity curve is reduced at long wavelengths. There is an increased blue sensitivity associated with reduced red sensitivity (François, Verriest, & Israel, 1966). Verriest (1970b) showed that the deformation of the relative spectral luminosity curve is more pronounced at a lower illumination level. Marré (1973) reported that the blue CVM is reduced in some cases. Hansen (1974c) found a blue Stiles mechanism and an aberrant green one peaking at about 500 nm (rhodopsin-shaped).

Stargardt disease is not necessarily limited to the macular area but may be associated with a peripheral tapetoretinal dystrophy (François, Verriest, & de Rouck, 1962). In such cases the results of color vision examination reflect the macular lesion, but the red–green deficiency is less evident in peripheral involvement (Pinckers, 1971b). The peripheral involvement is expressed by the ERG and the EOG and in the visual field defects. The type I red–green defect is present in the retinal periphery, although peripheral color discrimination may be less affected than foveal color discrimination (François, Verriest, & Metsälä, 1964). Scotopization is restricted mostly to 6° eccentricity, although in some cases it reaches 20° eccentricity (Verriest & Uvijls, 1977a). In its classical form Stargardt disease remains limited to the posterior pole, while the progressive cone dystrophies spread over the whole retina (Perdriel, Lanthony, & Chevaleraud, 1975a).

FUNDUS FLAVIMACULATUS

Fundus flavimaculatus is characterized by the presence of yellow or yellowish-white pisciform dots. Their localization is usually deep but sometimes superficial. The dots are distributed in the central part of the retina and seldom reach as far as the retinal periphery. Franceschetti and François (1965) made a subdivision of fundus flavimaculatus into three forms:

1. Pure form, in which dots are distributed in or around the posterior pole of the eye. In this subtype all of the visual functions are normal or nearly normal; visual acuity sometimes drops if the dots invade the foveola.
2. Associated form, in which the flavimaculatus dots are combined with Stargardt disease, or hemeralopia.
3. Atypical forms.

In the four cases described, color vision was normal. In Stargardt's (1909) original publication, the illustrations essentially show yellowish-white dots, similar to the dots in fundus flavimaculatus. Deutman (1971) admits that the central and pericentral type of Stargardt disease is sometimes indistinguishable from fundus flavimaculatus. The inheritance of both diseases is autosomal recessive.

The associated form is identical to the "form with foveal dystrophy" of Klien and Krill (1967). Krill and Deutman (1972a) subdivided the associated form into (1) a group with an atrophic macular degeneration (in subgroup A including the majority of patients, there is no evidence of electroretinographic cone abnormality; in subgroup B there is evidence of diffuse severe cone disease on the ERG), and (2) a group with progressive deterioration of peripheral retinal function as well as an atrophic macular degeneration.

François, Turut, Puech, and Hache (1975) observed that flavimaculatus dots with perimacular or peripheral localization coexist in the same family. They conclude from 62 personal observations that the same disease may present in three different forms: (1) pure Stargardt disease; (2) Stargardt disease with perimacular flavimaculatus crown; and (3) Stargardt disease with peripheral fundus flavimaculatus. Another clinical classification of fundus flavimaculatus, however, was proposed by Fishman (1976) and Fishman, Buckman, and Van Every (1977). The most remarkable feature of their four-category classification is that the authors do not use color vision discrimination as a clinical parameter.

In the pure form described by Franceschetti and François (1965), color vision is normal [Franceschetti & François (1965), 30 cases; Babel (1972), 20 cases; François (1974)]; the EOG is subnormal in 75 percent of cases (Klien & Krill, 1967). In the associated form an atrophic macular degeneration occurs. Color vision examination in such cases reveals a type I acquired red–green deficiency (Hollwich, 1963; Krill & Deutman, 1972a; Fiore, Korol, & Babel, 1975; Schiffer & Busse, 1975). Pinckers (1971b) observed six patients: One subject had a congenital red–green defect, and in the remaining five cases visual acuity was 0.2 or less. The anomalous quotient (Nagel model II) was 0.46 or less. The FM 100-hue test total error score was more than 168, and the error accumulations were on protan–deutan axes (six eyes), deutan axis (one eye), scotopic region (two eyes), or chaotic (one eye). The author noted that fundus flavimaculatus with Stargardt disease appears functionally like Stargardt disease.

Carr (1965) examined five cases of fundus flavimaculatus. Performance of the AO HRR was difficult or impossible because of a central scotoma. With the Farnsworth Panel D-15 there were minor errors (one eye) or no errors (four eyes). It is interesting to note that Fiore, Korol, and Babel (1975) observed fundus flavimaculatus and tritanopia in a family. Imaizumi, Takahashi, Mita, and Hoshi (1976) reported blue–yellow defects. Such papers or reports emphasize the need for extensive family studies and long-term studies in fundus flavimaculatus and Stargardt disease. Without any doubt, there are diseases that present a Stargardt-like macular involvement together with flavimaculatuslike flecks (Notting & Pinckers, 1978).

VITELLIFORM DYSTROPHY OF THE FOVEA

In vitelliform macular dystrophy the results of color vision examination differ. Normal color vision was reported by Zanen and Rausin (1950) (using the Ishihara and color perimetry), François (1971; 1974), Dran (1973), Brink (1974), and Miller (1977). A mild defect without predominant confusions was reported by Falls (1949) (using the Ishihara and FM 100-hue test), Verriest (1964; 1974a), Turut, Hache, and François (1972), Dran (1973), Brink (1974), Benson, Kolker, Enoch, Van Loo, and Honda (1975), and Miller, Bresnick, and Chandra (1976). A type III blue–yellow defect was reported by Zanen and Rausin (1951), Remky and Kölbl (1971), Deutman (1971) (AO HRR, Farnsworth Panel D-15), and Krill and Deutman (1972a) (FM 100-hue test). A red–green defect was reported by Remky, Rix, and Klier (1965) and Deutman (1971) (AO HRR, Farnsworth Panel D-15).

The color vision defect is correlated with the deterioration of visual acuity (Krill, Morse, Potts, & Klien, 1966; Dorne, 1970). The presence of a color vision abnormality therefore has a diagnostic value (Turut, Hache, & François, 1972). François and Turut (1975) examined 29 cases with the FM 100-hue test—2 cases were classified as normal, 27 as slightly defective or strongly defective. The confusion directions were discordant. The degree of color vision defect is related to the decline of visual acuity; color vision defect, however, is observed in cases with visual acuity 0.9 or 1.0 (Turut, 1972). The authors concluded that there is cone pathology in an early stage of the disease.

Color vision is significantly abnormal if visual acuity drops to 0.5 or worse (Krill & Deutman, 1972a); there is a shift of the Rayleigh equation toward red, and the matching range is greater than normal [Deutman (1971), two cases; Krill & Deutman, (1972)].

Dorne (1970) observed that in early stages the results of plates and anomaloscope are normal but the FM 100-hue test shows a loss of chromatic discrimination without predominant confusions. The spectral luminosity curve, however, is not scotopized as in Stargardt disease (Falls, 1969). Deutman (1971) showed that color vision can return to normal if visual acuity does so. There are vitelliform lesions with a normal EOG (Fishman, Trimble, Rabb, & Fishman, 1977); the two cases tested showed a type III blue–yellow defect without pseudoprotanomaly.

DOMINANT DRUSEN

Drusen or hyaline structures of Bruch's membrane can generally be divided into degenerative drusen and hereditary drusen. Drusen frequently manifest themselves as a result of primary hereditary dystrophy of the posterior pole of the retina with an autosomal dominant mode of inheritance; they are known variously as Hutchinson-Tay choroiditis, Holthouse-Batten superificial chorioretinitis, Doyne honeycomb degeneration, or malattia levantinese (Remky, Rix, & Klier, 1965).

Color vision is usually normal until the fovea is affected (Deutman, 1971; François, 1974), but sometimes one can find an acquired blue–yellow defect in cases with normal visual acuity (Franceschetti, François, & Babel, 1963). Acquired blue–yellow defect is reported by Pinckers (1971a) (23 cases), Raudrant-Mathian (1972), and Bonnet (1972).

Deutman and Jansen (1970) examined eight cases—color vision was normal in five, in two there was diminished red sensitivity measured on the anomaloscope [combined with a mild red–green (AO HRR test) in one of the two], and in the eighth case there were combined red–green and blue–yellow defects. In a further study Deutman (1971) concluded that if the fovea is affected the first sign is an anomaloscopic diminished red sensitivity, followed later by a red–green defect (AO HRR). In advanced stages a type III blue–yellow defect is possible.

In an investigation of 60 eyes (Pinckers A: Personal communication) color vision was normal in 15 eyes, 3 eyes showed a slight disturbance without prominent confusion, in 13 eyes there was a red–green deficiency (4 being congenital and 2 a type I defect), and in 17 eyes there was a type III blue–yellow defect, only 2 of them showing an anomaloscopic pseudoprotanomaly, in 8 eyes there was a combination of an acquired red–green defect with a type III acquired blue–yellow defect, and the 4 remaining eyes had severe acquired color vision defects without predominant axes.

Degenerative changes in the macular area as a sequel to chronic vascular insufficiency give rise to intracellular and extracellular accumulations and finally result in atrophy (Naumann & Lüllwitz, 1975). Such a condition seems to be present in the new "dominant progressive foveal dystrophy" described by Frank, Landers, Williams, and Sidbury (1975). The disease develops from scattered drusen with pigment dispersion, via confluent drusen with or without pigment clumping, toward choroidal atrophy. The color vision of 19 affected and 20 nonaffected family members was examined with the AO HRR and Farnsworth Panel D-15 by Frank, Landers, Williams, and Sidbury (1975); only one affected member showed a type III blue–yellow defect. The ERG was normal.

BUTTERFLY-SHAPED DYSTROPHY

This dominantly inherited fundus abnormality was first mentioned as "pseudoangioid streaks" accompanied by peripheral pigment alterations (Franceschetti, François, and Babel, 1963). The ERG is normal. The defect occurs sometimes in juvenile macular degeneration and the condition resembles that in two observations made by Behr (1920). Deutman, Van Blommenstein, Henkes, Waardenburg, and Solleveld–Van Driest (1970) described a similar picture and called it butterfly-shaped pigment dystrophy of the fovea. In the four cases they examined, color vision was normal. Deutman (1971) concluded that the normal color vision results are consistent with other findings in foveal dystrophies, in which color vision was disturbed only when visual acuity was distinctly diminished. The four cases described by Deutman, Van Blommenstein, Henkes, Waardenburg, and Solleveld–Van Driest (1970) were reexamined 8 years later: visual acuity was 0.8 or more, the ERG was normal, the EOG was normal (three eyes) or subnormal (five eyes), and color vision was normal in five eyes but in three eyes there was an elevated FM 100-hue test total error score, two of them showing a type III blue–yellow defect (Pinckers A: Personal communication).

MYOPIA

Köllner (1907b) demonstrated that artificial myopia (using positive spectacle lenses) has no influence on color matches. According to Chapanis (1950) in artificial myopia the majority of the plate tests are correctly interpreted even if visual acuity is reduced to 0.2. In corrected myopia without ophthalmoscopic signs of degeneration Verriest (1964) observed a FM 100-hue test error accumulation in the region of cap 74.

Comberg (1941) and Gaillard (1962) reported a type III blue–yellow defect in advanced cases of myopic degeneration. The confusions are similar to congenital tritanopia, the FM 100-hue test error accumulation being situated near cap 4 [Bozzoni (1959), 21 cases] or similar to the tetartan type (Cox, 1960; 1961a, b). The chromatic thresholds for blue are elevated (Zanen, 1953); the spectral luminosity curve is normal or shows a selective lowering of the sensitivity to longer wavelengths, although not reaching scotopization (Verriest, 1964; 1970).

The characteristic feature of malignant myopia is a type III acquired blue–yellow defect, the Rayleigh equation being displaced toward red (François & Verriest, 1957a). Verriest (1964) stated that an acquired red–green defect is an exception, but a red–green confusion often complicates the type III blue–yellow defect. Nevertheless, normal color vision can be found, as can a type I red–green defect (François & Verriest, 1968). The characteristic type III acquired blue–yellow defect is a late event in malignant myopia, since according to Verriest (1964) it occurs only if visual acuity drops to 0.1 or less; this perhaps is the reason that Pinckers (1971a) found only five type III blue–yellow defects in 38 eyes in which visual acuity was 0.1 or more. In malignant myopia, as in Wagner syndrome (see above) a type III blue–yellow defect is encountered as soon as a nuclear cataract becomes evident (Pinckers, 1970a; Pinckers & Jansen, 1974; Pinckers, 1975a).

BENIGN CONCENTRIC ANNULAR MACULAR DYSTROPHY

Deutman (1974a) described four members of a family with an autosomal dominant concentric annular macular dystrophy resembling a bull's-eye picture. This dystrophy probably forms a specific nosologic entity. Visual acuity is normal or only slightly affected. On the AO HRR there were minimal to mild red–green defects, twice combined with a strong blue–yellow defect. On the Farnsworth Panel D-15 results were normal in three cases and showed a blue–yellow defect in one case. The FM 100-hue test showed a type III defect. Anomaloscope examination revealed a widened equation shifted toward the red end in three cases.

CENTRAL AREOLAR PIGMENT EPITHELIAL DYSTROPHY

Fetkenhour, Gurney, Dobbie, and Choromokos (1976) described a central areolar pigment epithelial dystrophy in three generations. The disease has its onset in childhood and is asymptomatic; retinal function studies were normal, revealing the benign nature of the dystrophy. Color vision was normal in three eyes (AO HRR, FM 100-hue test) and disturbed in one eye due to macular hemorrhage. Although this disease occurred in three consecutive generations, there was no inheritance from father to son.

DYSTROPHIA RETICULARIS LAMINAE PIGMENTOSA RETINAE
OF SJÖGREN

Sjögren (1950) reported a disease characterized in its earliest stage by a peculiar netlike structure of the pigment epithelial layer and in its further stage by the gradual disintegration and disappearance of the retinal pigment, whereas the inner layer of the retina remains intact. In the eight cases examined, visual acuity varied from 1.0 to finger counting. Color vision was defective only in one case, the seven other cases being normal. Deutman and Rümke (1969) described two cases in which color vision was normal. Benedikt and Werner (1971) reported another family in which color vision, examined in one affected member (Ishihara, Farnsworth Panel D-15, Nagel anomaloscope), was normal. Chopdar (1976) reported a case with normal plate test results.

SORSBY FAMILIAL PSEUDOINFLAMMATORY
MACULAR DYSTROPHY

Sorsby, Joll-Mason, and Gardener (1949) described an autosomal dominant macular dystrophy of late onset; there is a macular lesion of abrupt onset with the appearance of an inflammatory process. After healing of the lesion the process extends slowly, leaving areas of choroidal atrophy and pigment deposition. Color vision, tested with the Ishihara, was abnormal in one case. Cox (1960; 1961a, b) examined four cases; two showed normal color vision and two a type III acquired blue–yellow defect.

Franceschetti, François, and Babel (1963) reported an acquired red–green defect in one case and Verriest (1964) in two cases. Fraser and Wallace (1971) performed color vision tests (B-K charts, Ishihara, AO HRR, Farnsworth Panel D-15, FM 100-hue test, Nagel model I anomaloscope) among younger descendents of affected members still at risk of developing the dystrophy. They found an unusual mild red–green defect in 10 of the 30 examined relatives, perhaps representing an early manifestation of the dystrophy.

CHOROIDAL DYSTROPHY (SCLEROSIS OR ATROPHY)

Choroidal dystrophy can be subdivided into a diffuse or generalized form, a central areolar form, and a peripapillary form. In choroidal dystrophy François and Verriest (1968) (14 eyes) and Pinckers (1971a) (20 eyes) observed normal color vision (7 eyes), slight defects (6 eyes), unspecified red–green defects (3 eyes), type I defects (2 eyes), type III blue–yellow defects (12 eyes), achromatopsia (2 eyes), and congenital deficiency (2 eyes).

Generalized choroidal dystrophy is characterized by a diminished red sensitivity that according to Verriest (1964) (six eyes), may be considered either as a type III acquired blue–yellow defect similar to retinitis pigmentosa or as a type I acquired red–green defect, similar to juvenile macular degeneration. In individual cases the progression can be rapid. One case deteriorated from normal color vision to a type III acquired blue–yellow defect with a tendency to become achromatic (Ishihara, F_2, AO HRR, Farnsworth Panel D-15, FM 100-hue test, Nagel model I) within 4 years.

In central areolar choroidal dystrophy, color vision examination disclosed normal color vision [Deutman (1971), three eyes; Takki (1974b) two cases], a type III acquired blue–yellow defect, and sometimes an acquired red–green defect (Franceschetti, François, & Babel, 1963). Color vision in a few cases was unrecordable (Deutman, 1971; Takki, 1974b; Bonnet, 1975). Choriocapillaris loss is an early finding in central areolar choroidal dystrophy, which supports the assumption of a primary dystrophy of the choriocapillaris. Noble (1977) observed a central areolar choroidal dystrophy in a 47-year-old man, his daughter, and his son—red–green plates of the AO HRR were missed, but the Farnsworth Panel D-15 showed nondiagnostic errors in the father and daughter and a normal result in the son.

Peripapillary choroidal dystrophy often occurs in malignant myopia. When the dystrophy invades the foveal area, this may influence color vision. Color vision examination in malignant myopia (above) has not yet been analyzed with respect to the extent of the peripapillary dystrophy.

DOMINANT CYSTOID MACULAR DYSTROPHY

Dominant cystoid macular dystrophy (DCMD) (Notting & Pinckers, 1977) is a dominantly inherited disease characterized by vitreous opacities, cystoid macular edema, and macular pigment alterations. There is often strong hyperopia and fine folding of the inner limiting membrane. The ERG is normal; the EOG may be disturbed. Color vision examination reveals a diminished red sensitivity; there is a type I red–green defect, but a fully developed central achromatopsia (including an electroretinographic cone dysfunction) is not observed. There is a slight to moderate concomitant blue–yellow defect, which appears when the AO HRR errors indicate a defect of moderate severity (Pinckers, Deutman, & Notting, 1976). Recent observations (Pinckers, Notting, & Lion, 1978) reveal that in an ultimate stage DCMD can manifest itself as an atrophic macular dystrophy with an atypical pigmentary dystrophy, sometimes even as a pericentral retinitis pigmentosa. In such cases the ERG is diminished, but there is no selective cone or rod impairment.

PATTERNED DYSTROPHY OF THE
RETINAL PIGMENT EPITHELIUM

Patterned dystrophy is used as a collective noun for diseases affecting the retinal pigment epithelium, including conditions such as butterfly-shaped dystrophy and dystrophia reticularis of Sjögren (discussed above) as well as conditions such as macroreticular dystrophy, the reticular pigment dystrophy, and fundus pulverulentus.

Hsieh, Fine, and Lyons (1977) described a family in which reticular dystrophy, macroreticular dystrophy, and butterfly-shaped forms alternated. Is there one pattern dystrophy with various manifestations? The retinal functions are similar except for the EOG in the butterfly-shaped form. In three cases color vision was examined: one subject made mild red−green and blue−yellow errors with the AO HRR, but the other two subjects had normal color vision.

In three generations of one family, alterations in the retinal pigment epithelium occurred, varying from granular pigment dispersion beneath the fovea in younger individuals to a reticular pigment pattern in older ones (Marmor & Byers, 1977). There was a mild visual disturbance and a subnormal EOG but normal visual fields, dark adaptation, ERG, and color vision.

OTHER MACULAR DEGENERATIONS*

Senile Macular Degenerations

Choroidal pathology is a basic feature of senile macular degeneration. The clinical picture of the senile macular degenerations is variable; the same choroidal disturbance may lead to the ophthalmoscopic picture of an atrophic, cystic, or colloidal (hyaline) macular degeneration, a subdivision made by Campbell and Rittler (1972). These authors made a comparison between the results of color vision examination in these three subgroups with respect to the age of occurrence and the visual acuity (Table 8.3). In both atrophic and colloidal groups the percentage of eyes with type III blue−yellow defects is far less for juvenile than for senile macular degeneration. In senile macular degeneration the incidence of type III blue−yellow defects approaches that of red−green defects. In the atrophic and colloidal group the incidence of type III blue−yellow defects in presenile and senile types does not differ. In the cystic group the age of onset is of little importance; there are more red−green than blue−yellow defects. If visual acuity has dropped to 0.4 or less there is a marked incidence of red−green as well as blue−yellow color defect; this finding is most marked in the juvenile group.

Sloan (1942) was the first to study color vision in senile macular degeneration. She observed that the readings of the Stilling tritan plates were defective. Zanen (1953) found elevated chromatic thresholds for blue even in aphakic patients. In a further study Zanen (1959) found elevated thresholds with a normal photochromatic interval; the anomaloscopic performance resembled the equation of a deuteranomalous subject. Bozzoni (1959) examined six cases (Farnsworth Panel D-15, FM 100-hue test); there was a blue−yellow axis with the FM 100-hue test errors accumulating at cap 3. Cox (1960; 1961a, b) reported 30 cases, 5 with normal color vision and 25 with a type III blue−yellow defect; the photopic luminosity curve was depressed in 1 case, depressed and shortened at both ends in 2 cases. The spectral wavelength discrimination curve was similar to that of congenital tritan defects. Verriest (1964) examined 18 subjects (22 eyes):

---

*Contributed by I. A. Chisholm, M.D., and A. J. L. G. Pinckers, M.D.

Table 8.3
Color Vision Defects on the AO HRR Test in Macular Degeneration*

	Atrophic (310 eyes)			Cystic (93 eyes)			Colloidal (167 eyes)		
	N	VA (>0.5)	VA (<0.4)	N	VA (>0.5)	VA (<0.4)	N	VA (>0.5)	VA (<0.4)
Juvenile	105			30			10		
Percent with blue–yellow defect		6	62		17	57		0	75
Percent with red–green defect		45	95		56	100		50	100
Presenile	97			20			38		
Percent with blue–yellow defect		50	62		14	33		18	94
Percent with red–green defect		66	88		50	83		36	100
Senile	108			41			119		
Percent with blue–yellow defect		64	81		29	56		58	93
Percent with red–green defect		75	95		61	82		70	90

*Data based on Campbell and Rittler, 1972.

there were type III blue–yellow defect with moderate concomitant red–green defect, and most cases displayed a blue–yellow defect or scotopic pattern. The Rayleigh equation was displaced toward red. Verriest (1964) stated that color vision disturbance is an early event because even in cases with normal visual acuity a severe color vision defect is possible. Peripheral color discrimination up to 20° also revealed blue–yellow defects. Color perimetry is normal or abnormal; if abnormal, it is characterized by a reduced blue and red sensitivity (François, Verriest, & Israel, 1966). A type III blue–yellow defect is also described by Kohler (1968), Kurata (1967b), Perdriel (1970), and Pinckers (1975a). A defect without predominant confusion was noted by Merin and Auerbach (1970). Helve and Krause (1972) have observed both types of color vision defects. Krill and Fishman (1971) found that the Rayleigh equation is more disturbed than the FM 100-hue test pattern, but Heinsius (1968; 1972) observed that the Rayleigh equation is normal in initial stages while the plate tests are already misread. According to Perdriel, Chevaleraud, Delpuget, and Bourgeois (1970) the examination of color vision in senile macular degeneration is of great importance from a prognostic point of view.

The atrophic form (or Haab and Dimmer type) shows a type III blue–yellow defect and according to Cox (1960; 1961a, b) is often associated with a concomitant red–green component, especially if visual acuity is reduced to 0.25; this agrees with the findings of Campbell and Rittler (1972) (Table 8.3). Recently, Singerman, Berkow, and Patz (1977) reported a family in which ten members displayed a slowly progressive macular dystrophy. Visual acuity remained good until the seventh decade. Macular changes included perifoveal pigment epithelial atrophy, posterior pole flecks, and fundus lesions resembling an atrophic form of senile macular degeneration. The authors suggest a hereditary predisposition to senile macular degeneration. Color vision (AO HRR or Farnsworth Panel D-15) was normal in the six cases examined. The EOG was normal in one case and subnormal in another case. The ERG was recorded in five patients; one showed a normal ERG, while the other four showed diminished cone and rod functions.

Serous detachment of the neuroepithelium may represent a beginning stage of the disciform senile form or Junius-Kuhnt (Coppez-Danis) type. In such cases of serous detachment there is an early color vision disturbance (Legras & Coscas, 1972). Bonnet (1974) studied color vision of central serous retinopathy progressing to senile macular degeneration: in one case with atrophy of the pigment epithelium as a result of central serous retinopathy, color vision was normal; in another case, at an early stage the Roth 28-hue test gave normal results but the contralateral eye presenting an advanced stage showed acquired achromatopsia. François and Verriest (1957a) observed that in the disciform type the type III blue–yellow defect is more pronounced than in the atrophic form. Table 8.4 summarizes the findings of François and Verriest (1968) and Pinckers (1971a) in senile macular degeneration.

Secondary Disciform Macular Degenerations

Secondary disciform macular degenerations may occur in several conditions; the most common include angioid streaks, myopic choroidal degeneration (Gass, 1967) and multifocal choroiditis (presumed histoplasmosis).

ANGIOID STREAKS

Angioid streaks cause a gap between the inner choroidal structure and Bruch's membrane. They often occur in combination with diseases such as pseudoxanthoma elasticum, Paget disease of the bones, sickle cell trait hemoglobinopathy, and hereditary

Table 8.4
Color Vision in Senile Macular Degeneration

	Eyes Examined	Normal Color Vision	Slight Defect	Type III	Achroma-topsia	Type I	Congenital
François & Verriest, 1968	47	8	6	28	—	5	—
Pinckers, 1971a	28	10	1	7	8	—	2
Haab type	17	8	1	5	1	—	2
disciform type	11	2	—	2	7	—	—

senile elastosis with acromegaly. There are often multiple drusen. In general there is a gradual loss of vision, but sometimes the loss is acute if hemorrhagic detachment occurs. Peau d'orange and salmon spots are precursors of angioid streaks (Krill, Klien, & Archer, 1973).

In angioid streaks, Krümmel (1950) observed a central scotoma for red and green. François and Verriest (1954) (four cases) found normal color vision (Ishihara) with normal visual acuity. Zanen (1959) examined one case with normal visual acuity and found normal foveal achromatic thresholds, the photochromatic thresholds for red being elevated. Verriest (1964) saw one case with normal color vision and one with a type III blue–yellow defect. Gerde (1974) examined a case with sickle cell trait hemoglobinopathy—the Farnsworth Panel D-15 was normal for the right eye but showed blue–yellow confusions for the left eye. In seven eyes of four cases (Pinckers A: Unpublished) color vision was normal (four eyes) or showed a type III blue–yellow defect (one eye) or a "congenital protanomaly" (one eye).

Preretinal Fibrosis (Jaffe Syndrome)

There are only a few reports on color vision examination in cases with preretinal fibrosis (Jaffe syndrome). In the stages preceding retraction Bonnet (1973) and Denden and Schröder (1976) observed normal color vision.

Once vitreoretinal retraction becomes manifest, there is an acquired color vision disturbance, in general without a predominant axis of confusion, but sometimes with an acquired red–green defect (Bonnet, 1973). The end result of the disease is a total achromatopsia (Denden & Schröder, 1976). Verriest and Uvijls (1977a) observed normal or, more frequently, uniformly depressed increment threshold spectral sensitivity curves.

Cystoid Degeneration

In peripheral cystoid degeneration Verriest (1964) observed normal color vision (two cases). In lamellar macular holes François and Verriest (1957a) saw one case with a slight color vision disturbance and another with a type III acquired blue–yellow defect. Cox (1960; 1961a, b) examined five cases and found normal color vision (two cases) or a tetartanlike defect (three cases). In dominant inherited macular cysts, according to Sorsby, Savory, Davey, and Fraser (1956), color vision and visual acuity are normal until the cyst ruptures. After age 40 years, when the cysts usually rupture, color vision may be normal (two cases) or disturbed without predominant axis (one case). In two cases the Ishihara plates were misread and the Rayleigh equation displaced to red. Similarly, Cox (1960; 1961a, b) observed three cases, two unruptured cysts with normal color vision and one ruptured cyst with an acquired red–green defect. Verriest (1964) examined one case; this disclosed a congenital color vision defect. Pinckers (1971a) saw one case with unruptured cyst and normal color vision.

VASCULAR AND HEMATOLOGIC DISEASE*

Disease processes affecting the blood elements or the containing vessel wall are manifested in the majority of cases by changes visible on funduscopy, which are an expression of a derangement of the retinal and optic nerve head circulation. The most

---

*Contributed by I. A. Chisholm, M.D.

common antecedent event is tissue hypoxia or anoxia clinically manifested by retinal venous engorgement and later by retinal edema, exudation, hemorrhage, and optic disc edema. The effect of breathing air with low oxygen concentration on the performance of healthy volunteers to the FM 100-hue response was studied by Smith, Ernest, and Pokorny (1976), who found an acquired blue–yellow defect at low photopic luminance. A study on patients receiving treatment in a hyperbaric chamber and breathing air at a pressure of 2 atm showed a similar deterioration of the FM 100-hue performance (Lewis R.D.H.: Personal communication).

Tissue anoxia or hypoxia may arise as a result of the following:

1. Reduced oxygen-carrying capacity of the blood; anemic anoxia as may be found in iron; vitamin B_{12}, and folate-deficiency anemias.
2. Raised venous pressure due to increasing resistance to blood flow or slowing of the circulation or both (stagnant anoxia). Slowed circulation may occur with increased blood viscosity, the result of an increase in the formed elements of the blood accompanying polycythemia and leukemia, or an increase in the protein content with plasma as in macroglobulinemia, multiple myelomatosis, and cryoglobulinemia. Slowing of the ocular circulation may be found to accompany congestive cardiac failure in conditions of the orbit in which there is increased intraorbital pressure, as in dysthyroid exophthalmos, and back pressure from cavernus sinus thrombosis.
3. Reduction in perfusion pressure to the globe as a whole; this is found in acute angle closure glaucoma, carotid occlusive disease, and profound systemic hypotension of recurrent blood loss.
4. Local arterial occlusion of retinal or choroidal vessels.
5. Diabetes.

Addisonian Perinicious Anemia

This form of macrocytic anemia is characterized by the presence of a megaloblastic bone marrow, reduced levels of vitamin B_{12} in the serum, reduced absorption of radioactive-labeled B_{12} in the body, an achlorhydria, and circulating antibodies to gastric mucosa or intrinsic factor. The anemia may be associated with a hereditary trait, a change in color of the body hair, a retrobulbar neuritis, or degenerative change in the spinal cord. Vitamin B_{12} deficiency may also be secondary to malabsorption states, and macrocytic anemia is known as part of folate deficiency.

A disturbance of color vision in megaloblastic anemia was reported by Adams, Chalmers, Foulds, and Withy (1967): 19 subjects were studied in the pretreatment phase of the anemia; 12 suffered from Addisonian pernicious anemia, 3 postgastrectomy steatorrhea, and 4 folate deficiency. Four or more errors on testing with pseudo-isochromatic plates under natural daylight conditions was taken as the criterion for color defect. Four of the Addisonian pernicious anemia patients were found to have color defect on screening; in three, color vision returned to normal following vitamin B_{12} therapy. The authors found that the older patients tended to show the color defects. No correlation was found between the hemoglobin concentration or serum vitamin B_{12} levels and the presence of color defect.

The deficiency of color discrimination experienced by patients suffering from Addisonian pernicious anemia was explored in greater depth by Chisholm (1972). His study was based on 58 patients, all of whom suffered from Addisonian pernicious anemia;

11 patients were in the acute pretreatment phase (group 2), and 26 had their hematologic deficits corrected and stabilized with cyanocobalamin (group 1). All of these patients had good visual acuity. The remaining 21 patients suffered in addition from bilateral retrobulbar neuritis of pernicious anemia (group 3). Color vision was investigated by the FM 100-hue test performed uniocularly under artificial daylight conditions; the results are summarized in Table 8.5.

The study showed that of those patients in the untreated phase the color discrimination when retinopathy was present was no different from when it was absent. In patients with no evidence of retrobulbar neuritis the color discrimination for treated and untreated patients was equally defective. The FM 100-hue test results obtained from those patients showed a characteristic violet-blue-green discrimination loss (Fig. 8.16 a) that differed markedly from the FM 100-hue test results obtained from those patients with the additional retrobulbar neuritis (Fig. 8.16 b).

By relating the FM 100-hue test error score to patient age for those patients without a field defect, a linear correlation was shown whereby the older pernicious anemia patients had poorer color discrimination $(r = + 0.57; p < 0.001)$. Although all the patients suffering from retrobulbar neuritis in the study smoked, Adams, Chalmers, Foulds, and Withy (1967) reported retrobulbar neuritis of pernicious anemia in a female lifelong nonsmoker. The color discrimination loss of the ten smokers suffering from uncomplicated pernicious anemia was significantly increased above that of the other nonsmoking patients $(t = + 2.106; p \partial 0.05)$. Chisholm (1972) concluded that there is a color disturbance associated with pernicious anemia that is permanent, increases with patient age, and is more obvious in the smoker than in the nonsmoker.

Systemic Hypertension and Atherosclerosis

Systemic hypertension from whatever cause and whether accompanied by sclerosis or not causes visible changes in the retinal vessels. The changes vary from alterations in vessel caliber and density of vessel wall to neuroretinal edema, focal retinal infarcts, and superficial retinal hemorrhages. The minor changes are universally present in those age 60 years or above and are part of the normal vascular sclerosis of aging.

Studies of color discrimination have recorded either a normal response or a type III blue–yellow defect. The earliest report was by Mauthner (1881), followed by reports by Simon (1894), König (1897), and Köllner (1908). Their findings were based on results

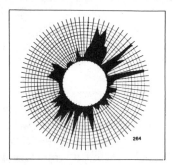 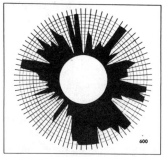

Fig. 8.16 (left) FM 100-hue test plot from a patient suffering from Addisonian pernicious anemia without optic neuropathy. (right) FM 100-hue test plot from a patient suffering from Addisonian pernicious anemia complicated by optic neuropathy. [From Chisholm, I. A. *Modern Problems in Ophthalmology*, 1972, *11*, 130–135 (reproduced with permission of S. Karger AG).]

Table 8.5
Color Vision in Patients With Addisonian Pernicious Anemia

Group	No. in Group	Male:Female	Mean Age (years)	Mean FM 100-Hue Test Error Score	No. of Smokers in Group
Pretreatment	26	12:14	62.57 ± 10.7	285.3 ± 134	6
Stabilized	11	1:10	58.36 ± 18.25	267.3 ± 143	4
Retrobulbar neuritis	21	20:1	68.40 ± 8.15	756.5 ± 234.5	21

Data of Chisholm, I. A. *Modern Problems in Ophthalmology*, 1972, *11*, 130–135, (with permission of S. Karger AG).

obtained with pigment or spectral matching tests. In more recent times, François and Verriest (1957a), Cox (1960), Verriest (1963), Koliopoulos, Chatzis, and Papgeoriou (1971), Pinckers (1972b), and Trusov (1972) all confirm the presence of a type III blue–yellow defect identified with plate tests, Farnsworth Panel D-15 (Fig. 8.17), FM 100-hue test, and anomaloscope.

All authors agree that the modification in color sense is confined to the central area of the visual field. François and Verriest (1957a) noted that the type III blue–yellow defect was to be found only in advanced stages of retinopathy (Keith and Wagner classification, stages 3 and 4). Trusov (1972) studied 118 patients using the AN 59 anomaloscope and found perception thresholds increased for all basic colors. In his study no correlation between high blood pressure, presence or absence of retinopathy, and extent of color defect was identified, but there was a correlation with visual acuity.

Posthemorrhagic Retinopathy

Although rare, severe recurring intestinal or uterine hemorrhage has been known for many centuries to cause visual loss. Gowers (1882) appreciated that damage to the nutrition of the retina could lead to the appearance of a "primary retinal inflammation." Pears and Pickering (1960) felt that the signs of neuroretinal edema, surface retinal hemorrhages, and "cotton wool" exudate were secondary to circulatory change following a hypotensive event rather than delayed anemia.

The vascular flow to the eye is dependent on the perfusion pressure, which is sensitive to changes in intraocular pressure (Best, Blumenthal, Futterman, & Galin, 1969) and thus accounts for the rapid deterioration of the visual field noted to follow hemorrhage in patients with chronic simple glaucoma (Perez, 1963; Blumenthal, Best, & Galin, 1971). Evidence of retinal neuroreceptor damage may be found following severe and recurring hemorrhage (Fig. 8.18). Chisholm (1969b) recorded the occurrence of similar findings in patients who during major thoracic surgery experienced a period of profound systemic hypotension.

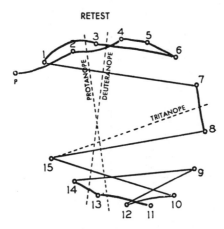

Fig. 8.17. Farnsworth Panel D-15 result from a patient with fulminating hypertensive retinopathy. [From François, J. & Verriest, G. *Annales d'oculistique* (Paris), 1957, *190*, 812–859 (reproduced with permission of Doin, Editeur).]

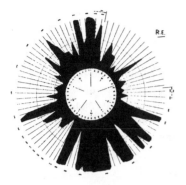

Fig. 8.18. FM 100-hue test plot from a 64-year-old male patient who suffered severe recurrent gastrointestinal hemorrhage resulting in profound visual loss. [From Chisholm, I. A. *British Journal of Ophthalmology*, 1969, *53*, 289-295 (reproduced with permission of the British Medical Journal).]

Local Vascular Occlusive Disease

The retinal blood vessels supply the inner two-thirds of the retina (nerve fiber layer, ganglion cells, inner nuclear layer); the outer third (neuroreceptors, outer nuclear layer, and pigment epithelium) is supplied by diffusion from the choriocapillaris of the choroid. Acute occlusion of the retinal arteriole will cause a localized retinal infarct involving the conductive apparatus, whereas acute occlusion of the posterior ciliary artery will result in death of the receptor apparatus in its segmental area of supply. The cause of vascular occlusion may be thrombosis, embolism, or one of the forms of arteritis.

RETINAL ARTERIAL OCCLUSION

Central retinal arterial occlusion, except where a cilioretinal artery supplies the macula, results in extinction of the light, form, and color senses. Branch arterial occlusion results in a permanent defect in field of vision. There are already signs of hypertensive or arteriosclerotic arterial disease; hence a preexisting type III blue–yellow defect may be identified. Branch and central retinal vein occlusion have been reported as causing a type III blue–yellow defect by François and Verriest (1957a), Cox (1960), and Pinckers (1972b). Lakowski and Begg (1976), in a study of patients with cystoid macular edema following chronic retinal vein obstruction, found reduced performance in testing with the FM 100-hue test and the Pickford-Nicolson anomaloscope. Anomaloscope defects were most marked for the yellow—blue and blue—green equations.

CHOROIDAL ARTERIAL OCCLUSION

Acute occlusion of the short posterior ciliary arteries results in an ischemic optic neuropathy with loss of vision completely or with a variety of residual field defects; in addition, there is a chorioretinal pigment degeneration visible on funduscopy. Perhaps chronic choroidal ischemia plays a role in the genesis of low-tension glaucoma, choroidal sclerosis, and senile macular degeneration. In their study of ten patients showing acute choroidal ischemia Foulds, Lee, and Taylor (1971), using the FM 100-hue test, demonstrated a residual type III blue–yellow defect in six and a residual red–green defect in one. Three patients examined in the initial acute phase showed a gross disturbance of color discrimination without dominant axis. The authors concluded that the color analysis was supportive of evidence of damage to the pigment epithelium and neuroreceptors.

Diabetes*

Inadequate insulin activity in patients with diabetes mellitus results in metabolic disturbance. Ophthalmoscopically visible changes in the retinal blood vessels are universally accepted as part of the overall pattern of diabetic retinopathy. The development of tissue anoxia from inadequate circulation is presumed to be the primary factor in diminishing visual function. The incidence of blindness due to diabetic retinopathy is about 8 percent in the U.S. and about 10 percent in Tasmania and Great Britain (Adams, 1963; Dube, 1963). This section outlines some of the changes in the deterioration of vision that can be detected by means of various tests of color discrimination.

STUDIES BEFORE 1963

Most of the early published results concerning the color vision of diabetics were included in papers dealing with many other pathologic conditions. It has been only in the last 30 years that diabetics have been tested in greater numbers. Table 8.6 summarizes the data of Zanen (1953), Dubois-Poulsen and Cochet (1954), Hong (1957), Zanen, Szucs, and Pirart (1957), Zanen (1959), Cox (1961a), and Yonemura (1962). It is important to note that the majority of patients were above age 50 years; within recent years Lakowski (1962), Verriest (1963), and Ruddock (1965a, b) have shown that normal color vision deteriorates with age, especially for the blue–yellow axis. In other words, a true assessment of the apparent loss of color vision can be made only by taking into account the normal changes taking place with increasing age.

STUDIES SINCE 1963

Verriest (1964) published the results of several tests of color vision, including the Ishihara plates, Farnsworth Panel D-15, FM 100-hue test, and Nagel anomaloscope, obtained from a group of 20 diabetics of whom only 3 were without ophthalmoscopic evidence of retinopathy; 4 of the patients were under 30 years of age, the rest over 40, and acuities ranged from normal to 0.1. Verriest (1964) concluded that only 2 of the patients could be classified as normal; half of the group had abnormal Ishihara responses, half revealed a blue–yellow axis with the Farnsworth Panel D-15 test, and 8 of the 14 tested with the FM 100-hue test also revealed a blue–yellow axis. The Rayleigh equation tended to be displaced toward red, suggesting the existence of an absorption system. The data of this survey and the others mentioned earlier leave little doubt that diabetics develop type III blue–yellow defects, but information about how soon such a deficiency could be detected after diagnosis of the disease and whether or not younger diabetics with ophthalmoscopically normal fundi could be affected remains unknown.

A survey of over 500 diabetics was made in Edinburgh in the early 1960s to clarify some of these points (Kinnear, Aspinall, & Lakowski, 1972; Lakowski, Aspinall, & Kinnear, 1973). A fairly even age distribution from 10 to 70 years was obtained, more than half the sample being less than 40 years old. Patients with poor reading acuity were excluded. The Ishihara test showed no differences between diabetics and the general population except for diabetics over 60 years old. However, the data for the FM 100-hue test (Fig. 8.19a) and the green-blue equation of the Pickford-Nicolson anomaloscope (Fig. 8.19b) showed that the diabetics had considerably poorer color discrimination than the general population and that diabetics with observable fundus changes had poorer color discrimination than those with normal fundi. Incidentally, the severity of the retinopathy

---

*Contributed by Paul Kinnear, Ph.D.

Table 8.6
Color Vision Studies of Diabetics up to 1963

Author(s)	Total Tested	Total With Impairment	Total Normal	Age <50	Age >50	Tests and Equipment
Zanen (1953)	3	3	0	0	3	Brief hue exposures
Dubois-Poulsen & Cochet (1954)	9	7	2			Various tests
Hong (1957)	1	1	0			Nagel anomaloscope
Zanen, Szucs, & Pirart (1957)	11	*	*	5	6	Brief hue exposures
Zanen (1959)	1	1	0	0	1	Brief hue exposures
Cox (1961a)	5	5	0	0	5	Various tests including FM 100-hue test
Yonemura (1962)	36	30	6			ERG

*Data presented as means.

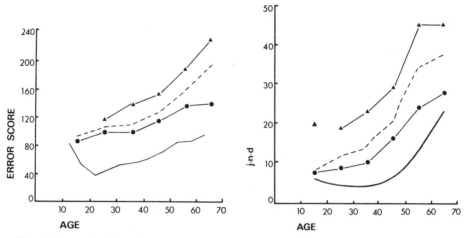

Fig. 8.19. (left) FM 100-hue test scores for categories of diabetics and for the general population. (right) Color discrimination data for categories of diabetics and for the general population expressed in units of just noticeable differences (jnd) for the green-blue equation of the Pickford-Nicolson anomaloscope. —, general population (Verriest, 1964); – – –, all diabetics (n = 467); ●—●, diabetics with apparently normal fundi (n = 324); ▲—▲, diabetics with signs of retinopathy (N = 143). [Data redrawn from Kinnear, Aspinall, & Lakowski (1972) and Lakowski, Aspinall, & Kinnear (1973).]

was generally very mild, since 65 percent of the group showed no more than a few microaneurysms. Attempts to predict color vision deterioration from clinical variables such as the duration of diabetes, the year of onset, and the level of blood-sugar control have not been successful. For example, many poorly controlled diabetics had good color discrimination, while many well-controlled diabetics did not. A full discussion is presented by Lakowski, Aspinall, and Kinnear (1973).

Barca and Vaccari (1978) tested 24 patients with diabetic retinopathy using the FM 100-hue test and reported that the diabetics had higher scores than the general population and that between 30 and 46 percent showed various degrees of type III blue–yellow defect.

In summary, diabetics are more liable than the general population to suffer a deterioration of color vision affecting the blue–yellow axis, indicative of neural deterioration within the retina. Furthermore, losses in color vision can occur before any ophthalmoscopic changes in the fundus are seen.

INFLAMMATORY CHORIOTAPETORETINAL DISEASE*

Anatomically, the ocular tissues on the inner side of the protective sclera envelope may be roughly separated into three zones, which from without inwards are as follows:

1. Tunica uvea—The larger part, lying posteriorly, is the choroid comprising blood vessels and pigment cells. Anteriorly is to be found the ciliary body and iris.
2. Tunica Ruyschiana—comprising the choriocapillaris, Bruch's membrane, and retinal pigment epithelium. This layer extends only as far as the choroid.
3. Tunica retina—comprising the retinal neuroreceptors and the neural conductive apparatus.

*Contributed by I. A. Chisholm, M.D.

Although each layer will be considered separately, this is a somewhat artificial division, since an inflammatory reaction in one layer will involve adjacent layers as well as distant parts of the same layer during the initial reaction or the late cicatricial stage.

Inflammation of the Choroid

Clinically, the most common indication of inflammation of the choroid is a round or oval soft-edged white or yellowish patch of exudation at a level deeper than that of the retinal vessels. There may be one or several discrete foci. The inflammatory reaction is manifested histologically by an aggregation of cells, fluid exudate, and vascular enlargement. The native pigmented cells become rounded and are displaced to the edge of the reaction, where they clump together or disintegrate with dispersal of pigment granules. Bruch's membrane acts as a barrier confining the reaction to the choroid, but perforation of this membrane allows migration of inflammatory cells and exudates into the retina (chorioretinitis) and vitreous fluid.

With subsidence of the acute phase, a flat white area with peripheral pigment clumping is left, indicating the former site of acute inflammation. At the points where Bruch's membrane was destroyed the retina and choroid adhere to one another, resulting in disorganization of the photoreceptors.

CHOROIDITIS

Choroiditis may accompany viral, bacterial, fungal, protozoal, or metazoal infection elsewhere in the body. The infecting agent may be carried by the bloodstream to the uveal tract, or the focus may be a manifestation of the allergically sensitized state of the choroidal cells to the toxic products of such a distant infection. On occasion, inflammation of the choroid may arise by extension of infection from the sclera (sclerouveitis) or retina (retinochoroiditis). The visual defect produced is variable, depending partly on the extent and the site of the inflammatory focus and partly on the presence of complicating edema of the macula or optic nerve head. An uncomplicated peripheral focus may pass unnoticed, while a focus at the macula will result in immediate central visual disturbance.

The presence of a type III acquired blue–yellow color defect arising in both the acute and cicatricial phases of choroiditis has been recognized since the studies of Galezowski (1868) and confirmed in recent times by François and Verriest (1957a), Cox (1960), Verriest (1964), François and Verriest (1968), Dubois-Poulsen (1972), Pinckers (1972b), and Legras and Coscas (1972) (see Table 8.7). Amongst the means of identifying the defect, plate tests, the Farnsworth Panel D-15 (Fig. 8.20), the FM 100-hue test, and the anomaloscope have been used. François and Verriest (1968) demonstrated that chorioretinal inflammation was responsible for not only a type III blue–yellow defect but also a type I red–green defect. The type I red–green defect could be identified only at an early stage of the process while good visual acuity was still retained.

Marré (1973), by examining the relative spectral sensitivity of the three CVMs (Chapter 6), found the earliest sign of choriotapetoretinal inflammation to be an isolated disturbance of the blue CVM. This can be recognized on the FM 100-hue test by a clustering of error scores into a monopolar or bipolar blue–yellow defect. At a later stage, the blue, green, and red CVMs were all affected, the blue mainly. With the FM 100-hue test, chromatic discrimination is severely impaired, resulting in high error scores without prominent axis.

Table 8.7
Acquired Color Vision Defects in Choroiditis

	Eyes Examined	Normal	Type I r-g Defect	Type III b-y Defect	Congenital and/or Unclassified Defects
François & Verriest (1957a)	15	4	—	6	5
Cox (1960)	6	2	—	4	—
François & Verriest (1968)	47	7	8	27	5
Pinckers (1972b)	27	13	—	11	3
Legras & Coscas (1972)	6	—	1	5	—

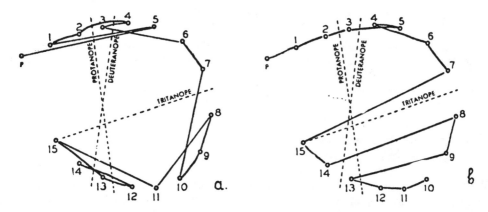

Fig. 8.20. Farnsworth Panel D-15 test results from a patient with chorioretinitis. (left) Acute clinical condition. (right) Healed clinical condition. [From François, J. & Verriest, G. *Annales d'Oculistique* (Paris), 1957, *190*, 894–943 (reproduced by permission).]

Verriest (1970b), studying the effect on the spectral curve of relative luminous efficiency in chorioretinitis, reported four normal curves, two with generalized flattening, and five with a sensitivity loss for long wavelengths. Verriest and Uvijls (1977a), studying increment threshold spectral sensitivity in five patients, found uniform sensitivity loss in the visible spectrum.

PERIPHERAL CHOROIDITIS—PARS PLANITIS—
CYCLITIS POSTERIOR

This clinical entity, orginally described by Schepens (1950), is characterized by an inflammatory reaction of the vitreous base, frequently bilateral and found in young adults. It is accompanied by the inflammatory stigmata of white gravitational deposits overlying the ora serrata, edema of the macula and optic nerve head, a vasculitis of the terminal retinal vessels, and an anterior uveitis. Sarcoidosis has been considered the most common underlying cause. In the series reported by Chester, Blach, and Cleary (1976) retinitis pigmentosa was associated in 12 percent and demyelinating disease in 14 percent of their patients. Although the initial visual loss may be severe, the prognosis in general is good regardless of therapy. The combination of vitreous haze and macular edema would be sufficient to cause the variable fall in visual acuity and type III acquired blue–yellow defect (Fig. 8.21).

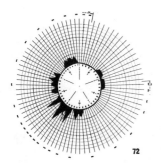

Fig. 8.21. FM 100-hue test plot from an 11-year-old girl with pars planitis.

Inflammation of the Pigment Epithelium

Under this heading are considered several conditions having common features in the acute phase. All show an initial inflammationlike reaction with focal exudation at the level of the choriocapillaris and retinal pigment epithelium. Subsequently, they show morphologic differences as the foci age. Fluorescein angiography is valuable in differentiating among the types.

ACUTE POSTERIOR MULTIFOCAL PLACOID PIGMENT EPITHELIOPATHY

This condition is characterized by acute visual loss coincident with the appearance of multiple yellowish-white plaques scattered over the posterior fundus and located at the level of the pigment epithelium. Rapid resolution of lesions occurs, with a permanent disturbance of the pigment epithelium and minimal upset to adjacent retina and choroid. Significant visual improvement occurs after apparent resolution of lesions. Reports of color vision studies, until recently, were confined to investigation in the late healed stage. Normal color vision on testing with plate test (Kirkham, Ffythe, & Saunders, 1972) and Farnsworth Panel D-15 (Laatikainen & Erkkila, 1973) have been reported. A type III acquired blue–yellow defect (Scuderi, Recupero, & Valvo, 1977) or elevated FM 100-hue test scores (Pinckers A: Personal communication) were found in the acute phase. Smith, Pokorny, and Ernest (1978) attribute the abnormal color match found at the anomaloscope to a physical disturbance of the photoreceptors.

SERPIGINOUS AND GEOGRAPHIC CHOROIDOPATHY

These are descriptive terms for an insidious disseminated choroidal inflammation characterized by multiple confluent foci of exudate and scar formation involving the choriocapillaris and retinal pigment epithelium. The acute lesion is a well-defined grayish-yellow area similar to acute posterior multifocal placoid pigment epitheliopathy and accompanied by overlying retinal edema. This is a slowly progressive condition that is not accompanied by prominent inflammatory signs within the eye. The condition is marked by recurring acute exacerbations over a period of years. Central vision is affected only when a lesion underlies the macula. In a study of six patients, color vision was within normal range in half the eyes examined; the FM 100-hue test error scores tended to be high normal without predominant axis (Pinckers A: Personal communication).

PIGMENT EPITHELIITIS

This is a self-limiting benign condition characterized by the finding of small black spots with a yellow halo and arranged in grapelike clusters (Krill & Deutman, 1972b). The spots are morphologically unique on fluorescein angiography. Attention is drawn to the condition by the complaint of blurred vision. These spots have been reported in association with central serous retinopathy and are considered by some to be healed pigment epithelial detachments (Gass, Norton, & Justice, 1966). As yet, no specific color vision disturbance has been reported in this condition. Normal color responses to testing with plate tests and Farnsworth Panel D-15 were reported by Deutman (1947b), and normal response to Ishihara and AO HRR plates, Lanthony's New Color Test, and the FM 100-hue test by Pinckers (Pinckers A: Personal communication).

CONGENITAL RUBELLA RETINOPATHY

This condition is characterized by collections of pigment varying from fine dustlike spots to clumps alternating with depigmented spots in either the central or peripheral fundus, often accompanied by optic disc pallor but not retinal vessel abnormality. A normal ERG response differentiates the condition from a congenital tapetoretinal degeneration, congenital syphilitic retinitis, or a pigmentary retinopathy secondary to radiation. Color vision studies using plate tests, the FM 100-hue test, and the anomaloscope were reported as normal (Krill, 1967; Franceschetti, François, & Babel 1974); Pinckers A (Personal communication).

Inflammation of the Retina

A series of conditions of the retina that show inflammatory signs and that are not retinopathies are grouped together under inflammation of the retina. These include retinitis secondary to inflammation of the walls of the retinal blood vessels—vasculitis, arteritis, or phlebitis.

RETINITIS

The retina is composed of two different types of tissue, the neural ectodermal tissue—comprising neurons, their connections, and neuroglia—and the mesenchymal tissue—composed of microglia and blood vessels. Each reacts differently to an acute inflammation. Local cell death, reactive hyperplasia, vasodilation, local tissue edema, and hemorrhage are found. The retinal pigment epithelium reacts to an acute inflammatory insult by cell death and release of pigment at the site. In more chronic inflammations the pigment cells proliferate and the blood vessels react by an endoarteritis.

On funduscopy the appearance of a healed retinitis is variable. Some instances may show multiple hyperpigmented spots, alternating hyperpigmented and depigmented spots (salt and pepper appearance), or demarcated geographic areas of retinal depigmentation with and without healed foci of choroiditis. All forms may be accompanied by sheathing of retinal vessels.

Primary retinitis, an uncommon event, is found when a blood-borne infection, bacterial, viral, fungal, or protozoal settles in the retina (acute suppurative retinitis, Roth septic retinitis). Such an inflammation can spread outward to involve the choroid. Secondary infections commonly arise in the uveal tract when the retina is involved by an inflammation already established in the eye. The visual deficit in both forms is identical, and the color vision abnormality makes no distinction between chorioretinitis and retinochoroiditis.

RETINAL PERIVASCULITIS

This is an inflammatory condition preferentially affecting the retinal veins (periphlebitis), more rarely the arteries (periarteritis), and sometimes both. The condition may not be associated with hemorrhage; nevertheless, a striking clinical feature is retinal and vitreous hemorrhage. When these are recurring (Eales disease), retinitis proliferans, retinal detachment, secondary cataract, and glaucoma may complicate the clinical picture. Retinal perivasculitis may be found secondary to uveitis in syphilis, sarcoidosis, Behçet disease, or pars planitis or in systemic disease in hemopoietic dysplasia, multiple connective tissue disorder, or neurologic disease such as multiple sclerosis, or as a primary perivasculitis (Eales disease).

Reports of color vision defects in retinal perivasculitis are few. François and Verriest (1968) reported normal responses in one eye, type III acquired blue–yellow defect in one eye, and a generalized depression of discrimination in two eyes.

CHORIOTAPETORETINAL HYPERPLASIA AND NEOPLASIA*

Benign Neoplasia and Hyperplasia

The various conditions under this heading can be subdivided into those that are accompanied by visual deficit and those that are not. The majority of these conditions do not cause visual disturbance. The benign neoplasias that do cause visual upsets do so by virtue of a pressure atrophy of adjacent neural tissue or an associated serous detachment.

BENIGN NEOPLASIA UNACCOMPANIED BY
VISUAL DISTURBANCE

Benign neoplasia and hyperplasia, which under normal conditions cause no upset in visual function, include solitary or grouped hyperplasia of the pigment epithelium (so-called bear-paw or cat-paw marks), diffuse choroidal melanosis as a part of melanosis bulbi or the nevus of Ohta, and benign choroidal melanoma.

BENIGN NEOPLASIA ACCOMPANIED BY
VISUAL DISTURBANCE

Benign neoplasia that may cause an upset in visual function due to their intrinsic growth include retinal or choroidal neurofibroma, which may exist alone or as part of Von Recklinghausen disease, choroidal hemangioma, which may be solitary or accompany glaucoma (Sturge-Weber syndrome), and racemose arteriovenous aneurysm of the retinal blood vessels, which can exist on its own or as part of the Wyburn-Mason syndrome.

Because of the lack of visual deficit, color vision analysis for many of these conditions has not been reported in the literature. Verriest (1964) and François and Verriest (1968) reported normal color responses in observers with benign choroidal nevi.

Malignant Neoplasia

Malignant neoplasias as part of their natural growth, lead to local retinal destruction and a serous retinal detachment. Among the conditions in this group may be found malignant melanoma of the choroid, secondary choroidal neoplasm, retinoblastoma, astrocytoma existing alone or as part of tuberosclerosis syndrome, and hemiangioblastoma as part of angiomatosis retinae or Von Hipple–Lindau disease. Visual function in an eye with a malignant neoplasm appears to depend on the size and location of the primary tumor and whether or not a serous detachment accompanies it (Fig. 8.22). A peripherally placed malignant tumor accompanied by a serous detachment will cause a type III acquired blue–yellow defect just as a peripherally placed rhegmatogenous retinal detachment does. The macular serous detachment caused by malignant choroidal melanoma gives rise to a variable color disturbance, including xanthopsia (Morax, 1925), a central scotoma for color objects (Kok–Van Alphen & Hagedoorn, 1960), and type III blue–yellow color vision defect (Verriest, 1964). François and Verriest (1968) analyzed the color responses from 15 eyes showing malignant choroidal melanoma and found in 8 a

---

*Contributed by I. A. Chisholm, M.D.

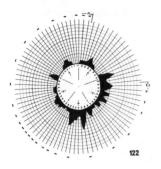

Fig. 8.22. FM 100-hue test result from an eye with a proven malignant melanoma of choroid before evidence of serous detached retina.

type III acquired blue–yellow defect. Kelecom (1963) reported a type III acquired blue–yellow defect in a patient suffering from carcinoma of the breast with metastatic involvement of the choroid.

GLAUCOMA*

During 1977 in Canada (population 22 million) there were 204 new blind registrations that were the result of "glaucoma" (Canadian National Institute for the Blind, 1977). The Ferndale Glaucoma Survey of 1965 (Hollows & Graham, 1966) showed an incidence of all types of glaucoma in the population aged 40 years and over of 0.84 percent—chronic simple glaucoma accounting for 0.43 percent—and nonglaucomatous ocular hypertension of 8.61 percent.

Elevation of the intraocular pressure above the normal range accompanied by functional change and structural damage to the eye is termed glaucoma. Sustained and prolonged elevation of the intraocular pressure may be accompanied by visual disturbance, sluggish pupil reaction, disturbance of dark (Ourgaud & Etienne, 1961) and color adaptation (Goldthwaite, Lakowski, & Drance, 1976), defects in the Bjerrum area of the visual field, color vision defect, lowering of the flicker fusion frequency (Campbell & Rittler, 1959), and an alteration in phase and amplitude of visually evoked responses (Cappin & Nissim, 1975). There are numerous causes of glaucoma (Table 8.8), each possessing its own special features in addition to those outlined above.

Table 8.8
Classification of Glaucoma

Congenital glaucoma	(Buphthalmos)
Primary glaucoma	Chronic simple glaucoma
	Angle closure glaucoma
Glaucoma secondary to:	Intraocular inflammation
	Intraocular neoplasia
	Ocular trauma
	Retinal vein occlusion
	Hypermature cataract
	Pseudoexfoliation of lens capsule
	Pigment dispension syndrome
	Raised intraorbital pressure
"Low-tension" glaucoma	
Corticosteroid-induced glaucoma	

*Contributed by I. A. Chisholm, M.D.

Ocular hypertension is present when elevation of the intraocular pressure is not accompanied by morphologic change of the optic nerve or glaucomatous visual field abnormality. Because a proportion of patients who show ocular hypertension undergo transition to chronic simple glaucoma, ocular hypertensive patients have been the focus of intensive clinical research in recent years. One subjective feature of chronic simple glaucoma, the most common of the primary glaucomas, is that of gradually failing vision. If the glaucoma is left untreated, the visual deterioration progresses to blindness. Acute angle closure glaucoma is a true ocular emergency in which the affected eye may become completely blind in a matter of hours. Even with prompt normalization of the intraocular pressure, evidence of functional damage to the eye is often found.

Color Vision Findings in the Glaucomas

The postulates of Köllner (1912) would lead one to expect a type II red–green color defect where the optic nerve was damaged by glaucoma. Examples of red–green defects have been reported (Engelking, 1925; Wessley, 1927; Köllner, 1929; Zimmerman, 1966) but are the exception rather than the rule; when present such defects are found in association with the late stage of glaucoma (Koliopoulos, 1978). Reduction in red sensitivity on perimetry (Rönne, 1911; Wessley, 1927), loss of the photochromatic interval for red (Pickard, 1938), and displacement toward the red in the Rayleigh equation (Verrey, 1926) have been recorded in glaucoma patients. Javal (1839–1907) suffered from red blindness long before he lost his sight completely from glaucoma—a clinical feature that Duke-Elder (1969) feels is atypical of glaucoma.

Numerous reports (François, Verriest, & DeRouck, 1957; François & Verriest, 1957a; 1959b; 1961b; 1968; Cox, 1960; Dubois-Poulsen & Mogis, 1961; Rey-Kokott, 1964; Verriest, 1964; LeGros, 1966; Kurata, 1967a; Ayres, 1967; Cvetkovic, 1967; Krill & Fishman, 1971) confirm that a type III blue–yellow defect with normal Rayleigh equation is the most common disturbance of color vision found in glaucoma from whatever cause. The spectral luminosity curve is normal. The evidence varies with the type of glaucoma and the sensitivity of the test used (Table 8.9). Next most frequently found is reduced color discrimination without prominent axis.

François, Verriest, and DeRouck (1957), in their study of functional parameters in 22 patients suffering from congenital glaucoma, found a significant incidence of type III acquired blue–yellow defect, testing with plate tests, Farnsworth Panel D-15 (Fig. 8.23), and Nagel anomaloscope.

A study of the pattern of visual damage after unilateral acute angle closure glaucoma by McNaught, Rennie, McClure, and Chisholm (1974) demonstrated significantly higher error scores on the FM 100-hue test for affected than for unaffected eyes (Fig. 8.24). The defect was type III blue–yellow defect, which was present only in 40 percent of the affected eyes studied. Only one affected eye revealed a type II red–green defect. The remaining affected eyes gave FM 100-hue test results within the normal range.

The detection of acquired dyschromatopsia in chronic simple glaucoma is test dependent. Most studies use the FM 100-hue test, and authors report a blue–yellow defect in over 30 percent of eyes examined and raised error scores without prominent axis in a further 30 percent. Numerous authors have their preference for a particular method of investigation—e.g., D and H color rule (Kalmus, Luke, & Seedburgh, 1974), Helmholtz-König color mixture apparatus (Grützner & Schleicher, 1972), Keely-Bristol plates (Marmion, 1978), FM 100-hue test (Fishman, Krill, & Fishman, 1974), and

Table 8.9
Color Defects in Glaucoma

		Reduced Color Discrimination (%)	Type I r-g Defect (%)	Type III b-y Defect (%)	Tests Used
Verriest (1964)	Chronic simple glaucoma	35	6	38	Plate tests, Farnsworth Panel D-15
	Angle closure glaucoma	49	4	30	FM 100-hue test, Nagel anomaloscope
Austin (1974)	Chronic simple glaucoma	13	—	49	FM 100-hue test
Kalmus, Luke, & Seedburgh (1974)	Chronic simple glaucoma	—	—	67	D & H color rule
	Angle closure glaucoma	—	—	57	

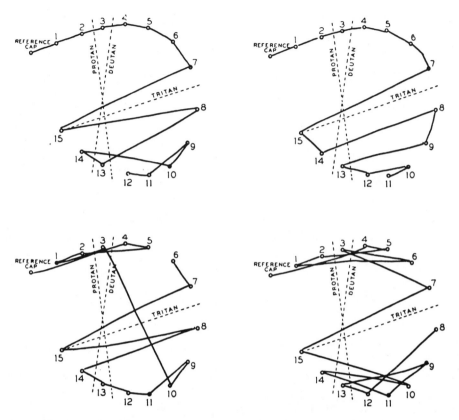

Fig. 8.23. Farnsworth Panel D-15 test results in congenital glaucoma. [From François, J., Verriest, G., & DeRouck, A. *Annales d'oculistique* (Paris), 1957, *189,* 81–107 (reproduced with permission of Doin, Editeur).]

Pickford-Nicolson anomaloscope (Lakowski, 1972)—and claim best results in their hands. Maione, Carta, Barberini, and Scoccianti (1976) studied the achromatic sensitivity of chronic simple glaucoma patients to red, green, and blue backgrounds and found a relative impairment for each mechanism similar to that found in optic neuritis. Glaucomatous field defects are more evident when the visual field is examined using a blue test object on a yellow background (Marré E: Personal communication).

Verriest (1964) and François and Verriest (1968) give extensive reviews of the literature in this field. In established chronic simple (open angle) glaucoma, Verriest (1964) reported normal color vision in 20 percent, moderate type III blue–yellow defect in 40 percent, severe type III blue–yellow defect in 32 percent, and a red–green defect in 6 percent.

Low-tension glaucoma is observed in elderly patients who show varying degrees of cardiovascular disease. Ocular examination shows the structural and some of the functional stigmata of glaucoma but in the presence of intraocular pressure within the normal range. This group forms a very small part of the pool of glaucoma patients. Color vision studies (François & Verriest, 1968) reported these patients to have a red–green defect (Fig. 8.25c).

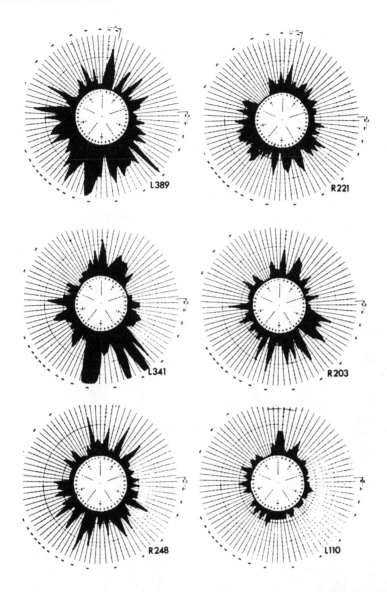

Fig. 8.24. Examples of FM 100-hue test patterns, following unilateral acute angle closure glaucoma. Affected eye (left) compared with unaffected eye. [From McNaught, E. I., Rennie, A., McClure, E., & Chisholm, I. A. *Transactions of the Ophthalmological Society of the United Kingdom,* 1974, *94,* 406–415 (reproduced with permission of the Ophthalmological Society of the United Kingdom).]

Modifying Influences on Color Vision in Glaucoma

The interpretation of the color vision screening results may be influenced by additional functional disturbances, which must be considered in the evaluation of the results.

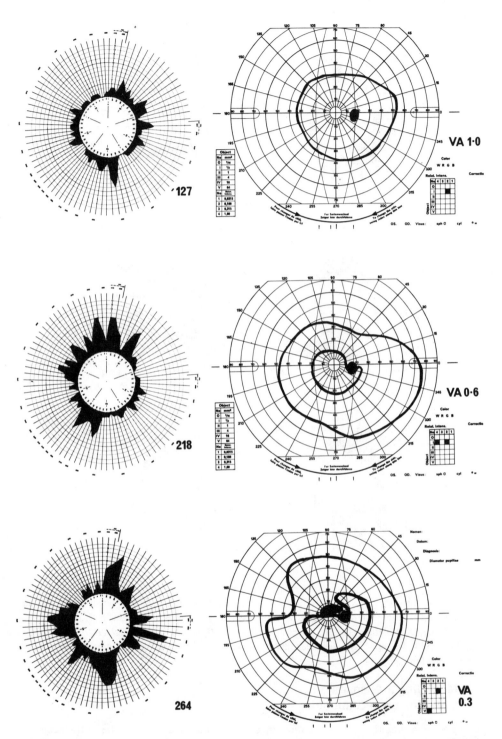

Fig. 8.25. Examples of visual fields and FM 100-hue test results from (top) ocular hypertension, (middle) mild–moderate chronic simple glaucoma, and (bottom) low-tension glaucoma.

AGE

The degree to which patient age influences individual test results has already been mentioned. Verriest (1964) showed that when age was taken into account the frequency of blue–yellow defects among the François and Verriest (1959b) patients was reduced.

VISUAL ACUITY

Untreated glaucoma results in progressive loss of vision. Such impairment of visual acuity may influence the result of color vision tests. Koliopoulos (1978) recommends a visual acuity of 0.6 or better for results to be meaningful. When visual acuity is lower, use of the Farnsworth Panel D-15 test is recommended.

PUPIL SIZE

Narrowing of the visual field by miosis (drug induced in glaucoma) can elicit a type III acquired blue–yellow defect recordable on the FM 100-hue test (Grützner & Schleicher, 1972; Marmion, 1978) or the Pickford-Nicolson anomaloscope (Lakowski & Oliver, 1974). A similar effect can be gained by lowering the luminance to a mesopic level. Vola, Leprince, Cornu, and Saracco (1978) found the average FM 100-hue test error score of 28 subjects to be 61.7 ± 26.9 at 2200 lux and 289.3 ± 170 at 0.2 lux. At 0.2 lux the error scores showed either a blue–yellow defect or a scotopic pattern.

Reversal of the miosis or increasing the illumination leads to improvement in the FM 100-hue test result and a less apparent type III acquired blue–yellow defect (Kurata, 1967a; Ourgaud, Vola, Jayle, & Daud, 1972) when present but has no influence on achromatic disturbances (Ourgaud, Vola, & Cornu, 1973). These features support the concept of mesopization of vision in glaucoma, as proposed by Ourgaud and Etienne (1961) and Verriest (1964). Additional support came from the report of Bessière, LeRebeller, Vallat, & Rougier-Houssin (1971), who found in early untreated glaucoma patients that the FM 100-hue test error score correlated with the loss in absolute sensitivity of mesopic visual acuity and visual field defect.

FIELD OF VISION

When color vision tests are administered it is central foveal vision that is being assessed; however, this is the last area of the field of vision to be affected by glaucomatous damage in chronic simple glaucoma. Several studies have shown a relation between the degree of color vison defect and amount of visual field loss in chronic simple glaucoma. The greater the loss of visual field, the greater the discrepancy in hue discrimination (Grützner & Schleicher, 1972; Fishman, Krill, & Fishman, 1974; Austin, 1974) (Fig. 8.25). This is not an invariable relationship; color vision defects may be apparent before visual field defects (Fishman, Krill, & Fishman, 1974; Lakowski, Bryett, & Drance, 1972) or the color sense may be normal in the presence of visual field defects (Legros, 1966; Koliopoulos, Mangouritsas, & Andreanos, 1975). In angle closure glaucoma no correlation between the degree of hue discrimination loss and duration of raised intraocular pressure or field loss could be elicited (McNaught, Rennie, McClure, & Chisholm, 1974).

Ocular Hypertension and Transition to Chronic Simple Glaucoma

In the population there exists a percentage of people over the age of 40 years [8.61 percent in the Ferndale Survey (Hollows & Graham, 1966)] with elevated intraocular pressure in the absence of any glaucomatous findings. A proportion of these subjects do

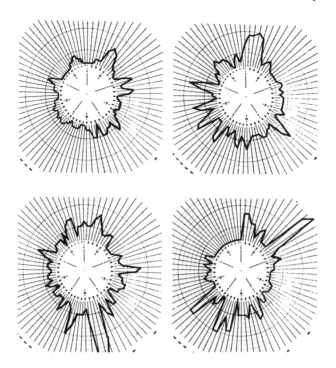

Fig. 8.26. Examples of FM 100-hue test patterns in ocular hypertension. [From Lakowski, R., Bryett, J., & Drance, S. M. *Canadian Journal of Ophthalmology,* 1972, 7, 86–95 (reproduced with permission of the Canadian Journal of Ophthalmology).]

develop chronic simple glaucoma after a number of years. The color vision characteristics of ocular hypertensive patients have been examined to evaluate their predictive value in determining which patients will develop chronic simple glaucoma. Type III blue–yellow hue discrimination losses have been identified (Lakowski, 1972; Lakowski, Bryett, & Drance, 1972; Fishman, Krill, & Fishman, 1974; Kalmus, Luke, & Seedburgh, 1974; Lakowski & Drance, 1978; Marmion, 1978) in ocular hypertensive subjects on testing with the FM 100-hue test (Fig. 8.26), Pickford-Nicolson anomaloscope (Fig. 8.27), or the D and H color rule. Test performance was significantly poorer then that of equivalent control subjects. The color vision tests indicated large variations in performance from near perfect to near achromatic. Lakowski and Drance (1978) suggest the FM 100-hue test and the Pickford-Nicolson anomaloscope to be the most sensitive of the clinical color tests. By their use they found 20 percent of 250 ocular hypertensives studied to possess an extensive color vision defect equivalent to that found in severe glaucoma; 9 of the patients studied over a period of 5 years developed chronic simple glaucoma. The color vision test results obtained from these patients while they were still ocular hypertensive showed discrimination losses. Lakowski and Drance (1978) consider large losses in color vision to be an important risk factor in the transition of ocular hypertension to chronic simple glaucoma.

Goldthwaite, Lakowski, and Drance (1976) carried out a study of dark adaptation using blue-green and yellow chromatic stimuli with normal and ocular hypertensive subjects. Deterioration of the dark-adaptation curve to blue-green and, to a lesser extent,

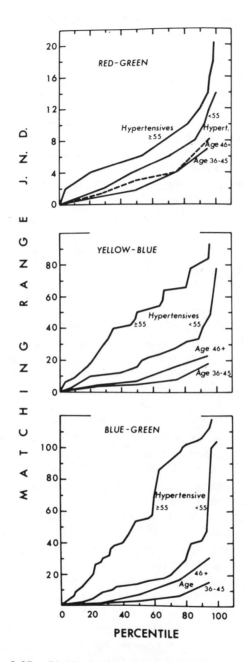

Fig. 8.27. Pickford-Nicolson anomaloscope findings. Comparison of matching ranges (discrimination) of ocular hypertensive subjects compared with various age groups of control subjects. [From Lakowski, R., Bryett, J., & Drance, S. M. *Canadian Journal of Ophthalmology,* 1972, 7, 86–95 (reproduced with permission of the Canadian Journal of Ophthalmology).]

yellow chromatic stimuli was found in the ocular hypertensive patients. There was also evidence of abnormal cone–rod transition among the ocular hypertensive subjects. Six glaucoma patients were also studied, and their adaptation curves were more abnormal.

Experimentally Induced Ocular Hypertension

The effect of raising the intraocular pressure in nonglaucomatous normal subjects on the field of vision (Drance, 1962), flicker fusion frequency (FFF)(Zuege and Drance, 1967), dark adaptation, and FM 100-hue test performance has been studied. Foulds, Chisholm, and Reid (1972) and Foulds, Chisholm, and Bronte-Stewart (1974) raised the intraocular pressure by suction cup or ophthalmodynamometer and produced a reversible type III acquired blue–yellow defect (Fig. 8.28) in a normal subject whose intraocular pressure had been raised to 40–50 mm Hg for 10 minutes. It was felt that the time taken for recovery may be of predictive value in indicating susceptibility to raised intraocular pressure.

DISORDERS OF THE VISUAL PATHWAYS AND HIGHER VISUAL CENTERS*

The nerve fibers comprising the optic nerves originate from the retinal neurones of the ganglion layer. At the optic chiasma there is a partial decussation of the fibers from each optic nerve (Fig. 8.29). The fibers arising from the nasal half of the retina (comprising 53 percent of the total in each nerve) cross, and they interdigitate with the fibers from the opposite temporal retina. The resultant blend of fibers constitutes the optic tract. Thus each optic tract contains nerve fibers bound for the ipsilateral cerebral hemisphere, conveying information arising from stimuli in the contralateral fields of vision of both eyes. Following a synapse in the lateral geniculate body, nerve impulses are conveyed to the striate cortex of the occipital cerebral cortex via the optic radiations. Because of the known anatomic arrangement of the visual fibers and their topographic representation in the visual field, examination of the patient's field of vision may yield information of a localizing value and thus of importance in a variety of neuroophthalmic conditions, as demonstrated by Traquair (1949).

Damage by compression or distortion to the visual pathways results in a disturbance of neural conductivity that is reflected by depressed visual function, which may include modification or abolition of color sensation. The color sensation for red was claimed more vulnerable than that for white (Wilbrand & Saenger, 1913; Traquair, 1949; Huber, 1961) but quantitative perimetry is more sensitive than the older forms of color perimetry in the investigation of visual pathway disease (Dubois-Poulsen, 1952) (see Chapter 6, Perimetry). This sort of disturbance of the color sensation frequently precedes the visible manifestations of atrophy at the optic disc and thus becomes of important diagnostic significance as an early sign of a retrobulbar disturbance of conductivity (Huber, 1961). Although peripheral disturbances of visual pathway conductivity are the principal causes of color vision defects in connection with intracranial tumors, color vision abnormalities are also observed in lesions of the visual cortex and higher visual centers.

Marré's (1973) analysis based on the CVMs (Chapter 6) in patients with nerve pathway disease demonstrated a disturbance of the blue CVM as an early transient stage. This was succeeded by combined disturbance of blue, green, and red CVMs (Chapter 6).

---

*Contributed by I. A. Chisholm, M.D.

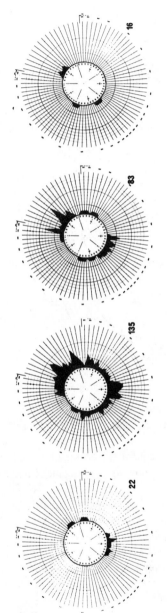

Fig. 8.28. Experimental elevation of intraocular pressure. Transient acquired blue–yellow defect following maintenance of intraocular pressure at 40 mm for 10 min. Note return of error score to subject's normal values. Sequence of patterns from left to right: hypertension; immediately after hypertension for 10 min; after 15 min; after 2 hours.

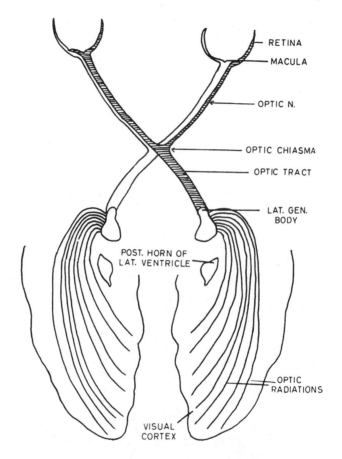

Fig. 8.29. Drawing of the visual pathways.

In the early blue CVM disturbance, wavelength discrimination is reduced throughout the spectrum, the luminosity curve is normal, and colorimetric purity discrimination is reduced for shorter wavelengths. In the combined disturbance of all three CVMs wavelength discrimination and colorimetric purity discrimination are both reduced and the luminosity curve varies from normal to showing displacement to either long or short wavelengths.

A history of visual hallucinations is of some significance in suspected neurologic disease. Unformed transient colored phenomena—"flashes of light," "showers of sparks" (phosphenes)—may arise from local retinal disease or cerebrovascular insufficiency, or as a prelude to a migraine headache. Formed colored hallucinations, on the other hand, are of definite significance—stories of "pink elephants" or "green men" are encountered in chronic ethyl alcohol toxicity and as part of the aura in temporal lobe epilepsy.

The afterimage of a color sequence following retinal stimulation by a white light, so called "flight of colors," has been used in the diagnosis of retinal and visual pathway pathology (Berry, 1927; Bender & Kahn, 1949). A high degree of correlation has been found between the presence of central color vision on both sides of the midline of an eye and the presence of "flight of colors." Disturbance of the visual pathways serving central vision on either side of the vertical meridian results in feeble or absent "flight of colors" (Feldman, Todman, & Bender, 1974).

Central color vision analysis does not have the localizing value that peripheral color vision analysis has, and its role is limited to exclusion of local ocular disorders in those neuroophthalmic conditions with visual symptomatology. The incidence of acquired color vision defects declines from 78 percent in optic neuritis and 67 percent in chiasmal syndromes to 57 percent in retrochiasmal disorders (Vola, Riss, Jayle, Gosset, & Tassy, 1972).

Serial color vision studies have been used in the followup assessment of patients recovering from optic neuritis: Chisholm, Bronte-Stewart, and Awduche (1970) studied the rate of recovery from the toxic optic neuropathy induced by tobacco (tobacco amblyopia) when treated with vitamin B_{12}, and Pinckers (1970) studied the treatment of acute optic neuritis with systemic corticosteroids. Both of these reports relied on the FM 100-hue test. Earlier, Riddell (1936) had followed recovery from tobacco amblyopia (with serial Ishihara plate readings) and noted that although visual acuity had apparently returned to normal levels, plate test errors were made.

Optic Nerve and Optic Disc

The optic nerve, some 2–3 inches long, passes backwards within the orbit from the eyeball through the optic foramen of the sphenoid bone to gain the middle cranial fossa and the optic chiasma. The nerve is enclosed in sheaths similar to and continuous with the meningeal sheaths of the brain. These sheaths blend with the sclera around the point of exit of the optic nerve from the eyeball. The optic disc marks the internal commencement of the optic nerve as viewed ophthalmoscopically.

PRIMARY HEREDITARY OPTIC ATROPHIES*

The primary hereditary optic atrophies include Leber hereditary optic atrophy, autosomal dominant optic atrophy, sex-linked recessive optic atrophy, congenital or infantile optic atrophy, and Behr optic atrophy. Table 8.10 summarizes the ophthalmoscopic findings and color vision defects in these primary hereditary optic atrophies.

Leber hereditary optic atrophy.   Leber hereditary optic atrophy (Leber disease, Leber optic atrophy, Leber hereditary optic neuritis) is a bilateral disease of unknown cause first recognized by Leber (1871a). Among whites the disease affects primarily males between the ages of 18 and 23 years; more rarely, females are affected, but with later age of onset. The mechanism of inheritance is unclear, since the disease does not follow classical patterns of X-chromosome–linked inheritance. A particular anomaly is that no daughter of an affected male has transmitted the disease (Lundsgaard, 1944; van Senus, 1963). Leber disease does not show linkage with deuteranomaly (Grützner & Schrapp, 1974). Went has emphasized the occurrence of mild neurologic symptoms in Leber disease (De Weerdt & Went, 1971; Went, 1972).

The disease usually has an acute onset with loss of vision to a visual acuity of 0.1 and a dense central scotoma. François, Verriest, François, and Asseman (1960; 1961), Verriest (1963), Grützner (1966), and Foulds, Chisholm, Bronte-Stewart, and Reid (1970) have reported that a type II defect accompanies the loss in acuity. Recently, Nikoskelainen, Sogg, Rosenthal, Fribert, and Dorfman (1977) have studied the color vision in a family with Leber optic atrophy and were able to observe the progress of the disease in its early stages. In their cases the onset was insidious. They described

*Contributed by Joel Pokorny, Ph.D., and Vivianne C. Smith, Ph.D.

Table 8.10

Color Defects in Primary Hereditary Optic Atrophies

Name	Inheritance	Symptoms	Eyegrounds	Visual Acuity	Color Defect
Leber hereditary optic atrophy	?	Headache, vertigo, loss of vision, mild neurologic symptoms	Initial papillitis followed by temporal optic atrophy	0.1, generally stationary	Type II
Autosomal dominant optic atrophy	Autosomal dominant	Reduced visual acuity noticed at school age	Temporal pallor	0.1–0.67, mild progression	Type III (most common); type II
Sex-linked optic atrophy	X-chromosome-linked recessive	Reduced vision, mild neurologic symptoms	Atrophy of entire disc	0.02–0.4, mild progression	Unclassified severe defect
Congenital or infantile optic atrophy	Autosomal recessive	Reduced visual acuity in infancy	Atrophy of entire disc	0.1, stationary	Type II or achromatopsia
Behr optic nerve atrophy	Autosomal recessive	Reduced acuity in infancy, psychomotor retardation pyramidal tract signs	Temporal optic atrophy	0.1–0.33, stationary	Type II or achromatopsia

Based in part on material presented by Smith, Pokorny, and Ernest: Primary hereditary optic atrophies. In *Krill's Hereditary Retinal and Choroidal Diseases, Vol. II. Clinical Characteristics*. A.E. Krill & D.B. Archer, (Eds.), Hagerstown: Harper & Row, 1977 (reproduced with permission of Harper & Row).

abnormalities of color vision, measured with the FM 100-hue test, that preceded visual acuity loss. Abnormalities of the visual evoked cortical potential paralleled the visual acuity loss. The authors confirmed that a type II acquired color defect occurs in Leber optic atrophy. In one of their patients, a 19-year-old male with Leber optic atrophy, the initial examination revealed the left eye to be affected with visual acuity of 0.1. The right eye had vision of 1.2 but showed an abnormal error accumulation above 100 on the FM 100-hue test. Three months later the visual acuity of the left eye had dropped to finger counting at 30 cm, that of the right eye to 0.07. On color vision examination there was a severe type II acquired color defect in the right eye. The test result on the FM 100-hue test is shown in Fig. 8.30.

Specialized psychophysical tests of wavelength discrimination and neutral-point matching were made by Grützner (1966). In one patient with Leber optic atrophy and a visual acuity of 0.2, the wavelength discrimination curve showed a U-shaped function with minimum at 490 nm. This result is comparable to that with congenital red–green defects. There was a wide neutral range for a 2° field extending from 520 to 650 nm. In a patient with seriously reduced vision (0.03) the neutral range for a 4° field extended from 460 to 700 nm. The neutral range findings differ from those in congenital red–green defect, where the neutral point is narrow and coincides with optimal wavelength discrimination. In acquired type II red–green defect the neutral range is wide and coincides with the spectral region of deficient chromatic discrimination.

The cause of Leber disease is unknown, although suggestions include an inborn error of cyanide metabolism (Adams, Blackwood, & Wilson, 1966) or a virus (Colenbrander, 1962). Biochemical studies (Chisholm & Pettigrew, 1970) have supported the concept of defective cyanide detoxification in Leber optic atrophy. Adams, Blackwood, and Wilson (1966) advocated treatment with vitamin B_{12}. Such treatments were performed by Fould, Chisholm, Bronte-Stewart, and Reid (1970) who found no improvement in 20 cases of long-standing atrophy; however, they reported an improvement in visual acuity coincident with start of treatment with hydroxycobalamin in five of six patients with recent Leber optic atrophy. Visual acuity improvement was paralleled by a reduction in error score on the FM 100-hue test. The acuity gains were modest: in the five patients showing improvement, the pretreatment acuities ranged from 0.016 to 0.05, posttreatment acuities from 0.05 to 0.17. Chisholm and Bronte-Stewart (1972) suggest that visual improvement may reflect the action of hydroxycobalamin in the regeneration of damaged neurons.

Autosomal dominant optic atrophy. This is a relatively benign disease of unknown pathology (Kjer, 1959). The diagnosis is made by evaluating several diagnostic criteria in the members of a suspected family. The major factors indicating a positive diagnosis

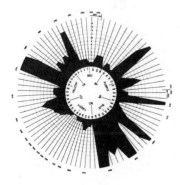

Fig. 8.30. FM 100-hue test errors from a patient with Leber optic atrophy. The visual acuity was less than 0.1. [From Nikoskelainen, E., Sogg, R. L., Rosenberg, ˙A. R., Friberg, T. R., & Dorfman, L. J. *Archives of Ophthalmology*, 1977, *95*, 969–978 (reproduced with permission of the American Medical Association, copyright 1977).]

include (1) the dominant inheritance pattern, (2) slightly to moderately reduced visual acuity, (3) temporal pallor of the optic disc, (4) color defect, and (5) subtle visual field abnormalities. As in many diseases of dominant inheritance, inter- and intrafamilial variability of symptoms is a keynote of the disease. The ophthalmoscopic finding is of optic disc pallor. There is variability in the degree and extent of the pallor. Pallor usually involves the temporal optic disc but may occasionally include the entire optic disc. Normal-appearing optic discs may occur in some family members. There is wide inter- and intrafamilial variability in the visual acuity. The visual acuity usually ranges from 0.67 to 0.1 but may be normal or as low as 0.02. It is possible to find pedigrees in the literature with acuities of affected members ranging from 1.2 to 0.05. Both eyes are usually affected to a similar degree, although there are numerous exceptions. The visual acuity loss may or may not be progressive.

A type III blue–yellow color defect occurs as the most usual color defect in autosomal dominant optic atrophy (Jaeger, 1954; Kjer, 1959; Cox, 1960; 1961a, b; Verriest, 1963; Grützner, 1963b; François, 1966; 1968; Krill, Smith, & Pokorny, 1970; 1971; Smith, 1972a, b, c). This defect can be observed in cases with minimal visual acuity defect (1.0–0.67) (Krill, Smith, & Pokorny, 1970; 1971). The color defect may precede evidence of optic disc pallor in young patients (Jaeger, 1954). Red–green discrimination may also be affected in the most severe cases when visual acuity is poor, resulting in almost complete color blindness (François, 1966; 1968). Thus when only pseudoisochromatic screening plates are used an apparent type II color defect may be reported (Jaeger, 1954; Kjer, 1959; François, 1966; 1968; Krill, Smith, & Pokorny, 1970; 1971). If blue–yellow screening plates are not available, the Farnsworth Panel D-15 test may be used. However, the most sensitive clinical test for establishing the existence of the type III color defect is the FM 100-hue test (Smith, 1972a).

Krill, Smith, and Pokorny's (1970; 1971) data are typical of the many reports of clinical color vision testing in autosomal dominant optic atrophy. On the FM 100-hue test seven of ten patients showed a clearcut blue–yellow axis. Three of ten patients, including two with visual acuities of 0.2 or worse, showed mixed blue–yellow and red–green axes. Typical error accumulations on the FM 100-hue test are shown in Fig. 8.31. The Rayleigh equations showed normal midpoints. The matching width was enlarged in two patients,

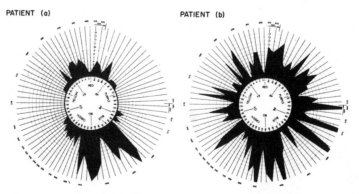

Fig. 8.31. FM 100-hue test errors from two patients in a single family with hereditary dominant atrophy. (a) Patient with visual acuity of 0.6 shows a blue–yellow axis. (b) Patient with visual acuity of 0.1 shows a mixed blue–yellow and red–green axis. [From Krill, A. E., Smith, V. C., & Pokorny, J. *Journal of the Optical Society of America,* 1970, *60,* 1132–1139 (reproduced with permission of the Optical Society of America).]

one of whom had a visual acuity below 0.1. On the AO HRR pseudoisochromatic plates nine of ten patients missed one or both of the B-Y screening plates. Four patients made errors on the R-G plates, including two patients with visual acuities of 0.2 or worse. Specialized psychophysical testing has included neutral-point and wavelength discrimination, spectral color matching, and color naming. Krill, Smith, and Pokorny (1970; 1971) found that six patients could match spectral wavelengths between 579 and 585 nm to a white light. The match ranges were 1–5 nm for five observers; one observer, with visual acuity of 0.1, had a wide match range of 13 nm. All of these patients showed confusion colors; they could match a spectral violet to a spectral green.

Grützner (1963a) also has reported wide neutral ranges for a 2° field in patients with autosomal dominant optic atrophy. The majority of his patients had severely impaired visual acuity. Grützner (1963b) measured wavelength discrimination for a 2° field in four families with autosomal dominant optic atrophy. The functions ranged from those appearing similar to functions obtained in tritanopia (Chapter 7) to those that showed a single minimum at 590–610 nm.

Using two patients with acuities of 0.67 or better and well-defined neutral points, Krill, Smith, and Pokorny (1971) measured color-matching characteristics and found them identical with those reported for congenital tritanopia (Chapter 7). Some autosomal dominant optic atrophy patients, with minimal visual acuity deficit, have the color vision characteristics of congenital tritanopia.

Smith, Cole, and Isaacs (1973) have reported color naming in two patients with autosomal dominant optic atrophy, one with good visual acuity (1.0) and one with poor visual acuity (0.1). The color-naming behavior showed a severe desaturation of the spectrum at short and middle wavelengths. For the patient with 0.1 vision, apparent desaturation was evident between 470 and 570 nm, indicative of a wide neutral zone comparable to the data of Grützner.

There have been reports that occasionally a type II red–green color defect may occur without a type III color defect. Waardenburg (1957), Kok–van Alphen (1960; 1970), François and Verriest (1968), Früh and Lauer (1971), and Jaeger, Früh, and Lauer (1972), have reported such red–green defects. Aulhorn and Grützner (1969) have reported a pedigree with red–green defect and long-wave luminosity loss similar to that of the protanope. The color defect is not comparable to the type I acquired color defect observed in cone degenerations (see Chapter 4), where the long-wavelength luminosity loss is between that of protanopes and achromats (Grützner, 1961). Jaeger, Früh, and Lauer (1972) suggested that autosomal dominant optic atrophy involves at least three separate types of color defect, which may represent separate genetic entities.

X-chromosome–linked optic atrophy.   Recently (Völker-Dieben, Van Lith, Went, Klawer, Staal, & de Vries–de Mol, 1974; Went, de Vries–de Mol, & Völker-Dieben, 1975) there were reports of a family in which optic atrophy was inherited with an X-chromosome–linked recessive pattern. The pedigree extended over four generations. The onset was early, with a severe reduction in visual acuity (0.1) evident in the youngest patient, age 8 years. The visual fields test showed an enlarged blind spot or paracentral scotoma. The optic discs were completely pale, and there were mild neurologic abnormalities. Ophthalmoscopic and neurologic examination was normal in the carrier female.

Color vision testing included the AO HRR and Ishihara plate tests, the Farnsworth Panel D-15, and the Nagel anomaloscope. The patients showed an unclassified strong color vision defect on the plate tests and the Farnsworth Panel D-15. Anomaloscope matches showed a wide matching range including the normal match.

Infantile optic atrophy. This (or congenital optic atrophy) is an extremely rare disease with autosomal recessive inheritance. Symptoms include nystagmus, sluggish pupils, pallor of the optic discs, and reduced vision evident at or soon after birth. The visual acuity is usually 0.1. François (1966; 1968) and Waardenburg (1956) have noted a severe acquired color vision defect. This defect may involve a type II dyschromatopsia or even complete achromatopsia.

Behr optic nerve atrophy. This (or Behr disease, complicated infantile optic atrophy) has autosomal recessive inheritance. It is associated with central nervous system signs (minimal psychomotor retardation and pyramidal tract signs of increased tendon reflexes, loss of coordination, spastic gait, muscular rigidity, Babinski sign, weakness of the sphincter of the bladder with incontinence, and often congenital deformity of the feet). There is severe psychomotor retardation initially, but this improves, and many of the affected individuals are eventually able to lead relatively normal lives. There may be nystagmus. There is a temporal pallor of both optic discs. The retinal vessels and retinae are normal. The visual acuity varies between 0.33 and 0.1. There is a gradual loss of visual acuity over several years, after which vision stabilizes and may even improve or appear to improve as the child's mental status becomes better. Franceschetti (1968) has reported presence of either a very severe type II color defect or complete achromatopsia. The type II color defect has also been noted by Dubois-Poulsen (1972).

ACUTE OPTIC NEURITIS*

Optic neuritis (retrobulbar neuritis and papillitis) refers to a group of diseases in which the optic nerve is primarily affected. As used clinically, the term does not necessarily mean that the diseases are inflammatory. Causes of optic neuritis do include inflammatory diseases (meningitis and sinusitis) but include also demyelinating diseases (multiple sclerosis, Devic disease) and vascular disease (giant-cell arteritis, metabolic disease). Generally, the visual acuity is reduced, and there is a central scotoma.

Most authors (François & Verriest, 1957a; Cox, 1960; 1961a, b; François & Verriest, 1968; Nikoskelainen, 1975) who have examined color vision in optic neuritis agree that a type II red–green color defect occurs no matter what the cause of the optic neuritis; however Ohta (1970) has reported blue–yellow defects. The Rayleigh equation and relative luminosity values are normal (Verriest, 1963). There is a large error accumulation on the FM 100-hue test with a predominant red–green axis. With severe visual acuity loss there is achromatopsia. In a disease such as multiple sclerosis that shows a fluctuating course, the color vision defects also fluctuate, paralleling the disease process (Cox, 1960; Wildberger & van Lith, 1976). Even after recovery of visual acuity to 1.0, there may be a persistent type II color vision defect (Cox, 1960; Scheibner & Thranberend, 1974; Wildberger & van Lith, 1976).

Specialized psychophysical tests of color vision in optic neuritis have included luminosity studies, neutral zone determination, and wavelength discrimination. Cox (1961b) has reported luminosity functions and wavelength discrimination in two patients with retrobulbar neuritis. The HFP luminosity curve was normal; the wavelength discrimination curve showed elevated thresholds for wavelengths above 490 nm. Grützner (1966) studied luminosity, wavelength discrimination, and neutral points in retrobulbar

---

*Contributed by I. A. Chisholm, M.D.

neuritis also, and Grützner noted normal luminosity, but Verriest (1970b), using heterochromatic flicker photometry (Chapter 6), has noted that some cases show a relative increase in sensitivity at short wavelengths. The wavelength discrimination function in a mild case shows poor overall chromatic discrimination, with a neutral zone near 550 nm; in a severe case the wavelength discrimination function is virtually unattainable through the majority of the spectrum, and large $\Delta\lambda$ steps may be obtained only in the regions of 480 and 590 nm. The neutral zone extends from 560 nm to the blue-green and to the long-wavelength spectral extreme. Scheibner and Thranberend (1974) measured wavelength discrimination in a patient 4 months after the onset of optic neuritis in one eye; the wavelength discrimination steps remained elevated for wavelengths above 490 nm in the affected eye, although the visual acuity had already returned to normal.

Although the shape of the luminosity curve may be normal, Verriest and Uvijls (1977a) have shown in eight of ten cases that the increment sensitivity is uniformly reduced at the fovea and at extrafoveal locations. In two of their cases they also noted a secondary peak at 450 nm 6° parafoveally, indicating sparing of the sensitivity to short wavelengths.

The Wald-Marré technique (Marré, 1970) has demonstrated an overall diminution in all three CVMs in optic neuritis. Zisman, Bhargava, and King-Smith (1977) used chromatic flicker detection on white backgrounds in two patients with optic neuritis. The first patient was unable to detect flicker rates above 25 Hz and showed greatly diminished sensitivity to rates between 7 and 25 Hz. With a 1 Hz repetition rate the sensitivity function resembled in shape the normal function obtained at 25 Hz. This patient showed no evidence of color-opponent response and had greatly reduced overall sensitivity. The second patient showed a normal 1 Hz function but reduced flicker sensitivity above 7 Hz. According to the authors, the data on this patient suggest a differential affect of the neuritis—large, fast-responding fibers mediating high-frequency achromatic response were more affected than the small, slow-responding fibers mediating the low-frequency color-opponent response.

Kurata (1965) felt that a red–green defect was atypical in the acute phase of optic neuritis but was typical in the atrophic stage. In this he was supported by Ohta (1970), who studied the patients with the Farnsworth Panel D-15 and Ohta 40-hue tests and found that patients showed a type III acquired blue–yellow defect more frequently than a type II acquired red–green defect. Enoch and Sunga (1969), in retrobulbar neuritis, found fatigue of retinal sensitivity when studied with quantitative perimetry. They referred to this as visual fatigue or saturation like syndrome and discovered that it was more obvious at high luminance levels.

CHRONIC OPTIC NEURITIS

Whereas acute optic neuritis tends to be unilateral, chronic neuritis may be bilateral. The slow onset and the gradual increase in the severity of symptoms with little tendency toward spontaneous recovery in chronic optic neuritis forms a sharp contrast with the features for acute optic neuritis. Essentially, the chronic condition presents in two ways—a peripheral constriction or a focal depression of the visual field. A generalized depression of optic nerve conduction characterized by peripheral constriction of the visual fields and optic atrophy is a clinical picture found in tertiary syphilis, mercury toxicity (Minamata disease), subacute myeloopticoneuropathy, and some instances of external compression of the optic nerve by neoplasm or osteitis deformans. Color vision studies in *tabes* involvement of the optic nerve have revealed a type II acquired red–green defect (Verriest, 1964; François & Verriest, 1968; Pinckers, 1971).

Ohta (1970), analyzing patients suffering from subacute myeloopticoneuropathy, noted a predominance of type II acquired red–green defect that differed from his findings in acute retrobulbar neuritis (see above). Matsuo, Okabe, Ueno, Takabatake, and Maeta (1971) studied 37 patients with subacute myeloopticoneuropathy: 10 patients showed optic atrophy, and of these, 8 had a type II acquired red–green defect and one a type III acquired blue–yellow defect; of the remaining 27 patients, 18 gave normal color responses to the Farnsworth Panel D-15 test and the FM 100-hue test, 5 showed a gradual color loss, 3 a type II acquired red–green defect, and 1 a type III acquired blue–yellow defect.

The focal depression of the visual field, characteristic of the toxic optic neuropathy (toxic amblyopia) in which there is specific depression of the central and centrocaecal areas of the visual field, is found in association with a variety of nutritional deficiencies and toxic agents. The clinical findings include reduced visual acuity, depressed sensitivity (greater for color than white) in the centrocaecal area of the field of vision, and a type II acquired red–green defect. Usually the eyes are unequally involved, and the central vision may be sufficiently depressed that vision is achromatic.

In Europe toxic optic neuropathy is frequently observed, mostly in tobacco amblyopia, which is almost exclusively a disease of the elderly, undernourished, tobacco-smoking male. The condition is associated with an altered vitamin B_{12} status and the presence of impaired cyanide detoxification. The retrobulbar neuritis of pernicious anemia and that of diabetes, when the patient is a smoker, are indistinguishable from tobacco amblyopia. Certain features in the clinical course of Leber hereditary optic atrophy and topical ataxic neuropathy are similar also, and they may be classed along with the toxic optic neuropathies. Chronic retrobulbar neuritis has been recorded in patients showing sensitivity to chloramphenicol (Begg, Small, & White, 1968), ethambutol (Carr & Henkind, 1962), Ibuprofen (Palmer, 1972), and monoamine oxidase inhibitors (Gillespie, Terry, & Sjoerdsma, 1959).

Galezowski (1868) was the first to draw attention to the color vision defect in tobacco amblyopia, and Groenouw (1892) pointed out how this acquired color defect differed from that found in the congenital dichromat. Defective red–green discrimination has been recorded by François and Verriest (1957a), Cox (1960), Verriest (1964) Saraux, Labet, and Biais (1966), Bouniq and Coscas (1966), Chisholm, Bronte-Stewart, and Awduche (1970), and Pinckers (1971a) in tobacco amblyopia. Bhargava (1973), using the Pickford-Nicolson anomaloscope, found the midmatching point was shifted to red and the matching range enlarged and on the basis of these findings concluded that the lesion in tobacco amblyopia was retinal rather than neuritic.

Chisholm, Bronte-Stewart, and Awduche (1970) analyzed 65 patients suffering from the toxic optic neuropathy associated with tobacco smoking. The FM 100-hue test mean error score for the group prior to therapy was 732 ± 236. The FM 100-hue test error score correlated with visual acuity $(p < 0.001)$ and patient age $(p < 0.01)$. The FM 100-hue test profile revealed a depression of color discrimination in most regions of the spectrum, but with a prominent red–green loss. By recording serial FM 100-hue test results, Chisholm, Bronte-Stewart, and Awduche (1970) demonstrated that with treatment an improved clinical state was accompanied by improved color discrimination. This was illustrated by a falling FM 100-hue test error score (Fig. 8.32) and a contracting profile, which often was slowest in the red–green area (Fig. 8.33). By plotting error score against time on therapy, the values fitted an exponential curve $(Y - Ae^{kt} + C)$. Converting to logarithms $[\log_e(Y - C) = \log(Ae - kt)]$, an inclined slope given by the value for k indicated the rate of recovery. By this technique those authors demonstrated differing recovery rates in differing types of toxic optic neuropathy (Fig. 8.34).

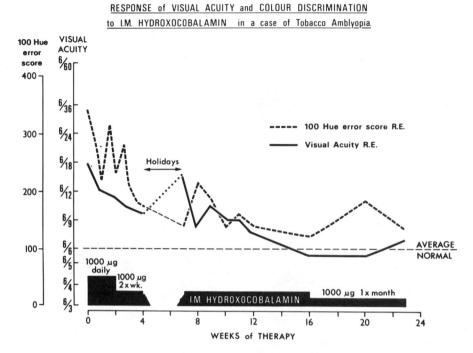

Fig. 8.32. Visual acuity and FM 100-hue test error score related to time of treatment with hydroxylcobalamin. [From Chisholm, I. A., Bronte-Stewart, J., & Awduche, E. D. *Acta Ophthalmologica,* 1970, *48,* 1145– 1156 (reproduced with permission of Acta Ophthalmologica).]

ISCHEMIC OPTIC NEUROPATHY

There is general agreement that the ocular changes seen in acute ischemia are determined by a multitude of hemodynamic factors, both local and general, on the one hand, and the intraocular pressure on the other (Table 8.11). The condition is characterized by a dramatic loss of vision, a swollen optic disc, scattered hemorrhages, usually close to the disc, and frequently an altitudinal loss of visual field. There is an accompanying type III acquired blue–yellow defect (Fig. 8.35). Clinical and experimental evidence suggests that while the optic disc shows dramatic changes, the choroidal circulation is the more severely compromised.

PAPILLEDEMA

Papilledema refers to edema of the optic disc caused by increased pressure in cerebrospinal fluid. There are many causes, including intracranial tumor, hemorrhage, systemic infections, or metabolic disease (e.g., hypertension). Visual acuity is usually near normal, and the visual field defect consists of an enlarged blind spot. The most frequently reported color defect is the type III acquired blue–yellow defect with normal Rayleigh equation (Verriest, 1963; François & Verriest, 1968). There is an accumulation of errors on the FM 100-hue test arranged on a predominantly blue–yellow axis.

Special psychophysical testing has included the Wald-Marré technique (Marré, 1970). Marré noted that in the majority of cases the blue CVM was reduced, with minimal reduction of the green and red CVMs. Verriest and Uvijls (1977a) have noted a uniform reduction of sensitivity in papilledema.

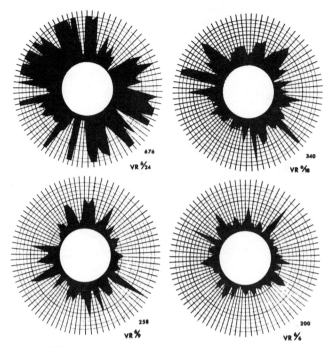

Fig. 8.33. Tobacco amblyopia showing improvement in the FM 100-hue profile with time of treatment. [From Chisholm, I. A., Bronte-Stewart, J., & Awduche, E. D. *Acta Ophthalmologica*, 1970, *48*, 1145–1156 (reproduced with permission of Acta Ophthalmologica).]

Optic Chiasma

The quadrilaterally shaped mass of nerve tissue known as the optic chiasma is a midline structure found in the middle cranial fossa. It is connected in front with each optic nerve and behind with each optic tract. It lies on the roof (diaphragma) of the sella turcica, which contains the pituitary gland. The stalk connecting the pituitary gland to the hypothalamus lies immediately behind the chiasma. Because of the complexity and

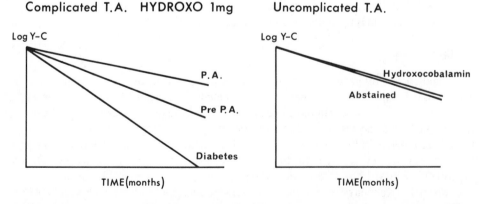

Fig. 8.34. Rate of visual recovery (log y-c) in various toxic optic neuropathies. [From Chisholm, I. A., Bronte-Stewart, J., & Awduche, E. D. *Acta Ophthalmologica*, 1970, *48*, 1145–1156 (reproduced with permission of Acta Ophthalmologica).]

Table 8.11
Hemodynamic Factors Resulting in Acute Ocular "Ischemia"

Decreased oxygen carrying capacity
    Sudden anemia—result of hemorrhage or hemolysis
    Reduced O_2 saturation—high altitude

Failure in perfusion pressure
    Acute systemic hypotension
    Local arterial disease (e.g., carotid stenosis)

Abnormal resistance to blood flow
    Elevation of intraocular pressure
    Venous stasis
    Increased whole blood viscosity (polycythemia, macroglobulinemia)
    Arteritis

proximity of surrounding structures the optic chiasma may be compressed or distorted by an expanding lesion from any direction. One in four intracranial tumors arise in its vicinity (Huber, 1961), the majority of which produce visual symptoms as their initial manifestations. The visual signs elicited may fall into one of three classical syndromes—anterior chiasmal, chiasmal, and retrochiasmal syndromes.

ANTERIOR CHIASMAL SYNDROME

Involvement of the intracranial portion of the optic nerve at its junction with the anterior chiasm may result in the following signs: (1) ipsilateral eye—reduced visual acuity; optic disc pallor and atrophy; a central scotoma in the field of vision accompanied by an acquired color vision defect; afferent pupil abnormality of Marcus Gunn; (2) contralateral eye—no abnormal findings if diagnosis is early enough; paracentral scotoma–junctional scotoma of Traquair. Involvement of the intracranial portion of the optic nerve thus results in subtle but subjectively obtrusive changes in vision. The afferent pupil abnormality of Marcus Gunn (swinging light test) and the striking color vision defect on testing with AO HRR pseudoisochromatic plates were noted by Knight, Hoyt, and Wilson (1972) to be prominent and early features. Possible pathologic processes giving rise to this syndrome include meningioma of tuberculum sellae or sphenoidal ridge, intrinsic glioma or astrocytoma, and demyelinating plaque. David and Hartmann (1935) had earlier reported a red–green defect in a patient with a sphenoidal meningioma.

CHIASMAL SYNDROME

Midline involvement of the body of the optic chiasm may reveal itself by the following:

1. Bitemporal hemianopia of peripheral or hemicentral situation. When the compression is from below the upper temporal quadrant of the visual field first shows a fall in sensitivity; when compression is from above the lower temporal quadrant is involved first.
2. Atrophic changes of the optic disc, if present, are equal in amount on each side.

Compression or distortion of the chiasm is more usual from below, and the cause is pituitary adenoma. The initial peripheral field loss progresses to the classical bitemporal hemianopia, but this is only found in 55 percent of patients (Smith, 1964). The craniopharyngioma is the most common expanding lesion compressing the chiasm from above. This condition is characterized by fluctuations in the clinical state and

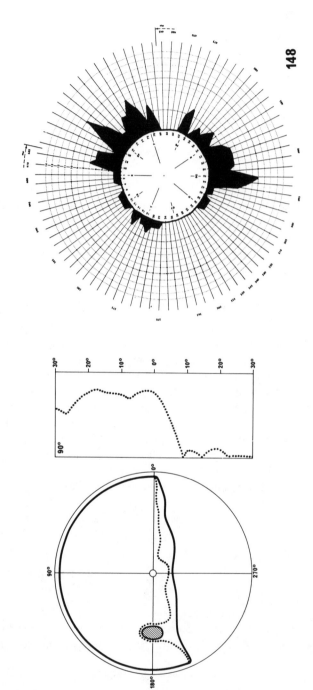

Fig. 8.35. Ischemic optic neuropathy: central visual field, and FM 100-hue test result.

pleomorphism of the visual field defects (Kennedy & Smith, 1975) and may give rise to any or all in succession of the three syndromes outlined earlier.

Color vision studies in the chiasmal syndrome reveal type II acquired red–green defects (Engelking, 1921; Dubois-Poulsen, 1952). Verriest (1964), Ohta (1970), and Pinckers (1971a), following investigation by pseudoisochromatic plates, Farnsworth Panel D-15, FM 100-hue test, anomaloscope, and spectral sensitivity tests, concluded that the red–green color vision defect in the chiasmal syndrome was a type II acquired red–green defect that progresses from a moderate stage to a severe one and finally to total color blindness (Fig. 8.36). Reporting their analysis of 28 eyes, François and Verriest (1968) found that 7 eyes gave normal responses, 18 eyes a type II red–green defect, and 1 eye a type III acquired blue–yellow defect. Bonamour, Bonnet, and Laffet (1971), in their case report of chiasmal syndrome accompanying pregnancy, noted that although the patient showed an upper temporal quadrantic hemianopia, color vision responses were normal.

From examples in Fig. 8.36 the FM 100-hue test plots show a type II acquired red–green defect when the field loss is peripheral, but once absolute scotomata to white are present in the central area the FM 100-hue test plot tends to become anarchic.

Optic Tract and Optic Radiations

Retrochiasmal lesions give rise to a lateral homonymous defect in the field of vision. The distortion of the visual pathways giving rise to this defect may be located anywhere from the optic chiasm to the optic radiations; thus the optic tract may be involved in chiasmal lesions, and the typical field defect of lateral homonymous hemianopia was found in 16 percent of pituitary tumors by Smith (1964) and 24 percent of craniopharyngiomata by Kennedy and Smith (1975). The most common cause of a lateral homonymous hemianopia is a cerebral vascular accident, but space-occupying lesions of the temporal and parietal cerebral lobes may also distort the visual pathways, although they are less common. A lateral homonymous hemianopia may be caused by pressure from an arterial aneurysm or injury, but these are both uncommon causes.

An acquired color vision defect in retrochiasmal lesions of the visual pathway was noted by François and Verriest (1968) in only one of seven eyes examined. Vola, Riss, Jayle, Gosset, and Tassy (1972) found a much higher incidence—57 percent of subjects showed a color vision defect on testing with AO HRR pseudoisochromatic plates, Farnsworth Panel D-15, and the FM 100-hue test. These latter authors found that an acquired color vision defect was relatively common when the visual field defect had an underlying vascular cause: 22 of 24 eyes examined, showed a red–green discrimination loss in patients suffering a stroke. They further observed that the eyes did not have equal color defects. In most instances it is not possible to differentiate between color defects due to lesions of the optic radiations and those due to lesions of the cerebral cortex.

Visual Cortex and Higher Cortical Centers

The visual cortex, Broca's area 17, is located at the tip of the occipital cerebral lobe and on the medial surface of the cerebral hemisphere above and below the calcarine sulcus. This area is characterized by the unique white line of Gennari, visible on its cut surface, lying in the gray matter. Possession of this white streak or line has conferred the name striate cortex on the visual area. Area 18, the parastriate cortex, and area 19, the

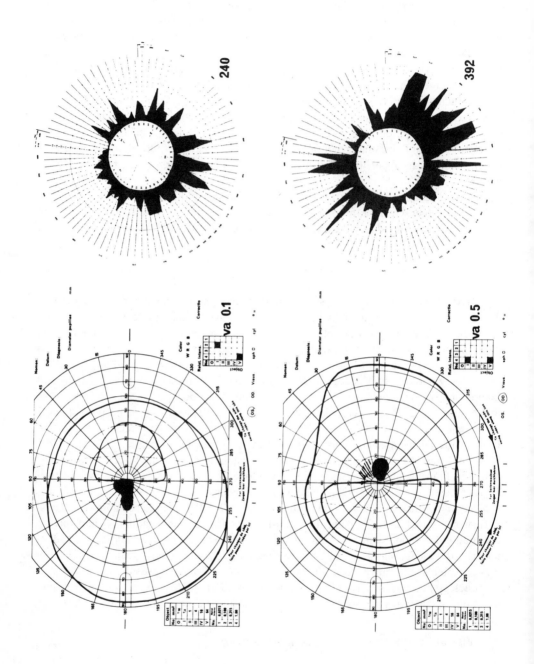

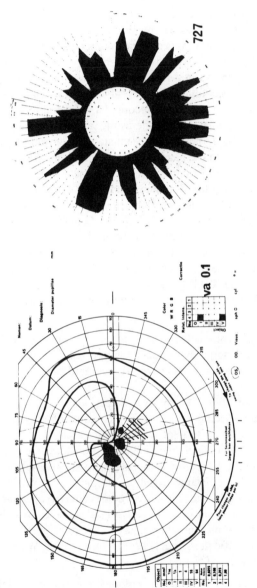

Fig. 8.36. Perimetric and FM 100-hue test examples from three patients with a pituitary tumor. Upper, 16-year-old female with pituitary tumor; FM 100-hue test shows anarchic plot; perimetry, paracentral scotoma. Center, 55-year-old male with pituitary tumor; FM 100-hue test shows a definite red–green defect; perimetry shows principally a temporal field loss. Lower, 55-year-old male with pituitary tumor; FM 100-hue test shows anarchic plot; perimetry shows temporal and lower field loss with paracentral scotomata.

peristriate cortex, function as higher integrating centers. The visual cortex is supplied by the posterior cerebral artery, with a small variable contribution at the tip of the occipital lobe, from the middle cerebral artery.

ACQUIRED COLOR DEFECTS OF CENTRAL ORIGIN*

Injury to the brain or visual pathway can result in loss of color perception. Several patients with acquired color defects of this nature were reported in the 19th century and included those suffering from vascular lesions of the cerebral cortex, concussion injuries, and specific lesions caused by gunshot wounds or tumors. For example, loss of color perception due to concussion sustained in a riding accident was described by Wilson in 1855, and "amnestic color blindness" following cerebral vascular lesions was reported by Brill in 1882, Wilbrand in 1884. In 1913 Abney recorded a unilateral loss of color vision following a stroke. These reports are both interesting and frustrating because the investigators did not possess the materials for an adequate color vision examination that are available today but had to rely on the patients' own descriptions. Even at the present time, interesting cases are still not reported in the detail that one might wish, since liaison between specialists in different disciplines is required, and there are ethical considerations to be examined before seriously ill patients are subjected to test procedures not directly related to treatment. The interest in this particular aspect of color vision investigation is the possibility of mapping the functional areas of the brain. In this context investigations of the anatomic structure and function of different areas of the cerebral cortex of the Rhesus monkey (whose visual system is most nearly similar to that of man) aids the understanding of the human system (Zeki, 1973).

Acquired color vision defects of cerebral origin may be of three different types and may appear singly or in combination.

1. The appearance of a specific color defect either similar to a congenital color defect or similar to an acquired defect normally associated with diseases of the eye. The most frequently reported cases are either severe type III acquired blue–yellow defects or complete color blindness.
2. Loss of wavelength discrimination. The ability to detect small wavelength differences is lost over the complete spectral range. A combination of a type III acquired blue–yellow defect and overall loss of wavelength discrimination may occur, especially if a lesion causing initially a specific blue–yellow loss deteriorates further.
3. Color agnosia is a condition that is often associated with aphasic symptoms such as alexia and prosopagnosia and is characterized by an inability to name colors or to select them by name alone, or to relate the correct color names to everyday objects. It appears that color agnosia can occur independently of either a specific color defect or loss of wavelength discrimination, but when aphasic symptoms are present adequate color vision examination is difficult (Stengel, 1948; Kinsbourne & Warrington, 1964; Oxbury, Oxbury, & Humphrey, 1969).

Although modern electrical techniques can pinpoint the site of specific cortical injuries, any lesion causes associated degeneration in the visual pathway and vice versa. Similar "backtracking" occurs in retinal and optic nerve lesions, especially after a period of time, and this makes it difficult to ascribe a particular color loss to the primary site only. It should be recommended that all patients with an acquired color vision defect attributed to a cerebral lesion should also be examined by an ophthalmologist and that a minimum investigation should include the measurement of visual acuity and visual fields,

---

*Contributed by Jennifer Birch, M.Phil.

together with a battery of color vision tests (the Ishihara test alone is not sufficient). A full investigation might include such measurements as dark adaptation, flicker fusion frequency, modulation transfer function, EOG, ERG, and fluorescein angiography. Coloring materials and outline pictures of everyday objects or sets of cards with familiar objects depicted in different colors are both useful in confirming color agnosia.

Disturbed perception of colors associated with localized cerebral lesions has been reviewed by Meadows (1974), and a large number of patients with hemianopic field defects have been examined with a battery of color vision tests by Llermitte, Chain, Aron, Leblanc, and Souty (1969). Meadows (1974) concentrates on lesions that have been reported as producing achromatopsia and includes all adequately described case histories since 1930. In these, heavy reliance is placed on the patient's own description of symptoms, and there are obvious differences among patients. However, in most cases the cerebral injury is vascular in origin and the disturbance of color vision occurs extremely rapidly and, in some cases, prior to any other symptoms. The descriptions of Pallis' patient are classic: "Everything appears in various shades of gray . . . I have difficulty recognizing certain kinds of food, and when I open a jar I never know whether I'll find pickles or jam" (Pallis, 1955). All the patients included in Meadows' survey have visual field defects, and there is a strikingly high incidence of bilateral defects affecting the upper quadrants. In addition, prosopagnosia is found in all but two patients, and these are taken from relatively early in the literature, when the condition may have gone unreported. Meadows (1974) concludes that the clinical evidence links the anterior inferior part of the occipital lobe with color perception and that bilateral lesions at this site may cause permanent impairment of color perception (achromatopsia) together with ← prosopagnosia and impaired topographic memory, while visual acuity remains intact. In support of this thesis Meadows (1974) describes a single patient (MH) with bilateral superior hemianopia and macular sparing following a cortical infarct. Slight aphasia and prosopagnosia are present, but although his color vision is severely impaired he is clearly not an achromat. A more detailed investigation of this patient, including isolation of Wald color mechanisms, reveals that he can describe all the spectral hues in terms of either pale blue or pale red and that his defect can be most nearly classified as a type III acquired blue–yellow defect together with overall impairment of chromatic discrimination (Birch-Cox, 1976). Similar profound loss of color perception can sometimes be found in patients with severe peripheral retinal diseases that result in gross field defects.

A similar patient with bilateral superior hemianopia following a stroke has been described by Critchley (1965). Again, prosopagnosia was present, but although the loss of color vision was extensive and the patient was led once again to describe a total loss, careful questioning revealed that he was not totally achromatic. An additional feature of this case, however, was a report of transient xanthopsia in which all objects appeared "covered with gold paint." The diagnosis of slight protanomaly obtained for this patient with the AO HRR plates is probably misleading and could be due either to his overall loss of hue discrimination or to a reduction in the relative luminous efficiency of the eye for long wavelengths. In the main the symptoms described by Critchley (1965) are similar to those of Meadows' (1974) patient MH (Birch-Cox, 1976). Yet another patient with superior hemianopia reported by Rondot, Tzavaras, and Garcin (1967) experienced a similar dramatic color loss that recovered somewhat with time but that included a period of erythropsia.

A bizarre symptom that sometimes occurs with coloropsia is perseveration. For example, the sensation of a particularly bright color may be retained for a period of time and pervade the whole environment after only a short viewing time, or the bright color of a dress may appear to spread out over the wearer's face and arms. There are also occasional reports of photophobia, but the most usual comment is that the environment appears dull and relatively colorless.

One of the characteristics of acquired color defects is fluctuation, and defects of cerebral origin illustrate this. The reports of achromatopsia are mostly subjective, and careful questioning on clinical testing usually reveals some chromatic discrimination. Whether this can be attributed to a degree of recovery rather than to an overemphasis by the patient is open to question. In a study of 42 patients with lateral hemianopias due to a variety of causes, Llermitte, Chain, Aron, Leblanc, and Souty (1969) find only two patients who may be tentatively described as monochromats by virtue of their responses to the AO HRR test. The test battery included both the Ishihara and AO HRR plates, the Farnsworth Panel D-15 test, and the FM 100-hue test. The results show that red–green discrimination remains intact but that frequent errors of the blue–yellow type are made with the AO HRR plates. In about one-third of cases blue–yellow errors were made with the AO HRR plates. In about one-third of cases a blue–yellow confusion axis was obtained with the FM 100-hue test, and the remaining two-thirds showed almost complete loss of overall chromatic discrimination, which was described as "pseudoachromatopsia." These data give support to the hypothesis that color deficiency and hue discrimination can be considered separately and that the total decline of discrimination occurs as a lesion producing a blue–yellow color defect deteriorates further. Most of the patients showing pseudoachromatopsia in this study had a tendency for the field defect to become bilateral, and some also exhibited color agnosia. No significant difference was found in the color vision results between left or right hemisphere–damaged patients.

This finding was confirmed by Assal, Eisert, and Hecaen (1969), who examined 155 patients with lateral hemianopias using the Farnsworth Panel D-15 test. However, in this study it is not clear if a specific color defect was found but only that overall test performance (or hue discrimination) was consistently inferior to that of a control group of patients. In contrast, a large group of patients with lateral hemianopias had normal color vision even when examined with the FM 100-hue test (Vola, Riss, Jayle, Gosset, & Tassy, 1972). The color-normal patients suffered either posterior occipital or temporoparietal lesions produced by tumors or compression, while color defects were consistently found in patients with diffused vascular lesions without regard to anatomic localization. Also using the FM 100-hue test, Scotti and Spinnler (1970) found that discrimination was more likely to be impaired in lesions of the right hemisphere than the left and that the right hemisphere plays the major part in chromatic discrimination has been confirmed by Davidoff (1976). In the description of a unique case of cranial trauma resulting in a pericentral field defect, Hansen (1972) also demonstrated a type III acquired blue–yellow defect. The inference is that the appearance of the color defect is related to the position, severity, and type of the field defect and that unilateral or sectional defects are possible. Destruction of the peripheral retina or the cortical area subserving the retinal periphery produces either a blue–yellow defect and/or loss of chromatic discrimination, and these data have implications for the way color information in coded in the normal visual system.

While there are groups of patients in the neurologist's clinic whose color vision defect might be more thoroughly investigated using colorimetric techniques, there are also occasional extensive reports of unique cases of color deficiency, without medical history, for which visual acuity or visual field data is lacking. These include patients who have significant monocular differences in color perception (Bender, Ruddock, de Vries—de Mol,

& Went, 1972; MacLeod & Lennie, 1976). In these so-called unilateral defects, the difference between the two eyes is usually a matter of degree, since the better eye does not have normal color vision (Cox, 1961c), and the defect is invariably deutan in character, one eye appearing deuteranomalous and the other deuteranopic. However, the defects are not always typical of congenital defects, and whether the differences between the two eyes has genetic or pathologic origin (or both) is open to question. In the case of a deutan defect the site of origin is more likely to be the optic nerve rather than the cerebral cortex, and measurement of the modulation transfer function together with visual fields might confirm whether or not such injury has taken place. However, if the defect is not entirely typical of deuteranopia, it is possible that an acquired blue–yellow defect has been superimposed upon congenital deuteranomaly.

Patients are rather unreliable in describing the onset of monocular differences, but definite reports of sudden onset without loss of visual acuity may implicate the visual cortex. In one such case, rapid onset, loss of hue discrimination, and the appearance of a blue–yellow defect surely indicates a cerebral lesion (King-Smith, Kranda, & Wood, 1976), and while this particular case is analyzed in terms of loss of the blue–yellow opponent color mechanism, a similar analysis could be applied to the patients with hemianopic field defects described previously. A characteristic of type III acquired blue–yellow defects is the appearance of a large neutral zone situated in the yellow region of the spectrum; this is much more extensive than in congenital defects of a similar type and has previously led to the conclusion that a fourth type of color deficiency exists (tetartanopia), since the sensation of yellow seems entirely absent. However, this feature always occurs with loss of blue perception, and the observation that "the local football team colors are yellow and blue but now they look black and white" is characteristic. The patient described by Sperling, Piantanida, and Garrett (1976) also shows extreme loss of sensitivity in the yellow region of the spectrum and poor overall chromatic discrimination coupled with failure of the F_2 plate. Spectral sensitivity functions measured using heterochromatic flicker photometry are anomalous, and suggestive of a cerebral lesion.

It may be considered that the appreciation of luminance differences as measured by the flicker fusion frequency is always impaired in color defects of central origin. This is confirmed in the study by Bender and Ruddock (1974). There is extreme loss of chromatic discrimination, anomalous flicker fusion frequency, and some photophobia for long wavelengths. The defect appears to be red–green in character (with a possible congenital component) rather than blue–yellow.

ACTION OF PHYSICAL AGENTS*

With the exception of trauma to the eyeball, the effect of a physical agent, be it ionizing radiation, light, sound, temperature, etc., may be unrecognized as injurious at the time of exposure, and its effects on retinal function may be delayed and of a subtle character. Much of our knowledge of our immediate environment, and almost all of our knowledge of the universe, comes from the study of photons (Ingram, 1962). A photon is a discrete package of energy discharged from a vibrating atom and propagated in an electromagnetic waveform, the wavelength of which will determine the sensation it creates (Fig. 8.37). Light, sound, and heat are sensations produced on stimulation of the receptors' appropriate sensory system. Although x-ray, ultrasound, and radio waves

---

*Contributed by I. A. Chisholm, M.D.

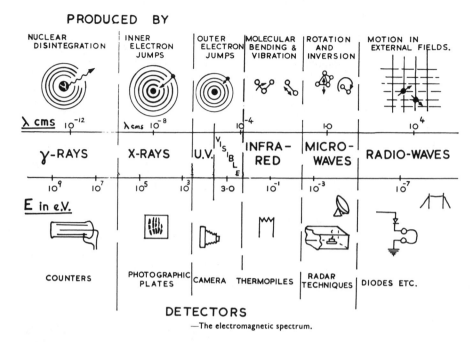

Fig. 8.37. Varieties of radiation within the electromagnetic spectrum. [From Ingram, D. J. E. *Advancement of Science,* 1962, *18,* 523–536 (reproduced with permission of the British Association for the Advancement of Science).]

produce no sensory percepts, absorption or reflection of their energy does occur, depending on the density of individual body tissues.

Sensory systems are designed to respond to a physiologic range of stimuli. Stimulation above this range results in exhaustion or even disorganization of the neuroreceptor. Electronic devices that compress photon energy in space and time exist (maser [Microwave Amplification by the Stimulated Emission of Radiation] and laser [used for a similar device operating in the visible wavelengths]), and accidental exposure to the amplified radiation is harmful.

The harmful effects of electromagnetic radiation will be discussed in three groups: ultravisible radiation, visible spectrum, and ultrasound and sound. The harmful effects of various forms of stress will then be discussed.

Ultravisible Radiation

COSMIC RADIATIONS

Cosmic radiations are composed of elementary particles that travel in interstellar space at the speed of light (approximately 2.99×10^8 m/sec). They are absorbed by the Earth's atmosphere and may be studied only from satellites. Astronauts describe "phosphenes," which arise when a retinal neuroreceptor that has been struck and stimulated by an elementary particle. No acute effects on visual function have been reported, and the long-term effects of exposure are unknown.

IONIZING RADIATIONS

Ionizing radiation is a term applied to the effect of x-ray, α β and γ radiation on cells. These radiations convert intracellular water (H_2O) into hydroxonium ion (OH_3^-) and other ions. In sufficient concentration they cause immediate cell death; in lesser concentrations a gradual degeneration occurs. In the retina this latter phase is marked by a pigmentary degeneration and vascular sclerosis.

These forms of radiation also cause phosphenes when the eye is exposed to the rays. Stenström (1946) made use of this fact when he used an x-ray technique to study axial length of the living eye.

Visible Spectrum

A proportion of the light entering the eye is absorbed by the visual pigments, thereby initiating the neurosensory process of seeing. Of the remainder a small amount is reflected back out of the eye, and the balance is absorbed by the pigment-containing cells of the retinal pigment epithelium and choroid. The energy of this absorbed light is degraded to thermal energy and conducted out of the eye by the choroidal blood flow. The intensity of the photon energy entering through the pupil initiates the protective mechanism of pupillary constriction when it is high and pupillary dilatation when it is low. Thus the pupil will be active as ambient light conditions vary. Exposure to an intense source of light results in bleaching of the photopigments followed by a sequence of positive and negative afterimages. When a colored source is viewed, visual recovery passes through a sequence of color change—flight of colors. This sequence of change is considered by some to be of diagnostic significance in optic nerve disease (Feldman, Todman, & Bender, 1974) and in macular edema.

The harmful effects of excessive light have been recognized from the recorded experience with eclipse observers and early astronomers. This knowledge guided Meyer-Schwickerath (1960) to develop his light coagulation apparatus and to alert ophthalmologists to the probable harmful effect of laser light (Kapany, Peppers, Zweng, & Flocks, 1963) and resulted in the evolution of a code of practice for laser use in clinical practice. Much interest has been channeled into research on the harmful effect of excessive visible radiation and the changes that occur in the neuroreceptors on exposure to light. These investigators have also considered the transparency of the ocular media to electromagnetic radiation (Geeraets, Williams, Chan, Hamm, Gerry, & Schmidt, 1960), absorption of radiation by the pigmented retinal and choroidal cells (Geeraets, Williams, Chan, Hamm, Gerry, & Schmidt, 1960), temperature conversion (Campbell, Noyori, Rittler, & Koester, 1963; Litwin & Glew, 1964), and rate of choroidal blood flow.

Continuous light has an early effect on the outer segment of the photoreceptor, characterized by morphologic change and separation (Kuwabara & Gorn, 1968), which is followed by phagocytosis by the pigment epithelium. Regeneration of outer segments will occur provided that the photic stimulus has not produced any significant lesion of the receptor cell body or pigment epithelium cell (Kuwabara, 1970). The sequence of change has been studied in experimental animals subjected to varying levels of light intensity for varying durations. Guignolo, Orzalesi, Castellazzo, and Vittone (1969) believe that the pigment epithelium and receptor cell bodies are more resistant to light than are the receptor outer segments, whereas Noell, Walker, Kang, and Berman (1966) and Hansson (1971) consider the outer segment degeneration to be secondary to pigment epithelial damage. Ultrastructural intracytoplamsic changes have been revealed at light levels known to cause reversible anterior segment degeneration, but researchers (La Vail, 1976; Marshall & Ansell, 1971) considered that these were an exaggeration of the normal diurnal shedding of receptor discs. Outer segment recovery following a photic injury is very slow; ERG responses do not show any tendency to recovery before 3 weeks and return to normal levels only 6 weeks after monochromatic (laser) exposure (Zwick, Bedell, & Bloom, 1973).

The efficiency of a source in producing photic retinal injury corresponds to its visual efficiency in terms of the experimental animal's spectral sensitivity (Gorn & Kuwabara, 1967; Anderson, Coyle, & O'Steen, 1972). Green and blue light stimuli are found to be equally effective, while ultraviolet light causes greater retinal change (Zigmann & Vaughan, 1974).

Harwerth and Sperling (1971) and Sperling and Johnson (1973) were able to induce reversible, spectrally selective dichromacy by exposure to monochromatic light. Recovery from photic injury required 30 days, and there was marked and permanent damage to the blue receptors. Harwerth and Sperling (1971) concluded that their results were a demonstration of the selective absorption by the photopigments. Zwick and Beatrice (1978) produced a similar prominent effect (with cumulative exposure) on conditioned monkeys.

Retinal damage is related to image size and radiance, both of which are dependent on and modified by the intensity of the light incident of the cornea, the area of the entry pupil, light scatter and absorption by the ocular media, and the focal length of the eye. Ophthalmologists now consider receptor damage to be possible in indirect ophthalmoscopy (T'so, Robbins, & Zimmermann, 1974) from the intraocular fiber optic light source used during vitrectomy (Fuller, Machemer, & Knighton, 1978), from accidental exposure to pulsed or continuous-wave laser sources operating in the invisible or infrared mode (Sliney, 1971), and from accidental, visual exposure to a welding arc (Filipiakowa, 1975; Romanchuk, Pollak, & Schneider, 1978).

Birch-Cox (1978) studied color vision responses in patients suffering from diabetic retinopathy but with good central acuity (0.5 or better) before and after photocoagulation (laser or xenon arc). The color responses were noted to plate tests, the City University color test, Farnsworth Panel D-15 test, and FM 100-hue test. Color matches were obtained using the Lovibond tintometer. Measurements of relative luminous efficiency and blue CVM (with selective chromatic adaptation) were also performed. Photocoagulation increased the type III acquired blue–yellow defect, abolished the blue CVM, and reduced the relative luminous efficiencies for both long and short wavelengths. After photocoagulation all patients reported a blue-green confusion and some additionally red-black, blue-black, or yellow-white confusions. Confirmation of loss of visual function following photocoagluation of diabetics has been produced by a study of the electroretinographic response of such patients (Schuurmatis, van Lith, & Oosterhuis, 1978).

Ultrasound and Sound

Sensory modalities, when influenced at the same time by different stimuli, often interact. For example, it has been recognized for many years that patients who are partially deaf hear better in the light than in darkness, and thus there has been interest in what effect, if any, sound has on visual function.

Kravkov (1936) found that auditory stimulation of moderate intensity heightened central sensitivity to white light, but that if monochromatic light was used the effect varied with the wavelength utilized, sensitivity to blue-green being increased and orange-red decreased. Letourneau and Zeidel (1971) confirmed these results, studying a greater number of subjects and having better control of the quality of the sound. Sensitivity to white and green (520 nm) increased under the influence of pure sound at 1000 Hz at intensities of 50, 70, and 90 dB. Sensitivity to red (610) nm) diminished when the intensity of sound reached 70 dB.

Auditory stimulation also has an effect on the flicker fusion frequency (CFF). A stimulation of 800 Hz at 85 dB reduced the FFF for green (520 nm) and raised the FFF for orange-red (630 nm). Auditory stimulation also affected FFF when using white light, the rate being heightened for central vision but lowered for peripheral vision (London, 1954).

In some individuals, strong acoustic stimulation preceding and accompanying light increased the brightness of the afterimage, which also faded sooner than without the sound. Sounds that were powerful enough to evoke intense auditory afterimages contributed more to heighten the brightness of the visual afterimage. The afterimage completely disappeared when an extremely loud tone was presented after the cessation of retinal illumination.

Lazarev had shown the sensitivity of peripheral vision is heightened when the subject is hearing sounds (London, 1954). Bogoslovskii and Kravkov (London, 1954) claimed that peripheral sensitivity falls by as much as 20 percent on stimulation from the prestimulation level (Grognot & Perdriel, 1961). Kekcheev and Ostrovoskii (London, 1954) report that exposure to ultrasonic frequencies (32,800 Hz) increased peripheral sensitivity. Kravkov (1936), however, has shown that this elevation was preceded by an initial fall in sensitivity.

Studies on experimental focused ultrasonic lesions of retina, choroid, and sclera have shown histologic evidence of receptor damage, similar morphologically to that produced by excessive light (Lizzi, Coleman, Driller, Franzen, & Jakabiec, 1978). The intensity at which these lesions were produced was far in excess of that used for routine diagnostic ultrasonic purposes. Absorption of ultrasound occurs diffusely within the retina and choroid. A mild chorioretinal lesion is often accompanied by extensive scleral reaction and degeneration (Lizzi, Coleman, Driller, Franzen, & Jakabiec, 1978).

Stress

ACCELERATION

The effect of a gravitation (g) acceleration has been recognized from the pioneer days of aviation. One of the features of a g force is temporary loss of vision. Centrifugal, or +g, and centripetal, or −g, accelerations are related to the position of the head to the point of application of the force. An increasing +g acceleration causes successively a "graying out" of vision, a "blacking out" of vision, and ultimately loss of consciousness, since g force is ischemic in origin. −g acceleration leads to vascular congestion and a "redout." The amount of g acceleration necessary to cause these visual disturbances varies with patient tolerance, duration of application, and measures taken to maintain circulation. Under a positive force of 3g the blood pressure falls to 50 mm Hg, equivalent to a "grayout." At 5.5g the blood pressure falls to a level equal to the intraocular pressure, and this constitutes a "blackout;" 0.6g higher than this would produce unconsciousness.

THERMAL

Under excessive temperature the body generates a series of physiologic mechanisms to combat the increased heat. These include vasodilatation and increased sweating with fluid and salt loss. Unless fluid and salt are replaced dehydration occurs, and this will be accompanied by a fall in intraocular pressure and probable visual disturbance.

The body's response to cold is marked mainly by shivering and a fall in body temperature. Cold eye lesions can occur on the eyelids and cornea on exposure to arctic temperatures at sea level or accidental exposure to the atmosphere at high altitudes. "Whiteout" occurs at sea level when the ground is snow covered, when there are no visual reference points in the environment. With a cloudy sky, everything is white. The subject is giddy and disorientated.

Photophthalmia may occur under snow conditions because of absorption of ultraviolet light if the eye is unprotected. Ultraviolet is absorbed both from above and from reflection off the snow; this condition is called snow blindness.

ELECTRICITY AND MAGNETISM

In modern industry, welding machines and electrosteel processes use strong low-frequency currents. The time-variable magnetic fields generated in these processes produce under certain conditions, well-established effects on the visual system (Brindley, 1955). Such magnetic fields in the frequency range 10–50 Hz produce magnetically induced flickering light phenomena (magnetophosphenes), with a maximum sensitivity at 20–30 Hz (Lövsund, Nilsson, & Öberg, 1978), but are influenced by the spectral content of the background light. Imamura (1975) made use of an alternating electric stimulus at 77 or 42.5 Hz, which he considers to stimulate the red or green processes. A long-term study on 198 subjects with dichromatism over a period of 2–7 years claimed improvement in their color vision responses on the anomaloscope or plate tests following stimulation at regular intervals.

ATMOSPHERIC PRESSURE

The finding of a reversible type III blue–yellow defect induced by hypoxia (Smith, Ernest, & Pokorny, 1976) at normal temperture and pressure was not repeated when the hypoxia was accompanied by hypobarism. Observations on nonacclimatized high-altitude mountaineers and skiers whose fundi showed the hemorrhagic retinopathy typical for high altitude revealed that they gave protanomalous responses to color vision testing (Kobrick, 1970). Acclimatized, experienced mountaineers, on the other hand, did not show any color upset (Wiedman, 1973).

Submariners, underwater swimmers,and caisson workers are exposed to varying degrees of increased atmospheric pressure for variable intervals. Hyperbarism is used therapeutically at 2 atm. Color discrimination by the FM 100-hue test in a group of patients undergoing hyperbaric therapy for various peripheral circulatory conditions revealed temporary significant increases in error score without characteristic pattern (Lewis R. D. H., Personal communication).

EMPTY VISUAL FIELD

The condition of empty visual field occurs when there is no detail in the visual field capable of being focused upon. Searching in such a field, the eyes cannot relax to the far point,and involuntarily there is approximately one diopter of accommodation exerted.

This means that in searching an empty visual field the emetrope, instead of being focused at optical infinity, is focused at a point about one meter from the eyes. This type of situation is met within whiteout (see above), in high-altitude myopia in which the aviator has no reference horizon, and in night myopia. The effect of an empty visual field is to reduce the maximum visual range and to impair judgment of a distant object's size and distance.

DRUG INTOXICATION AND HYPOVITAMINOSIS*

However beneficial a therapeutic drug may be, there is always the risk of side effects. Some side effects are tolerable, but others are so serious that they have to be balanced against the beneficial effect of the drug. For example, the dry mouth arising from the administration of the pupil dilator atropine is a tolerable side effect, whereas the sicca syndrome arising from practolol therapy is not. Unfortunately, the visual system is very susceptible to the side effects of drugs. Monitoring possible changes in color vision is a very convenient way of detecting whether or not a drug is affecting vision.

The symptoms of an intoxication appear mostly during drug therapy but can become manifest some time after withdrawal of the drug (e.g., chloroquine intoxication). After withdrawal of the drug the symptoms of intoxication may disappear (reversible effects), but it is possible that the symptoms remain unchanged or even progress (irreversible effects).

It is very difficult to establish an intoxication because it is often not possible to differentiate complications of the disease from the effects of drug therapy. In many diseases more than one drug is prescribed at the same time; it can be very difficult to find out which of the administered drugs causes the intoxication—perhaps a chemical interaction of both drugs or of their metabolites may be responsible. In some cases the matter is even more complicated; diet, the condition of the intestinal flora (vitamin synthesis, resorption), and the consumption of drugs, alcohol, or tobacco may play an important role.

This section reviews recent papers on the effects of drugs on color discrimination; data are summarized in Table 8.12. Other reviews to be consulted are those of Grant (1962), Verriest (1964), Brückner (1969), Crews (1969), Meier-Ruge (1972a, b, 1973), Hermans, Flerman, Van Oye, Watillon, Robe-Van Wyck, Dralands, & Garin (1972), and Lyle (1974).

Acquired Color Vision Defects and Acuity

Verriest (1963) says that an acquired color vision defect generally becomes evident as soon as the causal disease has reduced visual acuity below 0.6, but there is not necessarily a correlation between the extent of the acuity loss and the degree or type of color vision disturbance.

For example, Sakuma (1973) states that ethyl alcohol affects color vision more profoundly than it does acuity. Vérin, Pesme, Yacoubi, and Morax (1971) observed that the ethambutol-induced color vision defect persists after acuity has been regained.

Miscellaneous Disturbances

It is a well-known fact that vitamin therapy has a favorable effect in some cases of optic neuropathy (Perdriel, 1972; Foulds, Chisholm, & Pettigrew, 1974). Vitamin therapy is reported to have a favorable effect on color discrimination of normal subjects (Laroche

---

*Contributed by I. A. Chisholm, M.D., and A. J. L. G. Pinckers, M. D.

& Laroche, 1971). Laroche and Laroche (1970; 1972) reported an improvement of color discrimination (FM 100-hue test) during medication with trimethadione (Tridione), primaclone, spiramycin (Rovamycin), glybutamide, and carbutamide.

Trimethadione exerts its effect on the neural elements and causes nyctalopia (Brückner, 1969). The overall cone function becomes impaired (Dekking, 1950). There is erythropsia; color vision is impaired only at high intensities but improves somewhat after continued exposure. Viewed in an illumination of 215 lux, the Ishihara plates were read correctly by all patients (Sloan & Gilger, 1947). The FM 100-hue test reveals a type III acquired blue–yellow defect (Cox, 1960).

The psychotomimetics such as LSD and mescaline produce illusions of color or enhance or distort the color of objects.

No Influence on Color Discrimination

Extra vitamin A did not have any effect on color discrimination (FM 100-hue test) in patients with carotinemia (de Vries–de Mol, Went, & Völker-Dieben, 1974). No significant influence on color vision (FM 100-hue test) of a normal therapeutic dose is reported for phenobarbital, amobarbital, butobarbital, penicillins, tetracycline, oxytetracyline, oleandomycin, quinine, aspirin, and betamethasone (Laroche & Laroche, 1972).

Chromatopsias

Table 8.12 summarizes the occurence of chromatopsias as described by Sloan and Gilger (1947), Laroche (1967), Henkes (1968), Haut, Haye, Legras, Demailly, and Clay (1972), Dubois-Poulsen (1972), Hermans, Le Jeune, Van Oye, Watillon, Robe-Van Wyck, Dralands, and Garin (1972), Lyle (1974), and Saraux (1975).

Intoxications

Color vision examination as one of the methods used to detect intoxications is especially useful if the drug affects the macular region or the papillomacular-cortical pathway (Brückner, 1969). In the preclinical stage of toxic optic neuritis the FM 100-hue test is one of two methods able to detect any disturbance (Saraux, 1975). Color vision examination is also an important tool in followup examination of optic neuritis and other diseases (Pinckers, 1970b).

INTOXICATIONS LEADING TO A TYPE I
ACQUIRED RED–GREEN DEFECT

A type I acquired red–green defect is a symptom of (macular) cone damage; the combination of a type I defect with an electroretinographic cone dysfunction is a guarantee for the presence of impaired cone function.

The visual complaints in digitalis intoxication were often explained as symptoms of a retrobulbar neuritis. Robertson, Hollenhorst, and Callahan (1966a, b) believe that the scotomas most often are due to toxic effects on the receptor cells; they found elevated dark adaptation thresholds in three normal subjects given nontoxic doses of digitalis and concluded that digitalis can disturb the normal function of the receptor cells. Digitalis influences the π_5 mechanism of Stiles (Gibson, Smith, & Alpern, 1965). This agrees with the ERG measurements of Denden (1962). During a mass digitoxin intoxication in Veenendaal in the Netherlands, Cozijnsen and Pinckers (1969) found visual disturbances

Table 8.12

Color Vision Defects Associated With Various Drugs

Drug	Chromatopsias	Type I Acquired r-g Defect	Type II Acquired r-g Defect	Type III Acquired b-y Defect
Antidiabetics (oral)			+	
Chlorpropamide			+	
Tolbutamide			+	
Antipyretics			+	
Ibuprofen			+	
Phenylbutazone			+	
Salicylates	+			
Nitrofurane derivatives	+	+	+	
Furaltodone		+	+?	
Nalidixic acid	+		−	
Phenothiazine derivatives		+?		+
Thioridazine	+			
Quinoline derivatives	+	+	+	+
Atebrin	+			
Chloroquine derivatives			+	++
Clioquinol			++	+
Quinidine			+	
Quinine	+	+	+	
Sulfonamides	+		+	
Salazosulfapyridine		+		
Tuberculostatics			+	
Dihydrostreptomycin			+	
Ethambutol			+	
Isoniazide			+	
PAS			+	
Rifampin			+	
Streptomycin	+		+	
Adrenalin	+			
Amoproxan			+	
Amyl alcohol	+			
Arsenicals	+		+	
Barbiturates	+			
Cannabis indica	+			
Chloramphenicol			+	
Chlorothiazide	+			
Contraceptive agents (oral)		+		++
Cyanide			+	
Digitalis	+	++	+	+
Disulfiram			+	
Ergotamine	+		+	
Erythromycin				+
Ethanol	+		+	
Hexamethonium			+	
Indomethacin				+
Lead	+		+	
MAO inhibitors			+	
Mercaptopurine			+	

Table 8.12 (continued)

Drug	Chromatopsias	Type I Acquired r-g Defect	Type II Acquired r-g Defect	Type III Acquired b-y Defect
Penicillamine			+	
Strychnine	+			
Thallium			+	
Tobacco amblyopia			+	+ +
Trimethadione	+			+
Vincristine			+	

in 79 poisoned subjects, and during the initial 10 days red–green defects were detected on the AO HRR, Ishihara, and FM 100-hue tests (accumulation of errors at the protan site; Fig. 8.38). Verriest (1974) also observed a red–green defect. In digitalis poisoning the photochromatic intervals remain normal, thus indicating a retinal localization (Zanen, 1971; discussion by Babel & Stangos, 1972). A type III defect was reported by Grützner (1969a, b; 1970) and Babel and Stangos (1972). Examination of digitalis-poisoned subjects is difficult because of poor general condition. Anomaloscope examination is usually impossible because of the central scotomas.

In quinine poisoning the study of the photochromatic intervals revealed no abnormality; therefore Zanen (1971) concluded that the lesion was retinal. François, DeRouck, and Cambie (1972) reported three cases of acute quinine poisoning; they observed in the first instance involvement of the optic nerve and the ganglion cells, the bipolar cells and photoreceptors sustaining damage only after the retinal vascular changes appear.

Oral contraceptives caused an increased occurrence of "protanomaly" as well as a

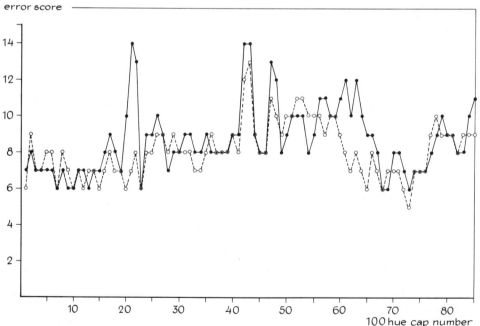

Fig. 8.38. FM 100-hue test error score in eight digitoxin-poisoned subjects during the intoxication (filled symbols) and 2 weeks later (dotted lines/open symbols); note the transient error accumulations at the "protan" sites.

reduced discrimination of blue as shown by the Ishihara, Nagel, Farnsworth Panel D-15, and 28-hue Roth tests (Neubauer, 1973). In a further study, Marré, Nemetz, and Neubauer (1974) observed that the occurrence of color defect effects depends on the duration of use of oral contraceptives (Anovlar, Eugynon 28, Lyndiol, Neogynon, Ovulen, Ovosiston). The longer the use, the more the risk that one will find a blue–yellow defect.

Siegel and Smith (1967) observed an acquired cone dysfunction during furaltodone (Altafur) therapy; the observed color vision defects, surprisingly, were type II.

Bhargava (1973), unlike most authors who agree that tobacco amblyopia (see also above) is an optic neuropathy with a type II acquired red–green defect, concluded that the origin was retinal because he obtained results with the Pickford-Nicolson anomaloscope that were similar to those of congenital extreme protanomaly.

Among subjects treated with pheniothiazine, there was an "abnormally high proportion of protanopes" (Boet, 1970).

INTOXICATIONS LEADING TO A TYPE II
ACQUIRED RED–GREEN DEFECT

A large number of papers have been published dealing with toxic optic neuropathy. A toxic optic neuropathy gives rise to a type II dyschromatopsia. As mentioned before, color vision examination is extremely important for the detection of a preclinical stage of optic neuritis and, of course, in toxic optic neuropathy. Once the diagnosis of this condition has been established, the effect of the therapeutic efforts can be easily followed by color vision examination. The FM 100-hue test, for example, enables one to follow the course of the type II defect by observing the changes in pattern of the errors plotted on the graph. Chisholm, Bronte-Stewart, and Awduche (1970) demonstrated that in tobacco amblyopia it is even possible to adjust the amount of therapeutic hydroxycobalamine intramuscularly to the FM 100-hue test total error score. Drugs and other chemicals that can cause toxic amblyopia, optic neuritis, optic atrophy, and related conditions are listed by Lyle (1974).

Antibiotics and chemotherapeutics. Tuberculostatics are toxic agents for the optic nerve (Brückner, 1969; Renard & Morax, 1977). The various types of tuberculostatics differ in their chemical structure, and as a result it is not easy to explain their neurotoxicity as a common trait. It is very difficult to implicate a maximum dosage or duration of therapy. It seems that toxicity often is not a direct but an indirect result, stemming, perhaps, from alterations of the intestinal flora and changes in the resorption capacity of the intestine (Pinckers, 1975b). Carroll (1966) suggested that nutritional amblyopia may be either primary or secondary to chronic alcoholism or that the use of tobacco as the centrocecal scotoma is the same in tobacco amblyopia as in alcohol amblyopia.

Paraaminosalicylic acid is reported to cause a toxic optic neuritis (Steiner, 1951; Crews, 1963).

Streptomycin is reported to cause optic neuritis (Crews, 1963). Laroche (1967) states that a type II acquired red–green defect even appears in congenital protanomalous and deuteranomalous subjects.

Ethambutol (Carr & Henkind, 1962; Bouzas, Kokkinakis, Papadakis, & Daikos, 1970; Vérin, Pesme, Yacoubi, & Morax, 1971; Orou, Sideroff, & Schabel, 1972; Thaler, Heilig, Heiss, & Lessel, 1974; Pinckers, 1975b). Koliopoulos and Palimeris (1972) followed 138 patients treated with ethambutol; 8 displayed a type II acquired red–green defect, and color vision remained normal in those cases who did not display an optic neuritis. Trusiewicz (1975) stated that the FM 100-hue test is particularly useful and reliable in the follow-up examinations of ethambutol-induced toxic optic neuropathy; in one case the acquired color vision defect was superimposed on a hereditary deficiency. Douche (1974) feels that the use of alcohol predisposes the patient to a toxic optic neuropathy during ethambutol therapy. Derka (1975), summarizing the results of 16 authors concerning 2,007 myambutol-treated subjects, concluded that the frequency of optic neuritis increases from zero for a dosage of 20 mg/kg/day to 32 percent for a dosage of 50 mg/kg/day.

Rifampin dihydrostreptomycin and isoniazid have been included in reports by François and Verriest (1961b), Crews (1963), and Laroche (1967).

Chloramphenicol. When this drug is systemically administered the risk is not only depression of the bone marrow followed by aplastic anemia but also the possibility of a toxic optic neuropathy (Crews, 1963; Kittel & Cornelius, 1969).

Sulfonamides. Toxic effects of the sulfonamides are transient myopia, xanthopsia, toxic optic neuritis with papilledema, and retinal hemorrhages (Henkes, 1968). In four patients with prolonged salazosulfapyridine therapy Pinckers (1975b) observed in one eye normal color vision, in four eyes disturbed color vision without prominent axis, and in three eyes a type II acquired red–green defect. Figure 8.39 shows the FM 100-hue test error score after withdrawal of the salazopyridine medication and therapy with hydroxocobalamin intramuscularly.

Nitrofurane derivatives. Siegel and Smith (1967) found an acquired cone dysfunction but type II acquired color vision defects during furaltadone (Altafur) therapy. Nalidixic acid (Negram) causes cyanopsia and ianthinopsia without defects of color discrimination (Haut, Haye, Legras, Demailly, & Clay, 1972).

Quinoline derivatives. The history of toxicology of the quinoline derivatives is described by von Jess (1969). The first derivative in this group found to cause blindness was quinine. In a recent report, François, DeRouck, and Cambie (1972) stated that

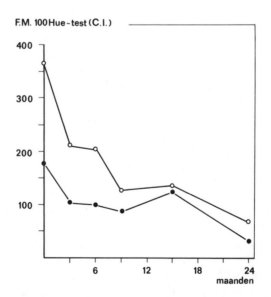

Fig. 8.39. FM 100-hue test error score in followup examination of a presumed salazosulfapyridinum toxic optic neuropathy. [From Pinckers, A. *Medikon*, 1975, *4*, 18–27]

involvement of the optic nerve is the first sign of pathology. During World War I, optochin and eucupin caused blindness. Quinidine gives rise to a toxic optic neuritis (Crews, 1963). After World War II the chloroquine derivatives (synthetic antimalarial agents) also turned out to be toxic, with essentially a type III acquired blue–yellow defect (Grützner, 1969a, b; Bec, Belleville, Arne, Philippet, & Secheyron, 1977), but a predominantly red–green defect sometimes is present (Grützner, 1969a, b). François, DeRouck, Cambie, and DeLaey (1972b) observed that of a total of 17 cases with chloroquine retinopathy, one red–green defect was observed. These observations may seem contradictory, but Pinckers and Van der Eerden (1973) followed 3 cases of chloroquine retinopathy, and they observed that the predominant type III blue–yellow defect becomes a predominant red–green defect as soon as the optic disc becomes atrophic (Fig. 8.40).

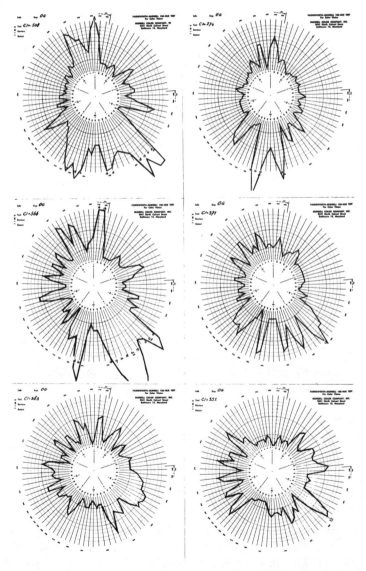

Fig. 8.40. FM 100-hue test "axis rotation" in followup examination of chloroquine-induced retinopathy.

Clioquinol intoxication is also known as subacute myeloopticoneuropathy (SMON). Matsuo, Okabe, Ueno, Takabatake, and Maeta (1971) examined 37 SMON cases; 10 had an optic atrophy. In the group of 27 without optic atrophy, 18 had normal color vision, 3 a red–green defect, 5 a nonclassified acquired defect, and 1 a type III acquired blue–yellow defect. In the group of 10 cases with optic atrophy, 8 had a red–green defect, 1 a type III acquired blue–yellow defect, and 1 an unclassified color vision disturbance. A type II acquired red–green defect is also described by Ohta (1968), Bron, Korten, Pinckers, and Majoor (1972), Boergen (1973), Thurn (1973), and others. Up to now, there is no report of intoxication on long-term therapy with glaphenine, which is also a quinoline derivative.

Antipyretics.   An optic neuritis can be caused by phenylbutazone therapy (Crews, 1963). Collum and Bowen (1971) observed 40 patients receiving Ibuprofen therapy; 2 developed cecocentral field defects and reduced visual acuity. There was a marked improvement when the drug was withdrawn. In 2 other cases a toxic reaction may have taken place, but the evidence was not conclusive. Pinckers (1975b) observed two additional patients developing cecocentral field defects, diminished visual acuity, and type II red–green defect. The symptoms disappeared after withdrawal of the drug.

Monoamine oxidase (MAO) inhibitors.   Gillespie, Terry, and Sjoerdsma (1959), Palmer (1963), and Joseph and Berkmann (1965) have described optic neuritis and type II acquired red–green color vision defects resulting from these drugs.

Oral antidiabetics.   Crews (1963) attributes an optic neuritis to medication with oral antidiabetics from the sulfonylureum group, such as tolbutamide and chlorpropamide.

Other drugs.   Thallium is said to be responsible for a toxic optic neuritis (Girot & Braum, 1929) with a type II acquired red–green defect (Pinckers, 1975b). During amoproxan (Mederel) treatment, optic neuritis and dermomucosal reactions are reported (François, Woillez, Guibert, & Carouges, 1971; Huriez, 1971; Saraux, 1971).

A chronic alcoholic, treated with disulfiram (Antabuse, Refusal), is again threatened by optic neuritis (Perdriel, 1966; Saraux & Biais, 1970) with concomitant type II acquired red–green defects.

Cyanide intoxication can cause optic neuritis (Foulds, Chisholm, Bronte-Stewart, & Wilson, 1969; Pinckers, 1975b), but there is no relationship between the cyanide content of various brands of tobacco and tobacco amblyopia (Darby & Wilson, 1967). An optic neuropathy due to lead poisoning is reported by Baghdassarian (1968). Vints (1975) examined 1045 workers exposed to increased lead content in the air and stated that the color fields were constricted, especially for green. An interesting fact is that 5.4 percent of the workers developed macular lesions. Crews (1963) observed optic neuritis during therapy with mercaptopurine, ergotamine, and hexamethonium; Saraux (1975) reported the same toxic effect occurring in penicillamine- and arsenic-treated patients.

INTOXICATIONS LEADING TO A TYPE III
ACQUIRED BLUE–YELLOW DEFECT

The diagnosis of a toxic type III acquired blue–yellow defect is not an easy one. It is much easier to diagnose a toxic optic neuropathy than a toxic maculopathy. Pinckers and Van der Eerden (1973), for example, observed the appearance of a type III acquired blue–yellow defect during hydroxychloroquine therapy, but careful examination revealed a central serous retinopathy that healed spontaneously.

Corneal deposits in general do not influence color discrimination, but once the deposits are dense, color vision will be affected to some slight degree (Lakowski & Davenport, 1968) but without a clear axis of confusion. The same holds true for iatrogenic cataract because only the "brown" cataracts cause a type III acquired blue–yellow defect (Pinckers, 1975). Table 8.13 summarizes some drugs causing corneal deposits or cataracts.

Synthetic antimalarial agents give rise to toxic retinopathy with a predominant type III acquired blue–yellow defect. This is particularly true for the chloroquine derivatives; there is, however, a much lower rate of incidence of retinopathy in hydroxychloroquine treatment. For 6 years Pinckers and Van der Eerden (1973) followed Plaquenil R–treated subjects (in total, about 300 cases) and never observed a Plaquenil-induced retinopathy. Accumulation of chloroquine in the choroid and the pigment epithelial layer does not necessarily mean that there is intoxication. At this moment there is no method of examination that can predict retinopathy, and we must therefore combine as much information as possible from different methods, including fundus examination and visual fields. In our opinion the value of the EOG in detecting an early stage of retinopathy is doubtful, since about 20 percent of untreated rheumatoid arthritics have a subnormal Arden ratio and since reactivation of rheumatoid arthritis simultaneously can diminish the Arden ratio (Kolb, 1965; Pinckers & Van Der Eerden, 1973). In only a few cases of chloroquine retinopathy is a type II acquired red–green defect observed; as suggested formerly, this may be interpreted as a sign of optic atrophy.

Indomethacin (Indocid) is implicated by Burns (1968) in causing corneal deposits and a maculopathy. A concomitant type III acquired blue–yellow defect is reported by Grützner (1969a) and Koliopoulos and Palimeris (1972) in two cases. Palimeris, Koliopoulos, and Velissaropoulos (1972) observed five patients in whom color vision became normal 6 months after withdrawal of the drug. Henkes, van Lith, and Canta (1972) and Carr and Siegel (1973) did not observe color vision defects.

Erythromycin, according to Laroche and Laroche (1971), gives type III acquired blue–yellow defects.

Table 8.13
Drug-induced Corneal Deposits and Cataracts

Corneal Deposits	Cataracts	
Alcian blue	Allopurinol	Galactose
Amiodarone HCl	Anticholinesterase eyedrops	Metals
Arsenicals	Beta-naphthol	Myleran
Bismuth	Busulfan	Naphthalene
Calcium	Carbromal	Penicillamine
Chloroquine derivatives	Chloroquine	Phenmetrazine
Clioquinol	Chlorpromazine	Phenothiazines
Cytarabine	Clomiphene	Piperazine
Epinephrine	Corticosteroids	Sulfonamides
Hydroxychloroquine	Deferoxamine	Thallium
Indomethacin	Dichlorisone	Trinitrotoluene
Metals	Dichlorobenzene	Triparanol
Phenothiazines	Dinitro-o-cresol	Vitamin A excess
Sympathicomimetics	Dinitrophenol	Xylose
Urethane	Echothiophate	Zyloprim
	Ergot	

From Lyle (1974).

There are an astonishing number of phenothiazine derivatives. The toxic effects of these agents on the eye may be interpreted as photosensitization of the eyelids and conjunctiva, cornea (deposits), lens (cataract), and retina (retinopathy). Connell, Poley, and McFarlane (1964) observed a young woman with thioridazine intoxication who showed a pericentral scotoma but tested normal on a plate test. Cameron, Lawrence, and Olrich (1972) examined an early thioridazine intoxication but did not undertake color vision testing. Davidorf (1973) noted complaints of erythropsia. Alkemade (1968) found no effects on the AO HRR performance, while Grützner (1969a, b) observed a predominant type III acquired blue–yellow defect. Phenothiazine retinopathy is frequently observed in psychiatric patients. A reliable color vision examination in these patients is not easy to accomplish.

As mentioned earlier, the use of oral contraceptives may result in a reduced discrimination of blue; prolonged application gives rise to pathologic blue–yellow defects.

Since Cogan (1965) posed the question of neuroophthalmologic complications during medication with oral contraceptives a mass of publications has appeared. Observed are retinal vascular disturbances including partial or total embolism of the central retinal artery, venous thrombosis, and (peri)vasculitis retinae, posterior cyclitis, retinal edema, optic neuritis, papilledema, retrobulbar neuritis, homonymous hemianopsia, diminished visual acuity without apparent cause, exophthalmos, paresis of the sixth cranial nerve, migraine ophthalmia, and reduced tolerance to contact lens wearing. In considering this list of complications one can easily conclude that during oral contraceptive use we may expect a type II defect for optic nerve involvement or a type III defect in most other cases. Eventually, a type I defect is observed in cases involving the receptors in the macular area. According to Levinson (1969) these side-effects are infrequent, varying, and difficult to document.

Hypovitaminosis

Vitamins are chemical compounds essential for proper metabolism. The body is unable to synthesize them for itself and as a consequence is dependent on dietary sources. Vitamins fall into two broad groups—the "fat-soluble" vitamins (vitamins A, D, and E) and the "water-soluble" vitamins (vitamin B group and vitamin C). The relative or absolute reduction of the body levels of any vitamin may occur because of specific dietary deficiency, defective absorption, impaired transport, or storage. The impairment of visual function does not appear as the sole manifestation of a reduced body level of any of the vitamins but may take the role as the presenting symptom.

HYPOVITAMINOSIS A

A subnormal level of vitamin A in the blood is associated with night blindness, reduced dark adaptation, a diminished ERG rod response, death of photoreceptors—abnormal keratinization of mucous membranes (Bitot spots and conjunctival xerosis)—and, in severe depletion, keratomalacia. The full spectrum of change in hypovitaminosis A is more often found in underprivileged countries associated with major nutritional problems. In European and North American societies a depletion of vitamin A is most often found in association with a form of retinitis pigmentosa, with hepatic cirrhosis, or in fat malabsorption syndromes.

Levy and Toskes (1975) observed normal color vision in a case of fundus albipunctatus and reversible vitamin A deficiency with steatorrhoea (AO HRR test).

Reddy and Vijayalaxami (1977) reported a color vision study of children in India (ages 4–12 years) who suffered from night blindness and conjunctival xerosis and who had subnormal levels of vitamin A in their sera. Color vision responses to testing with AO HRR plates were recorded before and after supplemental vitamin A therapy for 15 days; there was improvement in the night blindness, but the color vision, originally normal, remained so.

Since the bulk of the body vitamin A store is located in the liver, it is understandable that in chronic hepatic disease such as cirrhosis the serum vitamin A level may be depressed. Cruz-Coke (1964; 1965) recorded abnormal color vision to testing with AO HRR plates in subjects showing hepatic cirrhosis due to chronic alcoholism. Although the disease was thought originally to be related to genetically inherited red–green color defects, more recent evidence (reviewed by Cruz-Coke, 1972) indicates a blue–yellow defect. Sandberg, Rosen, and Berson (1977) measured tvr curves in vitamin A deficiency with chronic alcoholism and showed selective abnormalities of the blue (π_1) cone mechanism.

Numerous researchers have demonstrated abnormal color vision responses from patients suffering from chronic nonalcoholic hepatic disease—plate tests (Fialkow, Thuline, & Fenster, 1966) and the FM 100-hue test (Klein & Dressel, 1970; Bronte-Stewart & Foulds, 1972; Rothstein, Shapiro, Sacks, & Weis, 1973). The acquired defect recorded has been both blue–yellow and red–green (Dittrich & Neubauer, 1967; Neubauer & Dittrich, 1970) and anarchic on testing with FM 100-hue test. In acute hepatitis, Lukaszewicz, Wysocki, and Wozmy (1972) recorded constriction of the visual field to a blue target. The patients recorded by Bronte-Stewart and Foulds (1972) are of special interest because the color vision defect was reversible. The FM 100-hue test results and visual acuity improved significantly with vitamin A therapy (Fig. 8.41). The earlier findings of Fialkow, Thuline, and Fenster (1966) and Smith and Brinton (1971), who recorded improving responses to plate tests after specific therapy for cirrhosis, were thus confirmed.

HYPOVITAMINOSIS B₁₂ (COBALAMIN) AND B₁₁ (FOLIC ACID)

Deficiency of either vitamin leads to megaloblastic anemia (see above) and in exceptional instances to neurologic deficit (see above). A color vision defect on testing with Ishihara plates was reported by Adams, Chalmers, Foulds, and Withy (1967) in patients suffering from megaloblastic anemia to either B₁₂ or B₁₁ deficiency. A type III acquired blue–yellow defect was reported by Chisholm (1972) in a series of patients suffering from Addisonian pernicious anemia that persisted after correction of the avitaminosis. This was interpreted by Chisholm as representing an acceleration of a normal aging process but by Foulds (1969) as indicating a permanent ischemic change. Rothstein, Shapiro, Sacks, and Weis (1973), when analyzing patients suffering from cirrhosis, concluded that the poor color response to the FM 100-hue test was related to the subnormal serum folic acid levels of their patients.

ALCOHOLISM

Ethyl alcohol (ethanol, C_2H_5OH) is metabolized to carbon dioxide (CO_2) and water, with release of energy, in a manner similar to that of pyruvate. This breakdown takes place in the microsomal ethanol oxidizing system, principally located in the liver but also present in the muscle and to a small amount in the retina. Chronic alcohol addiction is recognized to be associated with a variety of systemic conditions—malnutrition, cirrhosis, encephalopathy, and peripheral neuropathy. Alcohol intake correlates with several biochemical and hematologic disturbances (Whitehead, Clarke, & Whitfield, 1978).

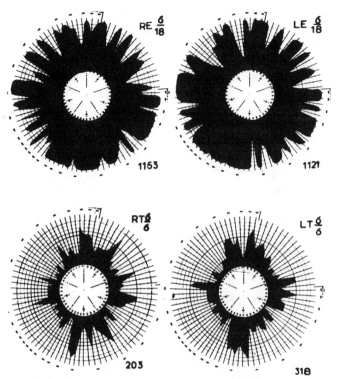

Fig. 8.41. FM 100-hue test profile before and after vitamin A therapy for a female patient suffering from cirrhosis of the liver and hypovitaminosis A.

Ingestion of ethyl alcohol produces disturbances of accommodation, diminution of the flicker fusion frequency, alteration in color vision, slowing of dark adaptation (Walsh & Hoyt, 1969), a decrease in resistance to glare (Verriest & Laplasse, 1965), and impaired visual search speed (Bertera & Parsons, 1978).

Methyl alcohol (wood alcohol or methanol, CH_3OH) is highly poisonous, and consumption in some individuals leads to a rapid loss of vision. Neural tissue shows changes such as edema with scattered hemorrhages and edema of neural cells followed by degeneration. The changes in the retina appear first in the ganglion cells, followed by the inner nuclear layers and lastly the neural receptors (Fink, 1943). Methyl alcohol is metabolized differently and more slowly than ethyl alcohol. It is oxidized in a series of stages to formic acid, in which form it is excreted in the urine. An intermediary form is formaldehyde, and this has been considered by many authorities to be the constituent that causes the widespread neurologic deficits and acidosis (Rϕe, 1946; Potts & Johnson, 1952). The earliest changes in the visual fields are due to loss of sensitivity to color. Initially, this occurs for green, followed by red, yellow, and, finally, blue. There is a central scotoma that is reversible in mild cases of poisoning; the peripheral field remains full even when optic atrophy is present (Rϕe, 1946). A type III acquired blue–yellow defect with neutral zone from 567 to 569 nm in methyl alcohol poisoning is described by Jaeger (1955).

Cruz-Coke (1964; 1965) found a significant association between color vision defect (AO HRR plates) and chronic alcoholic cirrhosis of the liver. Further research showed that the defect was a type III blue–yellow defect (Varela, Rivera, Mardomes, & Cruz-Coke, 1969). Cruz-Coke felt that a genetic explanation suggested that a sex-linked gene may control some metabolic pathway in the pathogenesis of the cirrhosis and the incidence of the color defect. Later workers (Swinson, 1972; Saraux, Labet, & Biais, 1966) were unable to confirm his findings; further, they found improvement in the color defect with therapy. Thuline (1967), studying patients with plate tests, found no association between the color defect and alcoholism unless the patient was acutely ill.

There seems little doubt that chronic alcoholism, with or without cirrhosis or psychosis, causes a disturbance in color discrimination, either blue–yellow or red–green, in spite of earlier reports to the contrary. Gorrell (1967) claimed that there was no color upset in alcoholism on the basis of his investigation with Ishihara plates. He gained support from Riffenburgh and Shea (1970) and Cinotti, Stephens, and Kiebel (1970). Sasson, Wise, and Watson (1970) confirmed the presence of a blue–yellow defect on testing with the Farnsworth Panel D-15 in 22 percent of alcoholics and a significant incidence in nonalcoholic relatives of alcoholics. Sakuma (1973) examined 56 eyes of chronic alcoholic males and 58 eyes of alcoholic psychotic males, making use of Ishihara plates, Farnsworth Panel D-15, the FM 100-hue test, and the anomaloscope. He found that an acquired defect of color vision was present in 80 percent of all cases of chronic alcoholism. The defect was principally a type II red–green defect, which he felt indicated a disturbance to the visual pathway.

FUNCTIONAL AMBLYOPIA*

The pattern of color vision defect in amblyopia secondary to strabismus (squint) is exceptional among the acquired color defects because it does not fall within the Verriest classification. It is part of a very complex disturbance of visual function that includes disorders of spatial summation, contrast, visual acuity, differential luminance thresholds, and dark adaptation. The etiology of these disturbances may be understood partly as a passive inhibition of functional development and partly as an active suppression by the visual cortex (perhaps extending centrifugally towards the retina). The first description of color vision defects in strabismic amblyopia was that of Javal (1868; 1871). Parinaud (1899) pointed out the relation between color vision defect and visual acuity and Wald and Burian (1944) the relation to the "lateralization" of vision. An excellent historical review up to 1965 was given by Roth (1968).

Clinical Tests

The usual clinical tests for color vision examination are suitable for detecting middle- and high-grade disturbances in functional amblyopia; however, the majority of results indicate only reduced chromatic discriminative ability.

PSEUDOISOCHROMATIC PLATES

Amblyopes with foveal or parafoveal fixation* will read pseudoisochromatic plates without error in most cases. With increasing eccentricity of fixation the number of errors increases, but a specific defect is not indicated (Verriest, 1964; Pajor & Medgyaszay,

---

Terminology of the central retina (Spitznas; 1975). Foveola: 20' (in the center of the fovea); fovea: 0°–3° eccentricity (diameter of 6°); parafovea: 3°–5.3° eccentricity; perifovea: 5.3°–11.3°eccentricity. *Terminology of the fixation mode.* Foveolar: steady fixation with the foveola, normal case of fixation; parafoveolar: outside the foveola but within the fovea; parafoveal: outside the fovea but within the parafovea; perifoveal: outside the parafovea but within the perifovea; peripheral: outside the perifovea; eccentric: all kinds of fixation outside the foveola.

*Contributed by Marion Marré, M.D.

1965; Roth, 1968; Krebs & Hubbe, 1969; Laszczyk & Szubinska, 1973). Simultaneous disturbance of form vision may influence the results. Zanen (1951) reported an excessive local adaptation so that Ishihara plates were not recognized after a few seconds of observation. By means of Rabkin's plates Giessmann (1966) found increased thresholds for chromatic discrimination and normal thresholds for purity discrimination.

NAGEL ANOMALOSCOPE

Typically the Rayleigh equation is normal when measured for amblyopic eyes of observers (Oppel, 1963; Saraux, 1963; Verriest, 1964; Frey, 1968; Krebs & Hubbe, 1969), but when middle- or high-grade amblyopia is present with eccentric fixation a broadened matching range (see Minor Color Deficiencies, Chapter 7) is found compared with the fellow dominant eye (Frey, 1968; Krebs & Hubbe, 1969). Occasionally, a shift of the Rayleigh equation to red has been reported (Pajor & Medgyaszay, 1965; Frey, 1968; Carvalho, 1973; cited by Verriest, 1974a).

ARRANGEMENT TESTS

Frey (1968) noticed that poor coordination of eye and hand can impair correct performance of arrangement tests.

On the FM 100-hue test, amblyopic observers with foveolar fixation have error scores within the limits of a corresponding age-matched control group (Bozzoni & Lumbroso, 1962; Lumbroso & Proto, 1963; Roth, 1968; Frühauf, Klein, & Ritter, 1973), but often the number of errors for the amblyopic eyes are higher than for the corresponding dominant eyes. Usually FM 100-hue test errors measured for amblyopic eyes with foveolar fixation show no predominant axis. Roth (1968) reported some predominance of a type III bipolar blue–yellow axis. There is a distinct growth of the numbers of errors with increasing eccentricity of fixation, but the character of these disturbances is not uniform. In the majority of cases the distribution of errors is without predominant axis, expressing a generally reduced chromatic discriminative ability. However, cases have been reported in which errors are predominant in the blue region (Bozzoni & Lumbroso, 1962) or in the red–green region (Lumbroso & Proto, 1963), and sometimes all kinds of defects are found in the patients in a single report (Verriest, 1964; Lasagni, De Molfetta, & Miglior, 1964; François & Verriest, 1965; 1966; Roth, 1968). No correlation between the distribution of errors and visual acuity or fixation mode could be demonstrated. Frühauf, Klein, and Ritter (1973) found significantly higher error scores even in the dominant eyes of persons with strabismic amblyopia than in a control group. Error scores in the dominant eye increased with the increasing eccentricity of fixation in the amblyopic eye, and error scores were higher on binocular than monocular testing.

On the Farnsworth Panel D-15 test, amblyopes with foveolar, parafoveolar, and parafoveal fixation show normal results. With perifoveal or peripheral fixation of increasing eccentricity, first minor errors are made; later confusions show a predominant scotopic pattern (François & Verriest, 1967) or a blue–yellow axis (Roth, 1968) and, finally, results of anarchic character.

On the Roth 28-hue test, amblyopes with foveolar or parafoveolar fixation show normal results or few errors. With parafoveal and peripheral fixation some results are within the norm and some show a scotopic axis. With increasing eccentricity of fixation, confusions become more frequent, type III and scotopic being most common (Roth, 1968).

On the Trendelenburg test (Trendelenburg, 1940) modified according to Ahlenstiel (1951), Giessmann (1962), Köhler (1965), and Krebs and Hubbe (1969) found disturbance of hue discrimination in individuals with amblyopic eyes and eccentric fixation.

CONCLUSIONS

In the 1960s two important clinical studies established the essential features of color vision defects in functional amblyopia. François and Verriest (1967) reported that color vision test results were often abnormal in strabismic amblyopia when central visual acuity was less than 0.2. The color vision defect does not correspond to the Verriest classification but approaches that of a normal subject using eccentric retinal fixation. Roth (1968) also concluded that color vision of the amblyopic eye is normal, no matter what visual acuity, provided that the fixation is foveolar. He noted that if fixation is eccentric it ought to be compared with eccentric color vision of a normal eye. The color vision of the fovea remains normal when the fixation is eccentric (measured with the afterimage method).

Results of Laboratory Tests

Only precise laboratory examination methods allow measurement of color vision defects other than reduced chromatic discriminative ability.

RETINAL SENSITIVITY

Absolute threshold spectral sensitivity.   Researchers differ as to whether retinal sensitivity in squint amblyopia is affected or not. Differences in the fixation mode of the examined eyes may account for these discrepancies. Wald and Burian (1944), using a 1° stimulus field positioned in the foveolar or eccentric retina, noted approximately normal absolute thresholds in 4 of 5 patients with strabismic amblyopia. In the fifth the thresholds were lower at shorter wavelengths and higher at longer wavelengths relative to normal data, with a minimum near 545 nm; this individual complained of difficulties in fixing the test spot during examination. Burian (1967) concluded that the reduction in absolute threshold sensitivity, if it was not artifactual, was of an entirely different order of magnitude than the reduction of form vision. In an examination of 11 patients with amblyopia and visual acuity of 0.6–0.1, Zanen and Szucs (1956) found an elevation of the achromatic and chromatic thresholds for a 3' field that increased as wavelength increased; the photochromatic interval remained normal. Zanen (1969) reported on the relation between the elevation of thresholds and the visual acuity; the luminous energy required for absolute threshold in amblyopic eyes with visual acuity 0.5 is three times greater than in normal eyes, and in amblyopic eyes with visual acuity 0.5–0.3 the energy requirement is six times greater. Szucs (1966) found the absolute threshold most depressed in the center of the visual field and least depressed at 20°–30° eccentricity.

Marré and Marré (1978b; 1979) compared the absolute threshold spectral sensitivities of amblyopic and normal eyes. The mean curve of measurements taken with ten amblyopic eyes with foveolar fixation showed only a slight reduction of sensitivity without statistical significance. The mean curve of measurements taken on ten amblyopic eyes with parafoveal fixation showed values similar to the normal foveolar values in the spectral range of 400–450 nm and depressed sensitivity ranging from 0.1 log unit at 475 nm to about 0.6 log unit between 560 and 700 nm. By comparing the mean curve of the amblyopic eyes with the curve of an individual normal eye at 6° eccentricity, it was shown that the shapes of the curves generally corresponded but that the curve of the amblyopic

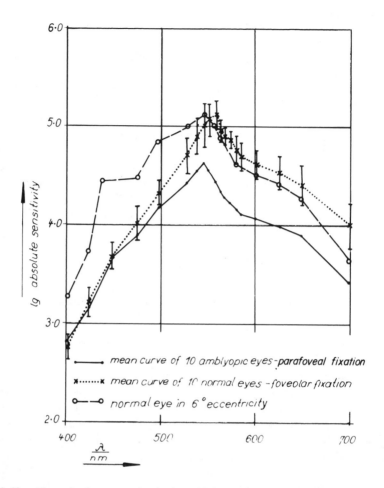

Fig. 8.42. Mean absolute spectral retinal sensitivity curves for amblyopic eyes with parafoveal fixation, ●—●; ten normal eyes with foveolar fixation, ×. . .×; and one normal eye at 6° eccentricity, ○—○. The mean curve of the amblyopic eyes resembles that of the normal eye at 6° eccentricity but is depressed across the entire spectrum by about 0.45–0.60 log unit. [From Marré, M. & Marré, E. *Modern Problems in Ophthalmology*, 1978, *19*, 248–252 (reproduced with permission of S. Karger AG).]

eyes was lowered rather regularly across the entire spectrum for about 0.45–0.60 log unit (Fig. 8.42). Thus in comparison with the normal sensitivity of the eccentric retinal area the sensitivity of the amblyopic eyes with parafoveal fixation was reduced.

Spectral curve of relative luminous efficiency. Verriest (1970b) reported that relative to the normal function the mean spectral relative luminous efficiency curve of five amblyopic eyes (visual acuity 0.4–0.05) showed a slight increase in sensitivity at short wavelengths and a slight reduction in sensitivity at long wavelengths. Marré (personal communication) found accordant results in ten amblyopic eyes with parafoveal fixation. The slight shift of the curves to the short-wave side of the spectrum corresponded to the eccentricities of the retinal fixation areas. In five amblyopic eyes with strong foveolar fixation the curves were normal.

Increment thresholds. Israel and Verriest (1972) measured achromatic increment thresholds for monochromatic blue and yellow lights on an achromatic background in the central visual fields of normal and amblyopic eyes by means of a Goldmann static perimeter. The fixation of the amblyopic eyes was "central or slightly eccentric." For the amblyopic eyes the mean yellow threshold was more reduced in sensitivity than the mean blue one.

Dark adaptation. Authors have described dark adaptation in squint amblyopia as normal (Wald & Burian, 1944; Jayle & Ourgaud, 1950; Oppel & Kranke, 1958) or as abnormal (Fujino, 1967; Flynn, 1968). Flynn and Glaser (1971) demonstrated that with foveolar fixation normal adaptation was observed but with eccentric fixation dark adaptation was not normal. Using Wald's colored filter technique these authors found threshold elevations in both cone and rod portions of the dark adaptation function.

INVESTIGATION OF COLOR VISION MECHANISMS BY
ADAPTATION TO CHROMATIC OR TO WHITE BACKGROUNDS

Two-color threshold technique. Hansen (1975) performed static perimetry during chromatic adaptation on 11 amblyopic eyes with foveolar or eccentric fixation using the Stiles' two-color threshold technique. In six patients with foveolar fixation no significant difference of threshold values was found between the amblyopic and dominant eyes. The perimetric profiles of the amblyopic eyes for which fixation was eccentric exhibited a central depression for the red and green sensitivity functions. The higher the degree of amblyopia, the more pronounced the depression relative to the data for the nonamblyopic eye. The blue sensitivity functions showed no corresponding depression.

Wald-Marré technique. Marré (1969) and Marré and Marré (1978a; 1979) determined the relative sensitivity of the three primary color vision mechanisms (CVMs) in squint amblyopia by the method described in Chapter 6. Amblyopic eyes with foveolar or unsteady foveolar fixation showed normal foveolar CVMs. For three cases in which fixation was parafoveolar, parafoveal, or perifoveal, the blue CVM was increased and the green and the red CVMs were decreased relative to those of the normal foveolar values (Fig. 8.43). The CVMs for amblyopic eyes with eccentric fixation corresponded to those of eccentric retinal areas in normal eyes, either at the same eccentricity or at a more central position than the amblyopic fixation area. Consequently, no reduction of the CVMs in comparison with the corresponding normal eccentric retinal area could be stated. Individuals in whom pathologic CVMs similar to those characterizing acquired color vision defects are observed (Marré and Marré, 1978b; 1979) are suspected to have organic lesions causing the amblyopia.

Increment threshold spectral sensitivity (white background). Harwerth and Levi (1977) determined increment threshold sensitivity curves using monochromatic test flashes superimposed upon an adapting white background at four different radiance levels. The sensitivity of the amblyopic eyes with unsteady central fixation was lower across the entire visible spectrum relative to the nonamblyopic eyes. This reduction in sensitivity was attributed to anisometropia, aniseikonia, or unsteady fixation. The amblyopic curves showed systematic differences in their relative shapes, especially in the position and depth of the dip in the yellow region (Fig. 8.44). For each amblyopic eye the dip was more

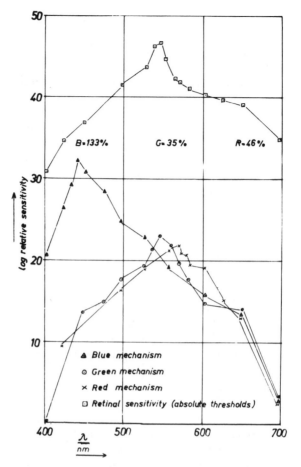

Fig. 8.43. Relative sensitivity curves for three CVMs from a patient with squint amblyopia, with fixation 2°–6° above the foveola. Eccentric CVM pattern: B mechanism increased, G and R mechanisms decreased. Absolute retinal sensitivity lowered, maximum lying at about 545 nm.

shallow and lay at a shorter wavelength than for the nonamblyopic eye. These differences were accounted for by anomalous lateral inhibition between the red and green cones in the amblyopic eye. At the highest background luminances the dip tends to be more like that of the normal eye.

WAVELENGTH DISCRIMINATION

Wavelength discrimination curves for 30 amblyopic eyes with known fixation mode were compared with those for normal eyes in foveolar and eccentric fixation by Marré (1972b) and Marré and Marré (1979). Hue discrimination in amblyopic eyes with foveolar or unsteady foveolar fixation may be normal, slightly reduced in the short-wave range, or slightly impaired over the whole spectrum. Similar hue discrimination findings were reported in color amblyopia (Grützner, 1971). In amblyopic eyes with parafoveal or perifoveal fixation, wavelength discrimination corresponded to that of eccentric retinal areas in normal eyes; the normal eccentric area does, however, have a more central

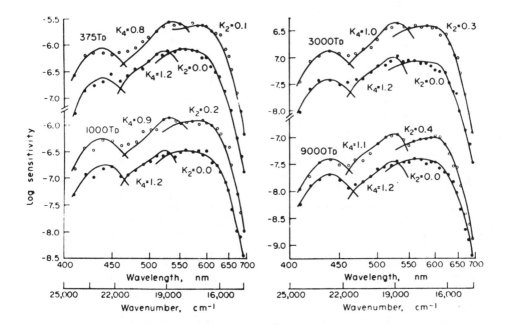

Fig. 8.44. Increment threshold spectral sensitivity curves showing those from amblyopic eye (filled circles) compared with the fellow nonamblyopic eye (open circles) from a patient with anisometric amblyopia. Curves are shown for the four background luminances indicated above each curve. The sensitivity of the amblyopic eye is lower across the entire visible spectrum and does not show the dip in the yellow region that is characteristic for the nonamblyopic eye. [From Harwerth, R. S. & Levi, D. M. *Vision Research,* 1977, *17,* 585–590 (reproduced with permission of Pergamon Press).]

position than the fixating area in the amblyopic eye (Fig. 8.45). Wavelength discrimination is better than could be expected with regard to the position of fixation. It is not clear if there is a real functional improvement in the fixating area or if the examination procedures themselves influence the fixation mode. François and Verriest (1965) stated that even amblyopes with visual acuity of less than 0.1 show only a slight deficiency, similar to that found in a normal subject whose vision is eccentric by a few degrees.

COLORIMETRIC PURITY DISCRIMINATION

In four cases of strabismic amblyopia with foveolar, unsteady foveolar, and parafoveolar fixation, Marré (1969; 1979) found normal sensitivity for colorimetric purity discrimination in a 12° field (Fig. 8.46).

Diagnostic Aspects

Normal foveolar or eccentric CVM patterns suggest functional amblyopia, whereas pathologic CVM patterns suggest invisible organic lesions (Marré & Marré, 1978b; 1979). Relatively normal chromatic discrimination distinguishes functional amblyopia from optic neuritis with its marked type II acquired red–green defect (Verriest, 1964). By means of color critical fusion frequency, Hokama (1968) could differentiate functional amblyopia from organic disease, especially from diseases of the optic nerve. Serial color vision

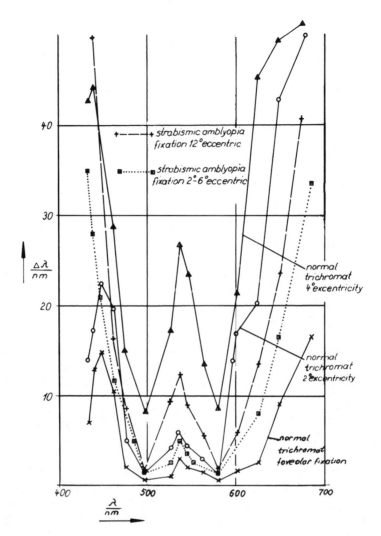

Fig. 8.45. Wavelength discrimination of two eyes with strabismic amblyopia and parafoveal and perifoveal fixation in comparison with the hue discrimination of a normal eye in foveolar vision, in 2° and in 4° eccentricity. The hue discrimination of the amblyopic eyes is better than could be expected with regard to the positions of their fixation areas. [From Marré, M. & Marré, E. *Modern Problems in Ophthalmology,* 1978, *19,* 248–252 (reproduced with permission of S. Karger AG).]

examination will be important before starting amblyopia reeducation, since it may be possible to detect cases in which the ambylopia is caused by ophthalmoscopically invisible organic damage. At present, available laboratory methods are still too complicated for the examination of very young children.

Prognosis

By means of the Roth 28-hue test and pseudoisochromatic plates, Roth (1968) demonstrated that color vision improves with amelioration of fixation during the course of amblyopic reeducation. Similar results were reported by Laszczyk and Szubinska (1973, Ishihara plates) and by Lumbroso and Proto (1963, FM 100-hue test).

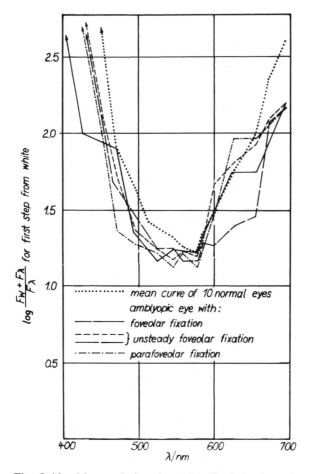

Fig. 8.46. Mean colorimetric purity discrimination of ten normal eyes (12° field foveolar fixation) compared with curves from four amblyopic eyes with foveolar, unsteady foveolar, and parafoveolar fixation. Discrimination of the amblyopic eyes is not significantly disturbed. [From Marré, M. & Marré, E. *Modern Problems in Ophthalmology*, 1978, *19, 248–252* (reproduced with permission of S. Karger AG).]

The practical consequence of color vision testing with regard to profession and traffic is limited. In squint amblyopia disturbances of visual acuity and binocular vision are more severe than the color discrimination loss, and as a rule the color vision of the dominant fellow eye is normal.

Conclusions

Color vision in eyes with functional amblyopia is dependent on the mode of fixation. With foveolar fixation the usual clinical tests give normal results, but spectral examination methods can detect depressions of the retinal sensitivity and slight reductions in wavelength discrimination ability. With increasing eccentricity of fixation, color vision undergoes an increasing deterioration. The usual clinical tests produce results resembling those of eccentric ·retinal areas in normal eyes. The spectral sensitivity measurements method shows a reduced retinal sensitivity for the eccentric fixation area. The relative luminous efficiency curve is shifted slightly to the short-wavelength side of the spectrum. Measurement of CVMs and wavelength discrimination give better results than could be expected with regard to the position of the fixating area as determined by visuscope. The values correspond to those obtained in retinal areas in normal eyes at least as close to the fovea as the amblyopic fixation point, but usually of an even more central position. Colorimetric purity discrimination is not disturbed.

Guy Verriest, M.D.

9

Vocational and Practical Implications of Defective Color Vision

Color vision deficiency can be a handicap in practical situations such as employment (Pierce, 1934; Bonnardel, 1936; Tiffin & Kuhn, 1942; Pickford, 1955; Dreyer, 1969; Taylor, 1971; Cole, 1972a, b; Fox, 1973; Verriest & Hermans, 1975; Voke, 1976; 1978). Apart from the obvious reduction in the ability to discriminate chromaticity differences, other visual skills such as matching metameric colors or naming shades may also be affected. Changes in the spectral curve of relative luminous efficiency of the absolute or increment threshold sensitivities may be important. Even changes in aesthetic judgement may have practical implications in a given situation.

ROADS AND HIGHWAYS

Early studies of the question as to whether or nor drivers with defective color vision are a potential hazard on roads and highways were inconclusive. The WHO recommendation of 1956 and some authors (for example, Harms, 1961; Zehnder, 1971; Kalberer, 1971b; Frey, 1973) suggested that color defectives should be granted a license to drive any kind of vehicle, while other authors (for example, Comberg, 1962; 1964; Hager, 1963; Schober, 1963; Nathan, Geoffrey, & Cole, 1964; Gramberg-Danielsen, 1965; Allen, 1966; Münchow, 1967; Broschmann, 1976) held that restrictions should be applied, especially in the case of protanopia. This uncertainty is reflected in the diversity of national regulations concerning the granting of licenses to protanopes. Some countries exclude them from driving any vehicle, others from professional driving, and others only from professional conveyance of passengers, while still others place no limitations at all. Some countries also exclude deuteranopes.

Gramberg-Danielsen (1976) anticipated the following possible difficulties for the color defective driver: (1) belated recognition of colored signals; (2) confusion of colored signals; (3) failure to see red signals owing to the shortening of the red end of the spectrum in protans. Experimental studies in simulated environments have confirmed that color defectives are significantly slower and make significantly more errors than normal observers in identifying the colors of signal lights, especially under conditions of lower intensity, shorter observation time, and greater distance (Ganter, 1955; Hager, 1963; Nathan, Geoffrey, & Cole, 1963; Cole & Brown, 1965; Spieker, 1965; Allen, 1966). More recently Verriest, Neubauer, Uvijls, and Sintobin (1978) have conducted a series of experiments reproducing as closely as possible the traffic conditions on a real road in the open and using both normal and red–green–defective persons as drivers. Their results were as follows:

1. The distance for noticing red octagonal "STOP" traffic signs was reduced to about 53 percent of the normal value in the case of color defectives. Other traffic signs indicating danger were seen at about 83 percent of the normal distance by color defectives. Experience during the experiment benefitted the normal observers to a greater extent than the defective observers (Fig. 9.1).
2. The distance for noticing stop lights especially in bright sunlight was reduced to between 39 and 73 percent of normal for protans and from 50 to over 100 percent of normal for deutans. In this case, the color defectives showed greater improvement in performance during the experiment (Fig. 9.2).
3. The distance for noticing rear red lights at night was reduced to 60 percent of normal for protans and 90 percent of normal for deutans (Fig. 9.3).
4. The ability to differentiate the colors of rear signal lights on vehicles in daylight such as red brake lights, orange direction indicators, and white backup lights was as follows: normals, no errors; anomalous trichromats, few errors; dichromats, more errors. Contrary to the results of other experiments, the deutans made twice as many errors as the protans.
5. In a second series of experiments these authors showed that deutans are as handicapped or more handicapped than protans in recognizing the colors of traffic lights (Fig. 9.4) and that in practice the defective individual identifies these signals using cues other than color, e.g., the position of lights on the post.

These results appear to contradict several statistical analyses of the causes of traffic accidents that showed that very few accidents could be traced to defective color vision (Sachsenwager & Nothaas, 1961; Gramberg-Danielsen, 1967; Zehnder, 1971). However, Neubauer, Harrer, Marré, and Verriest (1978) have pointed out that most of these papers are out-of-date and that traffic conditions have changed considerably in the last few years with the increase in traffic density and the expansion of the motorway system. They have also raised the following criticisms:

1. Not all drivers having accidents are included in the analysis.
2. The number of drivers having had a thorough ophthalmoscopic examination (before and after the accident) is too small.
3. Professional drivers, especially of emergency vehicles, should not be included.
4. Most authors have been concerned with whether or not a driver has confused the colors of traffic lights; this is unlikely, since color defectives can make use of brightness and position cues. What should be more closely examined are accidents where vehicles have collided with other vehicles either turning left or right or stopping or where drivers seem to have ignored red warning signs—a distinct

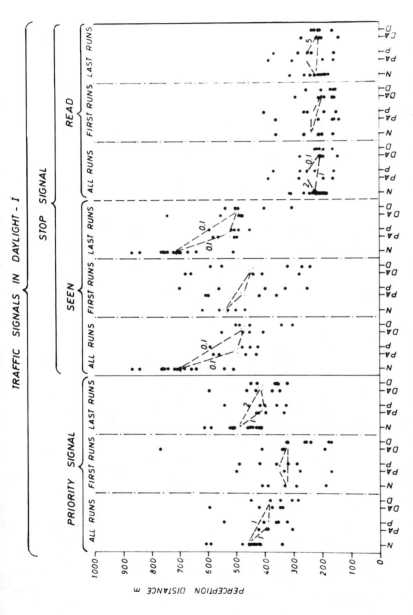

Fig. 9.1. Perception distances for traffic signals in daylight. N, normal; PA, protanomalous; P, protanopic; DA, deuteranomalous; D, deuteranopic. Each black dot represents the mean of the perception distances of one observer. Each triangle represents the mean of the means of the perception distances of the normal observers (left), of the protan (PA + P) observers (middle), and of the deutan (DA + D) observers (right). These triangles are connected by dashed lines, on which 0.1 indicates that the difference between two means is significant at the 0.001 level, while 1 indicates a 0.01 level, 2 a 0.02 level, 5 a 0.05 level, and no figure > 0.05. [Data of Verriest, Neubauer, Uvijls, & Sinotobin, presented at the second International Ergophthalmic Symposium at Nagoya, 1978.]

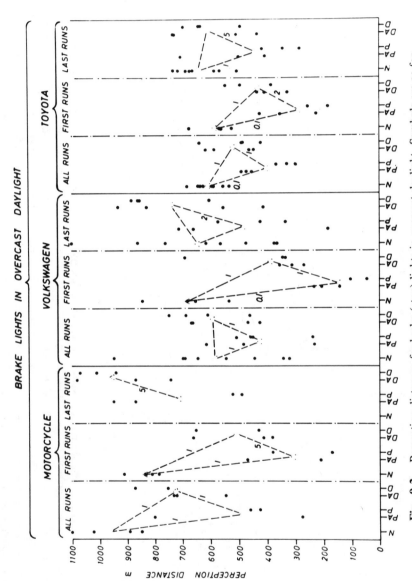

Fig. 9.2. Perception distances for brake (stop) lights in overcast daylight. Symbols are as for Fig. 9.1. [Data of Verriest, Neubauer, Uvijls, & Sintobin, presented at the Second International Ergophthalmic Symposium at Nagoya, 1978.]

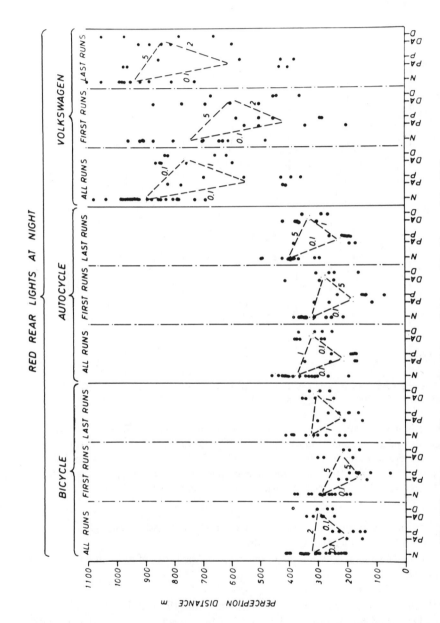

Fig. 9.3. Perception distances for red rear lights at night (those of the Volkswagen car were dimmed). Symbols are as for Fig. 9.1. [Data of Verriest, Neubauer, Uvijls, & Sintobin, presented at the Second International Ergophthalmic Symposium at Nagoya, 1978.]

353

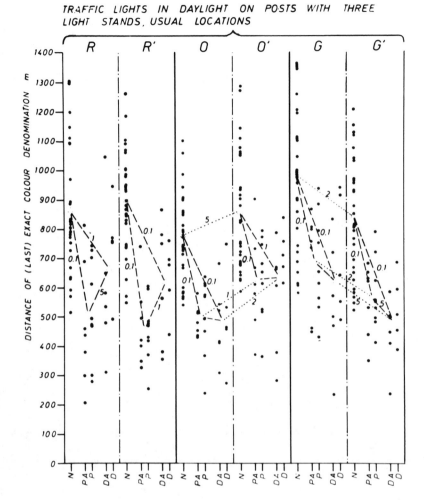

Fig. 9.4. Distances of (last) exact color denomination in daylight for traffic lights on posts with three light stands (red above, orange in the middle, green below). R, O, G: Futurit plastic cobweb red, orange, and green traffic light filters; R′, O′, G′: ATEA glass. Symbols as for Fig. 9.1. Significant differences between the results for the corresponding Futurit and ATEA filters are also indicated. [Unpublished data of Verriest, Neubauer, Uvijls, & Sintobin.]

possibility in protanopia. The use of red for both rear and brake lights can have problems for both normal and defective drivers.

5.   The statistics have generally not taken into account the types of red–green anomalies and defects.

Zehnder (1971), Hager (1963), and Gramberg-Danielsen (1976) did distinguish protans and deutans but found no significant differences. More recently, Marré (1978) showed that color defectives are not involved in more traffic accidents than normal drivers. An exception is rear-end collisions, which occur significantly more frequently for protan drivers. Possibly, persons with defective color vision take extra care in their driving.

There have been several suggestions about altering the current practice for signs and signals in order to aid color defectives. Broschmann (1970) pointed out the danger of a failure in one of the two lamps making up a double green signal as proposed by Allen. Gramberg-Danielsen (1967) proposed flashing red lights. Such special lights ought to be reserved for special cases such as traffic lights out of order, direction indicators, and priority vehicles, since Crawford (1963) has shown that irrelevant flashing lights slowed down the reaction to relevant flashing lights and only marginally shortened the response time as compared with a static light. Altering the shape of the visible color signal with triangular or square masks, as actually done in Swtizerland, tends to reduce the overall visibility of the lights. Allen (1970) even proposed changing the color of rear lights to green, but this is unacceptable because red and green in our culture have acquired distinct associations of "danger" and "proceed." Spiecker (1967) proposed the use of blue for brake lights; apart from the psychologic objection mentioned above, blue is badly recognized in fog (Gramberg-Danielsen, 1976) and at great distances.

Among the better solutions are the following: (1) improvements in the visibility of road signs and signals by making them bigger and more intense and by surrounding them with suitable contrasting material such as black boarding; (2) improving the conspicuousness of the backs of trucks with stripes or additional rear lights; (3) moving the chromaticity of green signal lights nearer to blue and avoiding exteme red lights within the CIE tolerance limits (CIE, 1975). Yellower reds are often identified as yellow rather than red by normal as well as color-defective observers. Thus yellower reds would be preferable for brake and tail lights than for traffic signals. A possibility might be to increase the irradiance of deep reds by using larger stands.

Two final points may be mentioned. (1) The reduced color discrimination of defective drivers may be further reduced by the wearing of tinted spectacles or contact lenses and by the use of tinted windshields, which are standard equipment now in many vehicles. (2) Various types of acquired color vision defects and the effects of excess noise, hypoxia, and fatigue on visual performance may need to be taken into consideration, although they are probably of only marginal importance.

RAIL, RIVER, AND SEA NAVIGATION; AVIATION

Possible dangers due to color vision deficiency have been virtually eliminated, since most countries have for many years excluded defectives from jobs in these modes of transport. It is ironic that the Swedish rail disaster of 1875, which led to the introduction of systematic testing of color vision for railway personnel, is now considered not to have been caused by the color vision defect of the driver (Frey, 1975a, b). Nevertheless, the exclusion of red–green defectives from rail and water navigation (personnel on deck) seems to be fully justified, since red and green are the predominant colors of the signals. Moreover, errors are hard to correct with a train, while on water the color signals often have to be identified under bad meteorologic conditions within a multitude of other point light sources.

The situation for air crews is slightly different, although many colors are used on cockpit instruments and at airports, since, in addition, instrumental guidance for landing and takeoff is becoming more important than visual guidance. Accordingly, the OACI norms are not very rigid, and the NATO Advisory Group for Aerospace Research and Development even proposed in 1972 that anomalous trichromats might be accepted as team pilots.

OTHER SITUATIONS

Color discrimination and color-naming situations occur in all walks of life, but poor discrimination or errors in naming are usually more inconvenient than dangerous. The housekeeper has to make chromatic discriminations when buying fruit and when choosing or repairing clothes, as does the child when drawing or learning modern mathematics. Espinda (1971) noted a definite trend to lowered grade point averages for color-deficient pupils. Nevertheless, there are some occupations, such as those already discussed, where color defectives have to be excluded; the sooner young people with color-defective vision showing an interest in such occupations are told of the position, the better. This allows them to consider other occupations and perhaps undertake the appropriate studies.

Verriest and Hermans (1975) classified occupations in which color deficiency can be a handicap into three groups:

1. Occupations requiring entirely normal color vision (color matching and color discrimination) either by the nature of the work or by regulations (rail, marine, etc.). Obviously, normal color matching is vital for dye matching, art restoration, tapestry, preparation of paints, inks, and papers, philately, color photography, and sorting of matters such as furs, tobaccos, fuel, fruit, pearls, cottons, etc. However, red–green defectives are not at a disadvantage when the colors to be distinguished lie exclusively on a blue–white–yellow axis of the chromaticity diagram (e.g., as for diamond grading) (Lakowski & Oliver, 1978). On the other hand, blue–yellow defectives are especially inept for specific jobs, such as the already mentioned diamond grading, sorting of meats, etc.
2. Occupations normally requiring normal color vision but in which instrumentation or the assistance of colleagues can help out with color problems. This group includes electronics, cartography, chemistry and associated biologic sciences, metallurgy, pharmacy, botany, zoology, and veterinary and human medicine, especially dermatology, pathology, anatomy, and bacteriology because of the Gram and Ziehl-Neelsen staining (Crone, 1966), and also endoscopy (Fletcher, 1978) and dentistry.
3. Occupations for which normal color vision is desirable but not essential, such as architecture, horticulture, landscaping, confectionery, fashion, drama, head-dress, decoration, teaching. According to Fletcher (1961) the protan subjects should be less apt for photography laboratory work because of their reduced sensitivity to the longer wavelengths. Details of appropriate testing procedures for persons considering occupations within these various groups can be found in Chapter 6. Practical performance tests should be done under the illuminant used at the job, as Lakowski and Oliver (1978) showed. Compared with daylight, industrial lighting reduces chromaticity discrimination more in color-defective than in normal subjects.

Concerning the norms of physical aptitudes to the jobs, there is still a dilemma; on the one side one is inclined to use severe criteria in view of increased performance and of prevention of accidents, while on the other side one is inclined to ease the criteria in view of maintenance of older workers and reclassification of handicapped persons.

ATTEMPTS TO IMPROVE THE COLOR PERFORMANCE OF COLOR DEFECTIVE PEOPLE

The only color vision defects that can be cured or at least reversed to a certain degree are those acquired as the result of disease. In some cases, treatment of the disease will cause an improvement in color vision. Attempts to improve the performance of congenitally defective people with drugs, vitamins, electrical stimulation, exercises, special illuminants (Thornton, 1974; Verriest, unpublished), and various types of visual aids have proved merely unsuccessful. Schmidt (1976) classified visual aids into three types:

1. Selective filters for successive comparison of brightness relationships. For example, a red and a green filter mounted side by side at the top of a spectacle lens enables the wearer to look at an object successively through the filters. A green object would appear much brighter when seen through the green filter than through the red filter, and vice versa for the red object.
2. Selective filters for immediate evaluation. For example, a magenta filter absorbing the part of the spectrum corresponding to a dichromat's neutral zone increases the saturation of the colors that can be seen.
3. Miscellaneous designs of filters. For example, the X-chrom lens combines the two preceding types with some binocular viewing effects.

Schmidt (1976) concluded that many red–green defectives can benefit from the extra clues for identifying colors, at least after intensive training, in everyday life but to a lesser extent in special work situations. Unfortunately, other errors may be introduced owing to the reduction in some contrasts and white being seen as colored.

References

The chapter numbers in italics following each reference refer to this book. Articles without credited authors are listed at the end of this section.

Abney WW: Researches in Colour Vision and the Trichromatic Theory. London, Longmans, Green & Company, 1913 *(Chapter 8)*

Abraham FA, Ivry M, Tsvieli R: Sector retinitis pigmentosa: A fluorescein angiographic study. Ophthalmologica 172:287–297, 1976 *(Chapter 8)*

Abraham FA, Sandberg MA: An unusual type of juvenile foveal dystrophy; Electrophysiological study. Doc Ophthalmol Proc Ser 11:75–83, 1977 *(Chapter 8)*

Adachi-Usami E, Gavriysky V, Heck J, Schenkel E, Scheibner H: Psychophysical and VECP examination of a rod monochromat and a cone monochromat. Doc Ophthalmol Proc Ser 4:179–186, 1974 *(Chapter 7)*

Adam A: Foveal red-green ratios of normals, colourblinds and heterozygotes. Proc Tel-Hashomer Hosp (Tel-Aviv) 8:2–6, 1969 *(Chapters 6 and 7)*

Adams AJ, Balliet R, McAdams M: Color vision: Blue deficiencies in children? Invest Ophthalmol 14:620–625, 1975 *(Chapter 5)*

Adams JH, Blackwood W, Wilson J: Further clinical and pathological observations on Leber's optic atrophy. Brain 89:15–26, 1966 *(Chapter 8)*

Adams P, Chalmer TM, Foulds WS, Withy JL: Megaloblastic anaemia and vision. Lancet 2:229–231, 1967 *(Chapter 8)*

Adams ST: Retina and optic nerve. Arch Ophthalmol 69:642–675, 1963 *(Chapter 8)*

Ahlenstiel H: Rot-Grün-Blindheit als Erlebnis. Göttingen, Musterschmidt Verlag, 1951 *(Chapter 8)*

Aitken J: On colour and colour sensation. Trans R Scot Soc Arts 8:375–418, 1873 *(Chapter 7)*

Alexander KR: Color vision testing in young children: A review. Am J Optom Physiol Opt 52:332–337, 1975 *(Chapter 5)*

Alkemade PPH: Phenothiazine-retinopathy. Ophthalmologica 155:70–76, 1968 *(Chapter 8)*

Allen MJ: Vision, vehicles and highway safety. Highway Res News 25:57–62, 1966 *(Chapter 9)*

Allen MJ: Vision and Highway Safety. Principles of Optometry Series. Philadelphia, Chilton Book Company, 1970 *(Chapter 9)*

Alpern M: What is it that confines in a world without color? Invest Ophthalmol 13:648–674, 1974 *(Chapter 7)*

Alpern M: Tritanopia. Am J Optom Physiol Opt 53:340–349, 1976 *(Chapter 7)*

Alpern M, Falls HF, Lee GB: The enigma of typical total monochromacy. Am J Ophthalmol 50:326–342, 1960 *(Chapters 6 and 7)*

Alpern M, Lee GB, Maaseidvaag F, Miller SS: Colour vision in blue-cone 'monochromacy.' J Physiol (London) 212:211–233, 1971 *(Chapters 6 and 7)*

Alpern M, Lee GB, Spivey BE: π_1 Cone monochromatism. Arch Ophthalmol 74:334–337, 1965 *(Chapter 7)*

Alpern M, Mindel J, Torii S: Are there two types of deuteranopes? J Physiol (London) 199:443–456, 1968 *(Chapter 7)*

Alpern M, Moeller J: The red and green cone visual pigments of deuteranomalous trichromacy. J Physiol (London) 266:647–675, 1977 *(Chapter 7)*

Alpern M, Pugh Jr EN: Variation in the action spectrum of erythrolabe among deuteranopes. J Physiol 266:613–646, 1977 *(Chapter 7)*

Alpern M, Torii S: Prereceptor colour vision distortions in protanomalous trichromacy. J Physiol (London) 198:549–560, 1968a *(Chapter 7)*

Alpern M, Torii S: The luminosity curve of the protanomalous fovea. J Gen Physiol 52:717–737, 1968b *(Chapter 7)*

Alpern M, Torii S: The luminosity curve of the deuteranomalous fovea. J Gen Physiol 52:738–749, 1968c *(Chapter 7)*

Alpern M, Wake T: Cone pigment in human deutan colour vision defects. J Physiol (London) 266:595–612, 1977 *(Chapter 7)*

Andersen KV, Coyle FR, O'Steen WK: Retinal degeneration produced by low-intensity colored light. Exp Neurol 35:233–238, 1972 *(Chapter 8)*

Arias S: Genetic hypotheses induced by unusual colour vision phenotypes. Mod Prob Ophthalmol 17:108–120, 1976 *(Chapter 7)*

Arias S, Rodriguez A: New families, one with two recombinants for estimation of recombination between the deutan and protan loci. Humangenetik 14:264–268, 1972 *(Chapter 7)*

Arias S, Rodriguez A: An informative large pedigree with four compound hemizygotes of three combinations of deutan and protan genes. Acta Cient Venezolana 24:44–52, 1973a *(Chapter 7)*

Arias S, Rodriguez A: Description of three different phenotypes for compound hemizygotes in various combinations of deutan alleles with an identical gene of the protan locus. Bol INDIO (Ven) 1:97–118, 1973b *(Chapter 7)*

Armington JC, Schwab GJ: Electroretinogram in nyctalopia. Arch Ophthalmol 52:725–733, 1954 *(Chapter 8)*

Aspinall P: An upper limit of non-random cap arrangements in the Farnsworth-Munsell 100 hue test. Ophthalmologica 168:128–131, 1974a *(Chapter 5)*

Aspinall P: Inter-eye comparison of the 100 hue test. Acta Ophthalmol 52:307–315, 1974b *(Chapter 5)*

Aspinall P, Adams A, Hayreh SS: Primary retinal pigmentary degeneration. II. Functional changes. IRCS International Research Communication System (73-3) 24-14-2, March, 1973 *(Chapter 8)*

Assal G, Eisert HG, Hecaen H: Analyse des résultats du test de Farnsworth D15 chez IS5 malades atteints de lésions hémispheriques droites et gauches. Acta Neurol Belg 69:705–717, 1969 *(Chapter 8)*

Atkinson WS: Retinitis punctata albescens; Report of two cases in which the dots disappeared. Arch Ophthalmol 8:409–413, 1932 *(Chapter 8)*

Aubert H: Ueber die Grenzen der Farbenwahrnemung auf den seitlichen Theilen der Retina. Albrecht von Graefes Arch Klin Ophthalmol 3:38–67, 1857 *(Chapter 6)*

Auerbach E, Kripke B: Achromatopsia with amblyopia. II. A psychophysical study of 5 cases. Doc Ophthalmol 37:119–144, 1974 *(Chapter 6)*

Auerbach E, Kripke B: Electrophysiological and psychophysical examinations of a family with progressive cone dystrophy. Doc Ophthalmol Proc Ser 10:371–387, 1976 *(Chapter 8)*

Auerbach E, Merin S: Achromatopsia with amblyopia. I. A clinical and electroretinographical study of 39 cases. Doc Ophthalmol 37:79–117, 1974 *(Chapter 7)*

Auerbach E, Wald G: The participation of different types of cones in human light and dark adaptation. Am J Ophthalmol 39:24–40, 1955 *(Chapter 6)*

Aulhorn E, Grützner P: Infantile optic atrophy with dominant mode of inheritance accompanied by an acquired protanopia, in Brunette J, Barbeau A (eds): Progress in Neuro-Ophthalmology, vol II, Proceedings of the Second International Congress of Neuro-genetics and Neuro-ophthalmology of the World Federation of Neurology. Amsterdam, Excerpta Medica Foundation, 1969 *(Chapters 6 and 8)*

Austin DJ: Acquired color vision defects in patients suffering from chronic simple glaucoma. Trans Ophthalmol Soc UK 94:880–883, 1974 *(Chapter 8)*

Ayres F: 0 Panel D-15 e o 100 Hue Test de Farnsworth no estudo das discromatopsias adquividas no glaucoma. Rev Brasil Oftal 26:45–60, 1967 *(Chapter 8)*

Babel J: Le fundus flavimaculatus; Étude clinicque, fonctionelle et génétique. Arch Ophthalmol (Paris) 32:109–121, 1972 *(Chapter 8)*

Babel J: Fréquence des complications rétiniennes dans la dystrophie myotonique. Contes rendues 3 ème Journée Européenne de Conseil Génétique (Genève): 167-171, 1975 *(Chapter 8)*

Babel J, Stangos N: Intoxication rétinienne par la digitale. Bull Soc Belge Ophtalmol 160:558–566, 1972 *(Chapter 8)*

Babel J, Tsacopoulos M: Les lésions rétiniennes de la myotonie dystrophique. Ann Oculist 203: 1049–1055, 1970 *(Chapter 8)*

Baghdassarian S: Optic neuropathy due to lead-poisoning. Arch Ophthalmol 80:721–723, 1968 *(Chapter 8)*

Bailey JE, Massof RW: In search of the physiological neutral point. Mod Prob Ophthalmol 13:135–139, 1974 *(Chapter 7)*

Baker HD: Single-variable anomaloscope matches during recovery from artificial red blindness. J Opt Soc Am 56:686–689, 1966 *(Chapter 7)*

Baker HD, Rushton WAH: An analytical anomaloscope. J Physiol (London) 168:31–33p, 1963 *(Chapter 6)*

Barca L, Vaccari G: On the impairment of color discrimination in diabetic retinopathy, a report of 24 cases. Atti Fond G Ronchi 32:635–640, 1977 *(Chapter 8)*

Barlow HB: Dark and light adaptation: Psychophysics, in Jameson D, Hurvich LM (eds): Handbook of Sensory Physiology, vol VII/4, Visual Psychophysics, Berlin, Springer-Verlag, 1972 *(Chapter 6)*

Bartleson CJ: Brown. Color Res Appl 1:181–191, 1976 *(Chapter 2)*

Baumgardt E: Un cas d'achromatopsie atypique. J Physiol (Paris) 47:83–87, 1955 *(Chapter 7)*

Baumgardt E, Magis C: Sur un cas exceptionnel d'achromatopsie. J Physiol (Paris) 46:237–240, 1954 *(Chapter 7)*

Beare AC: Color-name as a function of wavelength. Am J Psychol 76:248–256, 1963 *(Chapter 6)*

Bec P, Belleville D, Arne JL, Philippot V, Secheyron P: Intérêt de l'exploration du sens chromatique au Farnsworth 100 hue dans le dépistage de la maculopathie par antipaludéens de synthèse. Ann Oculist (Paris) 210:291–296, 1977 *(Chapter 8)*

Beckerman BL, Rapin I: Ceroid lipofuscinosis. Am J Ophthalmol 80:73–77, 1975 *(Chapter 8)*

Begg IS, Small M, White AM: Propionate and acetate excretion in chloramphenicol toxicity. Lancet 2:686–687, 1968 *(Chapter 8)*

Behr C: Die Heredodegeneration der Makula. Klin Mbl Augenh 65:463–505, 1920 *(Chapter 8)*

Belcher S, Greenshields K, Wright WD: A colour vision survey. Br J Ophthalmol 42:355–359, 1958 *(Chapter 5)*

Bell J: The Treasury of Human Inheritance, vol II. Anomalies and Disease of the Eye, London, Cambridge University Press, 1926 *(Chapters 4 and 7)*

Bender BG, Ruddock KH: The characteristics of a visual defect associated with abnormal responses to both colour and luminance. Vision Res 14:383–393, 1974 *(Chapter 8)*

Bender BG, Ruddock KH, de Vries-de Mol EC, Went

LN: The colour vision characteristics of an observer with unilateral defective colour vision: Results and analysis. Vision Res 12:2035–2057, 1972 *(Chapters 7 and 8)*

Bender MB, Kahn RL: After imagery in defective fields of vision. J Neurol Neurosurg Psychiatr 12:196–204, 1949 *(Chapter 8)*

Benedikt O, Werner W: Retikuläre Pigmentdystrophie der Netzhaut. Klin Mbl Augenh 159:794–798, 1971 *(Chapter 8)*

Benson WE, Kolker AE, Enoch JM, Van Loo JA Jr, Honda Y: Best's vitelliform macular dystrophy. Am J Ophthalmol 79:59–66, 1975 *(Chapters 6 and 8)*

Berry W: Color sequences in the after-image of white light. Am J Psychol 38:584–596, 1927 *(Chapter 8)*

Berson EL, Gouras P, Gunkel RD: Rod responses in retinitis pigmentosa, dominantly inherited. Arch Ophthalmol 80:58–67, 1968 *(Chapter 8)*

Berson EL, Gouras P, Gunkel RD, Myrianthopoulos NC: Rod and cone responses in sex-linked retinitis pigmentosa. Arch Ophthalmol 81:215–225, 1969 *(Chapter 8)*

Bertera JH, Parsons OA: Impaired visual search in alcoholics. Alcoholism 2:9–14, 1978 *(Chapter 8)*

Bessière E, LeRebeller M, Vallat M, Rougier-Houssin J: Acuité visuelle et explorations fonctionelles en luminance atténuée dans le glaucome debutant. Bull Mem Soc Ophtalmal Fr 71:877–881, 1971 *(Chapter 8)*

Bessière E, Verin P, Rougier-Houssin J, LeRebeller MJ: Evaluation de la fonction visuelle dans la maladie de Stargardt. Arch Ophtalmol (Paris) 29:463–478, 1969 *(Chapter 8)*

Best M, Blumenthal M, Futterman HA, Galin MA: Critical closure of intraocular blood vessels. Arch Ophthalmol 82:385–392, 1969 *(Chapter 8)*

Bhargava SK: Tobacco amblyopia and acquired dyschromatopsia: Anomaloscope tests. Acta Ophthalmol (Kbh) 51:822–828, 1973 *(Chapter 8)*

Bietti GB: Su alcune forme attipiche o rare di degenerazione retinica. Boll Oculist 16: 1159–1244, 1937 *(Chapter 8)*

Billmeyer FW, Saltzman M: Principles of Color Technology. New York, John Wiley & Sons, Inc., 1966 *(Chapter 2)*

Birch J: Dichromatic convergence points obtained by subtractive colour matching. Vision Res 13:1755–1765, 1973 *(Chapter 7)*

Birch J: New pseudoisochromatic plates for dichromats based on subtractive colour matches. Am J Optom 52:398–404, 1975 *(Chapters 5 and 7)*

Birch-Cox J: A case of acquired tritanopia. Mod Prob Ophthalmol 17:325–330, 1976 *(Chapter 8)*

Birch-Cox J: Defective colour vision in diabetic retinopathy before and after laser photocoagulation. Mod Prob Ophthalmol 19:326–329, 1978 *(Chapter 8)*

Bisantis C: La rétinopathie pigmentaire en secteur de G. B. Bietti. Ann Oculist 204:907–954, 1971 *(Chapter 8)*

Blackwell HR, Blackwell OM: Blue mono-cone monochromacy: A new color vision defect. J Opt Soc Am 47:338, 1957 *(Chapter 7)*

Blackwell HR, Blackwell OM: Rod and cone receptor mechanisms in typical and atypical congenital achromatopsia. Vision Res 1:62–107, 1961 *(Chapter 7)*

Blackwell HR, Blackwell OM: Spectral sensitivity mechanisms derived from studies of abnormal retinae. Color 69, Göttingen, Musterschmidt Verlag, 1970 pp. 131–137. *(Chapter 8)*

Blanck MF, Polliot L, Bernard P: La dégénérescence hyaloidéo-tapéto-rétinienne de Goldmann et Favre. Bull Mem Soc Ophtalmol Fr 86:242–245, 1973 *(Chapter 8)*

Bliss AF: The chemistry of daylight vision. J Gen Physiol 29:277–297, 1946 *(Chapter 3)*

Boergen KP: Opticusschäden durch oxychinolinhaltige Antidiarrhoica? Klin Mbl Augenh 163:217–219, 1973 *(Chapter 8)*

Boet DJ: Toxic effects of phenothiazines on the eye. Doc Ophthalmol 28:1–69, 1970 *(Chapter 8)*

Boles-Carenini B: Del comportamento del senso cromatico in relazione all'età. Ann Ottal Clin Ocul 80:451–458, 1954 *(Chapter 8)*

Bonamour G, Bonnet M, Laffay H: Contribution a l'étude du syndrome chiasmatique servenant au cours de la grossesse. Ann Oculist 204:235–256, 1971 *(Chapter 8)*

Bonnardel R: Vision et Professions. Paris, Publ Travail Humain, 1936 *(Chapter 9)*

Bonnet M: Les druses de la lame vitrée. Conf Lyonn Ophtalmol 113:1–56, 1972 *(Chapter 8)*

Bonnet M: Le syndrome de Jaffe. Arch Ophtalmol (Paris) 33:209–224, 1973 *(Chapter 8)*

Bonnet M: Choriorétinopathie séreuse centrale et dégénérescence sénile de la macula. Ann Oculist 207:1–13, 1974 *(Chapter 8)*

Bonnet M: Atrophie aréolaire de la macula. Arch Ophtalmol (Paris) 35:493–508, 1975 *(Chapter 8)*

Bouma PJ: Physical Aspects of Colour. Eindhoven, NV Philips, 1947 (revised by de Groot W, Kruithof AA, Ouweltjes JF, New York, St. Martins Press, 1972) *(Chapter 2)*

Bouman MA, Walraven PL: A study of normal and defective colour vision, in Visual Problems of Color, NPL Symposium 8, New York, Chemical Publishing Company, 1961, pp 97–107 *(Chapter 7)*

Bouniq C, Coscas G: Etude statistique et analytique de 164 cas de névrite optique alcoolo-tabagique. Ann Oculist 199:955–974, 1966 *(Chapter 8)*

Bouzas A, Kokkinakis K, Papadakis G, Daikos G: La toxicité oculaire de l'éthambutol. Ophthalmologica 161:361– 371, 1970 *(Chapter 8)*

Bowmaker JK, Dartnall HJA, Lythgoe JN, Mollon JD: The visual pigments of rods and cones in the rhesus monkey, Macaca mulatta. J Physiol (London) 274:329– 348, 1978 *(Chapter 3)*

Boynton RM: Contributions of threshold measurements to color-discrimination theory. J Opt Soc Am 53:165– 178, 1963 *(Chapters 3 and 6)*

Boynton RM: Implications of the minimally distinct border. J Opt Soc Am 63:1037– 1043, 1973 *(Chapters 2 and 3)*

Boynton RM: Vision, in Sidowski JB (ed): Experimental methods and instrumentation in psychology. New York, McGraw-Hill, 1966, pp 273-330. *(Chapter 1)*

Boynton RM, Gordon J: Bezold-Brücke hue-shift measured by color-naming technique. J Opt Soc Am 55:78– 96, 1965 *(Chapters 6 and 7)*

Boynton RM, Kandel T, Onley JW: Rapid chromatic adaptation of normal and dichromatic observers. J Opt Soc Am 49:654– 666, 1959 *(Chapter 7)*

Boynton RM, Scheibner H: On the perception of red by "red-blind" observers. Acta Chromatica 1:205– 220, 1967 *(Chapters 6 and 7)*

Boynton RM, Wagner M: Two-color threshold as test of color vision. J Opt Soc Am 51:429– 440, 1961 *(Chapters 6 and 7)*

Bozzoni F: Contributo alla conoscenza della dichromatopsie acquisite. Boll Oculist 38:297– 306, 1959 *(Chapter 8)*

Bozzoni F, Lumbroso BD: Ambliopia e senso cromatico. Boll Oculist 14:163– 168, 1962 *(Chapter 8)*

Brill NE: A case of destructive lesion of the cunens accompanied by color blindness. Am J Neurol Psychiatr 1:356– 368, 1882 *(Chapter 8)*

Brindley GS: The effects on colour vision of adaptation to very bright lights. J Physiol (London) 122:332, 1953 *(Chapter 3)*

Brindley GS: A photochemical reaction in the human retina. Proc Phys Soc 68B:862– 870, 1955a *(Chapter 3)*

Brindley GS: The site of electrical excitation of the human eye. J Physiol (London) 127:189– 200, 1955b *(Chapter 8)*

Brindley GS: Physiology of the Retina and Visual Pathway. London, Edward Arnold, 1960 *(Chapter 3)*

Brindley GS: Physiology of the Retina and the Visual Pathway (ed 2). Baltimore, Williams & Wilkins, 1970 *(Chapter 7)*

Brink JK: A family with vitelliform macular dystrophy. Acta Ophthalmol (Kbh) 52:609– 624, 1974 *(Chapter 8)*

Bron HLHM, Korten JJ, Pinckers AJLG, Majoor CLH: Subacute myeloopticoneuropathie na het gebruik van grote hoeveelheden joodchloorhydroxychinoline (Enterovioform). Ned T Geneesk 116:1615– 1617, 1972 *(Chapter 8)*

Brönte-Stewart J, Foulds WS: Acquired dyschromatopsia in vitamin A deficiency. Mod Prob Ophthalmol 11:168– 173, 1972 *(Chapter 8)*

Broschmann D: Zur Formenerbarkeit von Lichtsignalen. Verkehrsmed 17:260– 270, 1970 *(Chapter 9)*

Broschmann D: Sehstörungen und Kraftfahrtauglichkeit. Kongress der Augenärte der DDR, Berlin, 1976 *(Chapter 9)*

Brown KT, Murakami M: Rapid effects of light and dark adaptation upon the receptive field organisation of S-potentials and late receptor potentials. Vision Res 8:1145– 1171, 1968 *(Chapter 6)*

Brown PK, Wald G: Visual pigments in single rods and cones of the human retina. Science 144:45– 52, 1964 *(Chapter 3)*

Brown WRJ: Color discrimination of twelve observers. J Opt Soc Am 47:137– 143, 1957 *(Chapter 6)*

Brückner R: Frühdiagnose medikamentöser Schäden von Netzhaut und Sehnerv. Ophthalmologica 158:245– 272, 1969 *(Chapter 8)*

Brunner W: Über den Vererbungsmodus der verschiedenen Typen der angeborenen Rotgrünblindheit. Graefes Archiv Ophthalmol 124:1– 52, 1930 *(Chapter 7)*

Bucklers M: Spektrographische Untersuchungen über die Absorption des Lichtes durch die menschliche Linse (mit Demonstration). Ber Dtsch Ophthalmol Ges 48:234– 236, 1930 *(Chapter 8)*

Burian HM: The behavior of the amblyopic eye under reduced illumination and the theory of functional amblyopia. Doc Ophthalmol 23:189– 202, 1967 *(Chapter 8)*

Burian HM, Burns CA: Ocular changes in myotonic dystrophy. Am J Ophthalmol 63:22– 34, 1967 *(Chapter 8)*

Burns CA: Indomethacin, reduced retinal sensitivity and corneal deposits. Am J Ophthalmol 66:825– 835, 1968 *(Chapter 8)*

Campbell CJ, Noyori KS, Rittler MC, Koester CJ: Intraocular temperature changes produced by laser coagulation. Acta Ophthalmol (Kbh) Suppl 76:22– 31, 1963 *(Chapter 8)*

Campbell CJ, Rittler M: The diagnostic value of flicker perimetry in chronic simple glaucoma. Trans Am Acad Ophthalmol Otol 63:89– 98, 1959 *(Chapter 8)*

Campbell CJ, Rittler MC: Colour vision in retinal pathology. Mod Prob Ophthalmol 11:98– 105, 1972 *(Chapter 8)*

Cameron ME, Lawrence JM, Olrich JG: Thioridazine (Melleril) retinopathy. Br J Ophthalmol 56:131– 134, 1972 *(Chapter 8)*

Cappin JM, Nissim S: Visual evoked responses in the

assessment of field defects in glaucoma. Arch Ophthalmol 93:9–18, 1975 (Chapter 8)

Carlow TJ, Flynn J, Shipley T: Color perimetry parameters. Doc Ophthalmol 14:427–429, 1977 (Chapter 6)

Carr R: Fundus flavimaculatus. Arch Ophthalmol 74:163–168, 1965 (Chapter 8)

Carr RE, Henkind P: Ocular manifestation of Ethambutol. Toxic amblyopia after administration of an experimental antituberculous drug. Arch Ophthalmol 67:566–571, 1962 (Chapter 8)

Carr RE, Siegel IM: The vitreo-tapeto-retinal degenerations. Arch Ophthalmol 84:436–445, 1970 (Chapter 8)

Carr RE, Siegel IM: Retinal function in patients treated with indomethacin. Am J Ophthalmol 75:302–306, 1973 (Chapter 8)

Carroll FD: Nutritional amblyopia. Arch Ophthalmol 76:406–411, 1966 (Chapter 8)

Carvalho VL: Estudo do senso cromatico nas ambliopias refracional e estrabismica. Thesis, Belo Horizonte, 1973 (Chapter 8)

Cernea P, Constantin F: Discrimination chromatique dans les yeux amétropes. Ann Oculist (Paris) 210:383–386, 1977 (Chapter 8)

Chapanis A: Spectral saturation and its relation to color-vision defects. J Exp Psychol 34:24–44, 1944 (Chapter 7)

Chapanis A: Simultaneous chromatic contrast in normal and abnormal color vision. Am J Psychol 62:526–539, 1949 (Chapter 7)

Chapanis A: Relationship between age, visual acuity, and color vision. Hum Biol 22:1–33, 1950 (Chapter 8)

Chester GH, Blach RK, Cleary PE: Inflammation in the region of the vitreous base–pars planitis. Trans Ophthalmol Soc UK 96:151–157, 1976 (Chapter 8)

Chisholm IA: An evaluation of the Farnsworth-Munsell 100 hue test as a clinical tool in the investigation and management of ocular neurological deficit. Trans Ophthalmol Soc UK 89:243–250, 1969a (Chapter 5)

Chisholm IA: The optic neuropathy of recurrent blood loss. Br J Ophthalmol 53:289–295, 1969b (Chapter 8)

Chisholm IA: The dyschromatopsia of pernicious anaemia. Mod Prob Ophthalmol 11:130–135, 1972 (Chapter 8)

Chisholm IA, Bronte-Stewart J: Further observations on the therapy of the toxic amblyopias, in Cant JS (ed): The Optic Nerve, Proceedings of the 2nd William Mackenzie Memorial Symposium. London, Henry Kimpton, 1972 (Chapter 8)

Chisholm IA, Bronte-Stewart J, Awduche ED: Color vision in tobacco amblyopia. Acta Ophthalmol (Kbh) 48:1145–1156, 1970 (Chapter 8)

Chisholm IA, McClure E, Foulds WS: Functional recovery of the retina after retinal detachment.

Trans Ophthalmol Soc UK 95:167–172, 1975 (Chapter 8)

Chisholm IA, Pettigrew AR: Biochemical observations in toxic optic neuropathy. Trans Ophthalmol Soc UK 90:827–838, 1970 (Chapter 8)

Chopdar A: Reticular dystrophy of retina. Br J Ophthalmol 60:342–344, 1976 (Chapter 8)

Cibis P: Zur Pathologie der Lokaladaptation. Graefes Arch Ophthalmol 148:1–92, 1948 (Chapter 6)

Cinotti A, Stephens G, Kiebel G: The electroretinographic response and adaptation in chronic alcoholics. VIII ISCERG Symposium, Pisa, 1970, pp 269–270 (Chapter 8)

Cogan DG: Do oral contraceptives have neuro-ophthalmic complications? Arch Ophthalmol 73:461–462, 1965 (Chapter 8)

Cohen JD: Diagnosis of color vision deficiencies in learning-disabled children. Mod Prob Ophthalmol 17:364–367, 1976 (Chapter 5)

Cole BL: Visual standards for drivers of motor vehicles. Aust J Optom 55:135–142, 1972a (Chapter 9)

Cole BL: The handicap of abnormal colour vision. Aust J Optom 55:303–310, 1972b (Chapter 9)

Cole BL, Brown B: Optimum intensity of red road traffic signal lights for normal and protanopic observers. J Opt Soc Am 56:516–522, 1966 (Chapter 9)

Cole BL, Henry GH, Nathan J: Phenotypical variations of tritanopia. Vision Res 6:301–313, 1966 (Chapter 7)

Cole BL, Watkins RD: Increment thresholds in tritanopia. Vision Res 7:939–947, 1967 (Chapter 7)

Colenbrander MC: Observations on the heredity of Leber's disease. Ophthalmologica 144: 446–450, 1962 (Chapter 8)

Collins M: The Rayleigh colour equation with rotating discs. Br J Psychol 19:387–393, 1929 (Chapter 5)

Collins WE: The effects of deuteranomaly and deuteranopia upon the foveal luminosity curve. J Psychol 48:285–297, 1959 (Chapter 7)

Collins WE: Luminosity functions of normal deuteranomalous and deuteranopic subjects as determined by absolute threshold and CFF measurements. J Opt Soc Am 51:202–206, 1961 (Chapter 7)

Collum LMT, Bowen DI: Ocular side effects of Ibuprofen. Br J Ophthalmol 55:472–477, 1971 (Chapter 8)

Comberg D: Verkehrsgefahrdung durch Protanopie und Protanomalie. Verkehrsmed 9:113–117, 1962 (Chapter 9)

Comberg D: Zur Notwendigkeit der Belebung des Farbenuntuchtigen Kraftfahrzeugführers. Verkehrsmed 11:1–8, 1964 (Chapter 9)

Comberg W: Beziehungen zwischen Störungen des Farbensinnes und Ametropien. Klin Mbl Augenh 107:85, 1941 (Chapter 8)

Connell M, Poley BJ, McFarlane JR: Chorioretinopathy associated with thioridazine therapy. Arch Ophthalmol 71:816–821, 1964 *(Chapter 8)*

Conner JD, MacLeod DIA: Rod photoreceptors detect rapid flicker. Science 195:698–699, 1976 *(Chapter 7)*

Conreur L, Meur G: Influence de la longueur d'onde du stimulus lumineux dans les phénomènes de sommation spatiale rétinienne. Bull Soc Belge Ophtalmol 143:532–541, 1966 *(Chapter 6)*

Conreur L, Meur G, Zanen A: Utilisation de stimuli colorés dans l'étude de l'adaptation locale précoce (note préliminaire). Bull Soc Belge Ophtalmol 143:542–547, 1966 *(Chapter 6)*

Coren S, Girgus JS: Density of human lens pigmentation: In vivo measurements over an extended age range. Vision Res 12:343–346, 1972 *(Chapter 3)*

Coscas G, Legras M: Les perturbations de la vision chromatique au cours des chorio-rétinopathies séreuses centrales. Arch Ophtalmol (Paris) 30:491–496, 1970 *(Chapter 8)*

Cox J: Colour vision defects acquired in diseases of the eye. Br J Physiol Opt 17:195–216, 1960 *(Chapters 6, 7, and 8)*

Cox J: Colour vision defects acquired in diseases of the eye. Br J Physiol Opt 18:3–32, 1961a *(Chapters 7 and 8)*

Cox J: Colour vision defects acquired in diseases of the eye. Br J Physiol Opt 18:67–84, 1961b *(Chapters 6, 7, and 8)*

Cox J: Unilateral color deficiency—Congenital and acquired. J Opt Soc Am 619:992–999, 1961c *(Chapter 8)*

Cozijnsen M, Pinckers A: Oogheelkundige aspecten van digitoxine-intoxicatie. Ned Tijds Geneesk 113:1735–1737, 1969 *(Chapter 8)*

Crawford BH: The luminous efficiency of light entering the eye pupil at different points and its relation to brightness threshold measurements. Proc R Soc Lond B 124:81–96, 1938 *(Chapter 6)*

Crawford BH: The scotopic visibility function. Proc Phys Soc Lond 62:321–334, 1948 *(Chapter 8)*

Crawford BH: The Stiles-Crawford effects and their significance in vision, in Jameson D, Hurvich LM (eds): Handbook of Sensory Physiology, vol VII/4, Visual Psychophysics. Berlin, Springer-Verlag, 1972 *(Chapter 6)*

Crews SJ: Toxic effects on the eye and visual apparatus resulting from the systemic absorption of recently introduced chemical agents. Trans Ophthalmol Soc UK 82:387–406, 1963 *(Chapter 8)*

Crews SJ: Some aspects of retinal drug toxicity. Ophthalmologica 158:232–244, 1969 *(Chapter 8)*

Critchley M: Acquired anomalies of colour perception of central origin. Brain 88:711–725, 1965 *(Chapter 8)*

Crone RA: Clinical study of colour vision. Br J Ophthalmol 39:170–173, 1955 *(Chapter 5)*

Crone RA: Combined forms of congenital colour defects, a pedigree with atypical total colour blindness. Br J Ophthalmol 40:462–472, 1956 *(Chapters 5 and 7)*

Crone RA: Spectral sensitivity in color-defective subjects and heterozygous carriers. Am J Ophthalmol 48:231–238, 1959 *(Chapters 6 and 7)*

Crone RA: Quantitative diagnosis of defective color vision. A comparative evaluation of the Ishihara test, the Farnsworth dichotomous test and the Hardy-Rand-Rittler polychromatic plates. Am J Ophthalmol 51:298–305, 1961 *(Chapter 5)*

Crone RA: Kleurenzin en beroep. Tijdschr Voor Geneesk 44:327–331, 1966 *(Chapter 9)*

Cruz-Coke R: Colour blindness and cirrhosis of the liver. Lancet 2:1064–1065, 1964 *(Chapter 8)*

Cruz-Coke R: Colour blindness and cirrhosis of the liver. Lancet 1:1131–1133, 1965 *(Chapter 8)*

Cruz-Coke R: Defective color vision and alcoholism. Mod Prob Opthalmol 11:174–177, 1972 *(Chapter 8)*

Cvetkovic D: Color vision in glaucoma. Acta Ophthalmol Yugoslav 5:258–283, 1967 *(Chapter 8)*

Dain SJ: The Lovibond colour vision analyser. Mod Prob Ophthalmol 13:79–82, 1974 *(Chapter 5)*

Dalton J: Extraordinary facts relating to the vision of colours, with observations. Mem Lit Philos Soc Lond 5:28–45, 1798 *(Chapters 4 and 7)*

Dannheim F: Color perimetry in chiasmal lesions. Doc Ophthalmol 14:449–455, 1977 *(Chapter 6)*

Darby PW, Wilson J: Cyanide, smoking and tobacco amblyopia. Br J Ophthalmol 51:336–338, 1967 *(Chapter 8)*

Dartnall HJA: The interpretation of spectral sensitivity curves. Br Med Bull 9:24–30, 1953 *(Chapter 3)*

Dartnall HJA: The Visual Pigments. London, Methuen & Company, 1957 *(Chapter 3)*

Dartnall HJA: Photosensitivity, in Dartnall HJA (ed): Photochemistry of Vision. Berlin, Springer-Verlag, 1972, pp 122–145 *(Chapter 3)*

Dartnall HJA, Goodeve CF: Scotopic luminosity curve and the absorption spectrum of visual purple. Nature 139:409–411, 1937 *(Chapter 3)*

David M, Hartmann E: Les symptomes oculaires dans les méningiomes de la petite aide du sphénoide. Ann Oculist (Paris) 172:177–212, 1935 *(Chapter 8)*

Davidoff JB: Hemispheric differences in hue discrimination. Mod Prob Ophthalmol 17:353–356, 1976 *(Chapter 8)*

Davidorf FH: Thioridazine pigmentary retinopathy. Arch Ophthalmol 90:251–255, 1973 *(Chapter 8)*

Daw NW, Enoch JM: Contrast sensitivity, Westheimer function and Stiles-Crawford effect in a blue cone monochromat. Vision Res 13:1669–1680, 1973 *(Chapters 5, 6, and 7)*

Dekking HM: Visual disturbances due to tridione. Acta Cong Ophthalmol 1:465–467, 1950 *(Chapter 8)*

Denden A: Elektroretinografische Spektralsensitivität bei Farbigsehen nach Acetyldigitoxinbehandlung. Graefe Arch Ophthalmol 165:185–194, 1962 *(Chapter 8)*

Denden A: X-chromosomale vitreo-retinale Degeneration. Klin Mbl Augenh 166:35–43, 1975 *(Chapter 8)*

Denden A, Schröder GM: Beitrag zum Jaffe-Syndrom. Klin Mbl Augenh 168:235–241, 1976 *(Chapter 8)*

Derka H: Besteht Korrelation zwischen der Höhe der Myambutoldosis und der Häufigkeit der Neuritis Nervi Optici? Ophthalmologica 171:123–131, 1975 *(Chapter 8)*

Desvignes P, Legras M: Les expertises en ophtalmologie. Paris, Masson & Cie, 1973 *(Chapter 5)*

Deutman AF: The Hereditary Dystrophies of the Posterior Pole of the Eye. The Netherlands, Gorcum & Cie, 1971 *(Chapter 8)*

Deutman AF: Benign concentric annular macular dystrophy. Am J Ophthalmol 78:384–396, 1974a *(Chapter 8)*

Deutman AF: Acute retinal pigment epheliitis. Am J Ophthalmol 78:571–578, 1974b *(Chapter 8)*

Deutman AF, Jansen LMAA: Dominantly inherited drusen of Bruch's membrane. Br J Ophthalmol 54:373–382, 1970 *(Chapter 8)*

Deutman AF, Rümke AML: Reticular dystrophy of the retinal pigment epithelium. Arch Ophthalmol 82:4–9, 1969 *(Chapter 8)*

Deutman AF, Sengers RCA, Trijbels JMF: Gyrate atrophy of the choroid and retina with reticular pigmentary dystrophy and ornithine-ketoacid-transaminase deficiency. Int Ophthalmol 1:49–56, 1978 *(Chapter 8)*

Deutman AF, Van Blommenstein JDA, Henkes HE, Waardenburg PJ, Solleveld-Van Driest E: Butterfly-shaped pigment dystrophy of the fovea. Arch Ophthalmol 83:558–569, 1970 *(Chapter 8)*

DeValois RL: Physiological basis of color vision, in Richter M (ed): Color 69. Göttingen, Musterschmidt Verlag, 1970 *(Chapter 6)*

DeValois RL: Physiological basis of color vision. Farbe 20:151–169, 1971 *(Chapter 3)*

DeValois RL, Abramov I, Jacobs GH: Analysis of response patterns of LGN cells. J Opt Soc Am 56:966–977, 1966 *(Chapter 3)*

DeValois RL, DeValois KK: Neural coding of color, in Carterette ED, Friedman MP (eds): Handbook of Perception, vol V. New York, Academic Press, 1975 *(Chapter 3)*

Dieter W: Untersuchungen zur Duplizitatstheorie. III.

Die angeborene familiär-erbliche stationäre (idiopathische) Hemeralopie. Pflügers Arch Ges Physiol 222:381–394, 1929 *(Chapter 8)*

Dittrich H, Neubauer O: Störungen des Farbsehens bei Leber-Krankheiten. Münch Med Wochenschr 109:2690–2693, 1967 *(Chapter 8)*

Dodt E, Copenhaver RM, Gunkle RD: Electroretinographic measurement of the spectral sensitivity in albinos, Caucasians and Negroes. Arch Ophthalmol 62:759–803, 1959 *(Chapter 8)*

Donaldson GB: Instrumentation of the Farnsworth-Munsell 100 hue test. J Opt Soc Am 67:248–249, 1977 *(Chapter 5)*

Dorne PA: Le disque vitelliforme de la macula. Thesis, Lyon, 1970 *(Chapter 8)*

Dorne PA: La retinopathie séreuse centrale ou soulèvement séreux idiopathique de la retine maculaire; son diagnostic differentiel avec les décollements séreux secondaires et les maculopathies exsudatives et/ou disciformes. Conf Lyonn Ophtalmol 110:7–181, 1971 *(Chapter 8)*

Douche CC: A Propos de la toxicité oculaire de l'éthambutol. Ann Oculist (Paris) 207:557-561, 1974 *(Chapter 8)*

Dralands L, Evrard P, Pouchon P, Rommel J, Stanescu B: Les complications oculaires de l'hypoparathyroidie familiale chez l'enfant. Bull Soc Belge Ophtalmol 157:374–392, 1971 *(Chapter 8)*

Dran R: Cas familiaux de disques vitelliformes. Ann Oculist (Paris) 206:529–544, 1973 *(Chapter 8)*

Drance SM: Studies in the susceptibility of the eye to raised intraocular pressure. Arch Ophthalmol 68:478–485, 1962 *(Chapter 8)*

Drescher K, Trendelenburg W: Eine Lichtfläche zur Normierung der Helladaptation. Klin Mbl Augenh 76:776–778, 1926 *(Chapter 5)*

Dreyer V: Occupational possibilities of colour defectives. Acta Ophthalmol (Kbh) 47:523–534, 1969 *(Chapter 9)*

Drum BA: Chromatic saturation derived from increment thresholds for white and colored targets; A technique for projection of color perimetry. Mod Prob Ophthalmol 17:79–85, 1976 *(Chapter 6)*

Dube AH: Diabetic retinopathy. NY State J Med 63:2783–2786, 1963 *(Chapter 8)*

DuBois-Poulsen A: Le champ visuel, topographie normale, et pathologique de ses sensibilities. Paris, Masson & Cie, 1952 *(Chapters 6 and 8)*

DuBois-Poulsen A: Acquired dyschromatopsias. Mod Prob Ophthalmol 11:84–93, 1972 *(Chapter 8)*

DuBois-Poulsen A, Cochet P: Un cas de dyschromatopsie diabetique. Bull Soc Ophtalmol Paris 4:323–330, 1954 *(Chapter 8)*

DuBois-Poulsen A, Magis C: La dyschromatopsie du glaucome. Bull Mem Soc Fr Ophtalmol 74:23–31, 1961 *(Chapter 8)*

Duke-Elder S: Glaucoma and Hypotony. System of

Ophthalmology, vol XI, London. Kimpton, 1969 *(Chapter 8)*

Dunnewold CJW: On the Campbell and Stiles-Crawford effects and their clinical importance. Soesterberg, The Netherlands, Institute for Perception RVO-TNO, National Defence Research Organization TNO 1964 *(Chapter 6)*

Durup G, Piéron H: L'équation de Rayleigh et la dissociation des valences chromatique et lumineuse. Rev d'Opt 22:224–231, 1943 *(Chapter 6)*

Dvorine I: Improvements in color vision in twenty cases. Am J Optom 23:302–321, 1946 *(Chapter 5)*

Dvorine I: Quantitative classification of the color-blind. J Gen Psychol 68:255–265, 1963 *(Chapter 5)*

Ebrey TG, Honig B: New wavelength dependent visual pigment nomograms. Vision Res 17:147–151, 1977 *(Chapter 3)*

Eichengreen JM: A substitute for the Nagel anomaloscope. Mod Prob Ophthalmol 13:36–41, 1974 *(Chapter 5)*

Engelbrecht K: Grenzen und Grenzfälle der Farbenempfindung. Klin Mbl Augenh 110:630–637, 1944 *(Chapter 7)*

Engelking E: Über den methodischen wert physiologischer perimeterobjecte. Graefes Arch Ophthalmol 104:75–132, 1921 *(Chapter 8)*

Engelking E: Die tritanomalie, ein bisher unbekannter Typus anomaler Trichromasie. Graefes Arch Ophthalmol 116:196–244, 1925 *(Chapters 5, 7, and 8)*

Engelking E: Farbenschwäche und künstliche zeitweilige Farbenblindheit. Klin Mbl Augenh 90:9–21, 1933 *(Chapter 7)*

Engelking E, Eckstein A: Physiologische Bestimmung der Musterfarben für die klinische Perimetrie. Klin Mbl Augenh 64:88–106, 1920 *(Chapter 6)*

Engelking E, Hartung H: Spektraluntersuchungen über die Minimalfeldhelligkeiten des Tritanomalen und seine Unterschiedsempfindlichkeit für Änderungen der Helligkeit. Arch Ophthalmol 118:211–220, 1927 *(Chapter 7)*

Enoch JM: Amblyopia and the Stiles-Crawford effect. Am J Optom Arch Am Acad Optom 34:298–309, 1957 *(Chapter 6)*

Enoch JM: Further studies on the relationship between amblyopia and the Stiles-Crawford effect. Am J Optom Arch Am Acad Optom 36:111–128, 1959a *(Chapter 6)*

Enoch JM: Receptor amblyopia. Am J Ophthalmol 48:262–274, 1959b *(Chapter 6)*

Enoch JM: Optical properties of the retinal receptors. J Opt Soc Am 53:71–85, 1963 *(Chapter 6)*

Enoch JM: The current status of receptor amblyopia. Doc Ophthalmol 23:130–148, 1967 *(Chapter 6)*

Enoch JM: Photoreceptor orientation following retinal detachment. Am J Ophthalmol 67:603–604, 1969 *(Chapter 6)*

Enoch JM: The two-color technique of Stiles and derived component color mechanisms, in Jameson D, Hurvich LM (eds): Visual Psychophysics. Berlin, Springer-Verlag, 1972 *(Chapter 6)*

Enoch JM, Hope GM: An analysis of retinal receptor orientation. III. Results of initial psychophysical tests. Invest Ophthalmol 11:765–782, 1972a *(Chapter 6)*

Enoch JM, Hope GM: Analysis of retinal receptor orientation. IV. Center of the entrance pupil and the center of convergence of orientation and directional sensitivity. Invest Ophthalmol 11:1017–1021, 1972b *(Chapter 6)*

Enoch JM, Laties A: An analysis of retinal receptor orientation. II. Predictions for psychophysical tests. Invest Ophthalmol 10:959–970, 1971 *(Chapter 6)*

Enoch JM, Sunga R: Development of quantitative perimetric tests. Doc Ophthalmol 26:215–229, 1969 *(Chapter 8)*

Enoch JM, Van Loo Jr JA, Okun E: Realignment of photoreceptors disturbed in orientation secondary to retinal detachment. Invest Ophthalmol 12:849–853, 1973 *(Chapter 6)*

Enroth-Cugell C, Robson JG: The contrast sensitivity of retinal ganglion cells of the cat. J Physiol (London) 187:517–552, 1966 *(Chapter 3)*

Espinda SD: Color vision deficiency in third and sixth grade boys in association to academic achievement and descriptive behavioral patterns. Dissert Abstr Int 32/2-A:786, 1971 *(Chapter 9)*

Estévez O, Cavonius CR: Human color perception and Stiles π mechanisms. Vision Res 17:417–422, 1977 *(Chapter 3)*

Falls HF: Hereditary congenital macular degeneration. Am J Hum Genet 1:96–104, 1949 *(Chapter 8)*

Falls HF: The polymorphous manifestations of Best's disease (vitelliform eruptive disease of the retina). Trans Am Ophthalmol Soc 67:265–279, 1969 *(Chapter 8)*

Falls HF, Wolter JR, Alpern M: Typical total monochromacy. A histological and psychophysical study. Arch Ophthalmol 74:610–616, 1965 *(Chapter 7)*

Fankhauser F, Enoch JM: The effects of blur upon perimetric thresholds. Arch Ophthalmol 68:240–251, 1962 *(Chapter 6)*

Fankhauser F, Enoch J, Cibis P: Receptor orientation in retinal pathology. Am J Ophthalmol 52:767–783, 1961 *(Chapter 6)*

Farnsworth D: The Farnsworth-Munsell 100 hue and dichotomous tests for color vision. J Opt Soc Am 33:568–578, 1943 *(Chapter 5)*

Farnsworth D: The Farnsworth Dichotomous Test for

Color Blindness—Panel D-15. New York, Psychological Corporation, 1947 *(Chapters 5 and 7)*

Farnsworth D: The Farnsworth-Munsell 100 Hue Test Manual (revised ed). Baltimore, Munsell Color Company, 1957 *(Chapter 5)*

Farnsworth D: Let's look at those isochromatic lines again. Vision Res 1:1–5, 1961 *(Chapter 7)*

Farnsworth D, Paulson H, Connolly KT: Report on the evaluation of the Freeman Illuminant-Stable Color Vision Test. Unpublished report of the U.S. Naval Medical Research Laboratory, U.S. Submarine Base, New London, Conn. (undated) *(Chapter 5)*

Farnsworth D, Reed JD, Shilling CW: The effect of certain illuminants on scores made on pseudoisochromatic tests. Color Vision Report No. 4. New London, Conn., United States Naval Medical Research Laboratory, 1948 *(Chapter 5)*

Farpour H, Babel J: Les fossettes papillaries: Diagnostique differentiel, anomalies vasculaires et cas limités. Ann Oculist (Paris) 201:1–17, 1968 *(Chapter 8)*

Feldman M, Todman L, Bender M: "Flight of colours" in lesions of the visual system. J Neurol Neurosurg Psychiatr 37:1265–1272, 1974 *(Chapter 8)*

Ferree CE, Rand G: Effect of brightness of preexposure and surrounding field of breadth and shape of the color fields for stimuli of different sizes. Am J Ophthalmol 7:843–850, 1924 *(Chapter 6)*

Fetkenhour CL, Gurney N, Dobbie JC, Choromokos E: Central areolar pigment epithelial dystrophy. Am J Ophthalmol 81:745–753, 1976 *(Chapter 8)*

Fialkow PJ, Thuline HC, Fenster LF: Lack of association between cirrhosis and common types of color blindness. N Engl J Med 275:584–587, 1966 *(Chapter 8)*

Fick A: Zur Theorie der Farbenblindheit. Verh Physikal-Med Ges Würzburg 5:158–162, 1873–74 *(Chapter 7)*

Filipiakowa Z: Colour vision in electric welders. Klinika Oczna 8:933–938, 1975 *(Chapter 8)*

Fincham EF: Defects of the colour-sense mechanism as indicated by the accommodation reflex. J Physiol (London) 121:570–580, 1953 *(Chapter 7)*

Fink WH: The ocular pathology of methyl alcohol poisoning. Am J Ophthalmol 26:694–709, 802–815, 1943 *(Chapter 8)*

Fiore C, Korol S, Babel J: La valeur des examens fonctionnels dans la détection des dystrophies du pôle postérieur. Ann Oculist (Paris) 208:849–868, 1975 *(Chapter 8)*

Fischer FP, Bouman MA, ten Doesschate J: A case of tritanopy. Doc Ophthalmol 5-6:73–87, 1951 *(Chapter 7)*

Fishman GA: Fundus flavimaculatus. Arch Ophthalmol 94:2061–2067, 1976 *(Chapter 8)*

Fishman GA, Buckman G, Van Every T: Fundus flavimaculatus: A clinical classification. Doc Ophthalmol 13:213–220, 1977 *(Chapter 8)*

Fishman GA, Krill A, Fishman M: Acquired color defects in patients with open angle glaucoma and ocular hypertension. Mod Prob Ophthalmol 13:335–338, 1974 *(Chapter 8)*

Fishman GA, Trimble S, Rabb MF, Fishman M: Pseudovitelliform macular degeneration. Arch Ophthalmol 95:73–76, 1977 *(Chapter 8)*

Fletcher RJ: Ophthalmics in Industry. Aldwych, Hatton Press, 1961 *(Chapter 9)*

Fletcher RJ: A modified D-15 test. Mod Prob Ophthalmol 11:22–24, 1972 *(Chapter 5)*

Fletcher R: Confusion spot displays for endoscopy and other situations. Mod Prob Ophthalmol 19:95–96, 1978 *(Chapter 9)*

Flynn JT: Dark adaptation in amblyopia. Arch Ophthalmol 79:697–704, 1968 *(Chapter 8)*

Flynn JT, Glaser JS: Dark adaptation in strabismic amblyopia: The use of colored filters. Ophthalmol Res 2:1–15, 1971 *(Chapter 8)*

Fonta D: Correlations anatomiques et fonctionnnelles dans les chorioretinopathies séreuses centrales en periode d'activité. Marseille, Thèse, 1972 *(Chapter 8)*

Fouanon C, Ardouin M, Perdriel G, Dary J: Intérêt de l'examen génétique, fonctionnel, electrophysiologique angiographique dans la choroidérémie. Bull Soc Ophtalmol Fr 71:541–546, 1971 *(Chapter 8)*

Foulds WS: Visual disturbances in systemic disorders, optic neuropathy, and systemic disease. Trans Ophthalmol Soc UK 89:125–146, 1969 *(Chapter 8)*

Foulds WS, Chisholm IA, Bronte-Stewart J: Effects of raised intraocular pressure on hue discrimination. Mod Prob Ophthalmol 13:328–334, 1974 *(Chapter 8)*

Foulds WS, Chisholm IA, Bronte-Stewart J, Reid HRC: The investigation and therapy of the toxic amblyopias. Trans Ophthalmol Soc UK 90:739–763, 1970 *(Chapter 8)*

Foulds WS, Chisholm IA, Bronte-Stewart J, Wilson T: Cyanide induced optic neuropathy. Opthalmol Addit 158:350–358, 1969 *(Chapter 8)*

Foulds WS, Chisholm IA, Pettigrew AR: The toxic optic neuropathies. Br J Ophthalmol 58:386–390, 1974 *(Chapter 8)*

Foulds WS, Chisholm IA, Reid HCR: The effects of raised intraocular pressure on visual function, in Cant JS (ed): The Optic Nerve. London, Kimpton, 1972 *(Chapter 8)*

Foulds WS, Lee WR, Taylor WOG: Clinical and pathological aspects of choroidal ischemia. Trans Ophthalmol Soc UK 91:323–341, 1971 *(Chapter 8)*

Foulds WS, Reid HR, Chisholm IA: Factors influencing visual recovery after retinal detachment surgery. Mod Prob Ophthalmol 12:49–57, 1974 *(Chapter 8)*

Fox SL: Industrial and Occupational Ophthalmology. Springfield, Ill., Charles C. Thomas, 1973 *(Chapter 9)*

Franceschetti A: Die Bedeutung der Einstellungstreite am Anomaloskop für die Diagnose der einzelnen Typen der Farbensinnstörungen nebst Bermerkungen über ihren Vererbungsmodus. Schweiz Med Wochenschr 52:1273–1278, 1928 *(Chapter 7)*

Franceschetti A: Première observation d'une fratrie issue de deux daltoniens de type différent. Bull Schweiz Akad Med Wiss 5:227–232, 1949 *(Chapter 7)*

Franceschetti A: Acquisitions récentes concernant les troubles congénitaux du sens chromatique et leurs relations aver les aberrations chromosomiques. Archiv Julius-Klaus-Stiftung Versbungsfrich 35:322–412, 1960 *(Chapter 7)*

Franceschetti A: Congenital and hereditary neuro-ophthalmic diseases, in Beard C, Falls JF, Franceschetti A, et al (eds): Congenital Anomalies of the Eye, Transactions of the New Orleans Academy of Ophthalmology. St. Louis, The C. V. Mosby Company, 1968, pp 99–113 *(Chapter 8)*

Franceschetti A, François J: Fundus flavimaculatus. Arch Ophtalmol (Paris) 25:505–530, 1965 *(Chapter 8)*

Franceschetti A, François J, Babel J: Les hérédodégénérescences choriorétiniennes. Paris, Masson & Cie, 1963 *(Chapter 8)*

Franceschetti A, François J, Babel J: Chorioretinal Heredodegenerations. Springfield, Ill., Charles C. Thomas, 1974 *(Chapters 7 and 8)*

Franceschetti A, Jaeger W, Klein D, Ohrt V, Rickli H: Etude pathophysiologique et génétique de la grande famille d'achromates de l'île de fur (Danemark) (Description d'une nouvelle famille avec achromatopsie totale chez le fils aîné et achromatopsie incomplète chez le frère cadet). XVIII Concilium Ophthalmologicum 1958, Belgica, vol II, pp 1582–1588 *(Chapter 7)*

François J: Mode d'hérédité des hérédo-dégénérescences du nerf optique. J Genet Hum 15:147–220, 1966 *(Chapter 8)*

François J: (Infantile) optic atrophy with dominant autosomal heredity, in Gordom DM (ed): Genetic Aspects of Ophthalmology, International Ophthalmology Clinics 8: No. 4. Boston, Little, Brown & Company, 1968, pp 1004–1013 *(Chapter 8)*

François J: Vitelliform macular degeneration. Ophthalmologica 162:312-324, 1971 *(Chapter 8)*

François J: Dégénérescences maculaires juvéniles. Arch Ophtalmol (Paris) 34:497-512, 1974 *(Chapter 8)*

François J, De Rouck A, Cambie E: Retinal and optic evaluation in quinine poisoning. Ann Ophthalmol 4:177–185, 1972 *(Chapter 8)*

François J, De Rouck A, Cambie E: Dégénérescence hyaloidéo-tapéto-rétinienne de Goldmann-Favre. Ophthalmologica 168:81–96, 1974 *(Chapter 8)*

François J, De Rouck A, Cambie E, De Laey JJ: Visual functions in pericentral and central pigmentary retinopathy. Ophthalmologica 165:38–61, 1972a *(Chapter 8)*

François J, De Rouck A, Cambie E, De Laey JJ: Rétinopathie chloroquinique. Ophthalmologica 165:81–99, 1972b *(Chapter 8)*

François J, De Rouck A, Verriest G, De Laey JJ, Cambie E: Progressive generalized cone dysfunction. Ophthalmologica 169:255–284, 1974 *(Chapter 8)*

François J, Turut P: La dégénérescence vitelliforme de la macula. Arch Ophtalmol (Paris) 35:609–626, 1975 *(Chapter 8)*

François J, Turut P, Puech B, Hache JC: Maladie de Stargardt et fundus flavimaculatus. Arch Ophthalmol (Paris) 35:817–846, 1975 *(Chapter 8)*

François J, Verriest G: Les fonctions visuelles dans l'élastose rétinienne. Ann Oculist (Paris) 187:113–144, 1954 *(Chapter 8)*

François J, Verriest G: La détection à l'aide des tests de Farnsworth des dyschromatopsies acquises dans les dégénérescences tapéto-rétiniennes. Ann Oculist (Paris) 113:381–398, 1956a *(Chapter 8)*

François J, Verriest G: La détection à l'aide des tests de Farnsworth des dyschromatopsies acquises dans les dégénérescences tapéto-rétiniennes. Bull Soc Belge Ophtalmol 113:385–398, 1956b *(Chapter 8)*

François J, Verriest G: Les dyschromatopsies acquises. Ann Oculist (Paris) 190:713–746, 1957a *(Chapters 5 and 8)*

François J, Verriest G: Classification et symptomatologie des dyschromatopsies acquises. Bull Soc Belge Ophtalmol 116:351–392, 1957b *(Chapter 6)*

François J, Verriest G: Contribution a l'étude des dyschromatopsies congénitales a symptomes intermédiaires entre ceux des systèmes dichromatique classiques et ceux de l'achromatopsie typique: Observation personnelle et revue de la littérature. Ann Oculist (Paris) 192:81–120, 1959a *(Chapter 7)*

François J, Verriest G: Les dyschromatopsies acquises dans le glaucome primaire. Ann Oculist (Paris) 192:191–199, 1959b *(Chapter 8)*

François J, Verriest G: Functional abnormalities of the retina, in François J: Heredity in Ophthalmology. St. Louis, The C. V. Mosby Company, 1961a, pp 396–440 *(Chapter 7)*

François J, Verriest G: On acquired deficiency of color vision with special reference to its detection and classification by means of the tests of

Farnsworth. Vision Res 1:201–219, 1961b
(Chapter 8)

François J, Verriest G: Etude biométrique de la rétinopathie pigmentaire. Ann Oculist (Paris)
195:937–951, 1962 (Chapter 8)

François J, Verriest G: The visual functions in
strabismic amblyopia. J Pediatr Ophthalmol
2:59–64, 1965 (Chapter 8)

François J, Verriest G: Le funzioni visive nell'
ambliopia strabica. Proc Atti Giorn Europee
Studi Strabol, 25–26 April 1964, Parma, 3–11,
Torino, Minerva Medica, 1966 (Chapter 8)

François J, Verriest G: La discrimination chromatique
dans l'amblyopie strabique. Doc Ophthalmol
23:318–331, 1967 (Chapter 8)

François J, Verriest G: Nouvelles observations de déficiences acquises de la discrimination chromatique. Ann Oculist (Paris) 201:1097–1114,
1968 (Chapter 8)

François J, Verriest G: Paravenous pigmentary retinopathy. Doc Ophthalmol 10:281–289, 1976
(Chapter 8)

François J, Verriest G, De Rouck A: L'achromatopsie
congénitale. Doc Ophthalmol 9:338–424, 1955
(Chapter 7)

François J, Verriest G, De Rouck A: Les fonctions
visuelles dans le glaucome congénital. Ann
Oculist (Paris) 189:81–107, 1957 (Chapter 8)

François J, Verriest G, De Rouck A: Hérédo-
dégénerescence maculaire juvénile avec atteinte
prédominante de la vision photopique. Ann
Oculist (Paris) 195:1137–1191, 1962 (Chapter
8)

François J, Verriest G, De Rouck A, DeVos E: Contribution à l'étude statistique des déficits
fonctionnels dans le décollement rétinien. Bull
Mem Soc Fr Ophtalmol 75:104–109, 1962
(Chapter 8)

François J, Verriest G, De Rouck, Humblet M: Dégénérescence maculaire juvénile avec attente
prédominante de la vision photopique. Ophthalmologica 131:393–402, 1956 (Chapter 8)

François J, Verriest G, François P, Asseman R: Etude
comparative des dyschromatopsies acquises as-
sociées aux différents types d'atrophie optique
hérédo-familiale. Bull Soc Belge Ophtalmol
125:950–956, 1960 (Chapter 8)

François J, Verriest G, François P, Asseman R: Etude
comparative des dyschromatopsies acquises as-
sociées aux différents types d'atrophie optique
hérédo-familiale. Ann Oculist (Paris) 194:217–
235, 1961 (Chapter 8)

François J, Verriest G, Israel A: Périmétrie statique
colorée effectuée à l'aide de l'appareil de
Goldmann. Résultats obtenus en pathologie
oculaire. Ann Oculist (Paris) 199:
113–154, 1966 (Chapters 6 and 8)

François J, Verriest G, Matton-Van Leuven MT, De
Rouck A, Manavian D: Atypical achromatopsia

of sex-linked recessive inheritance. Am J
Ophthalmol 61:1101–1108, 1966 (Chapter 7)

François J, Verriest G, Metsälä P: La discrimination
chromatique latérale dans les dyschromatopsies
acquises. Ann Oculist (Paris) 197:425–440,
1964 (Chapter 8)

François P, Woillez M, Guibert MME, Carouqes J:
Une nouvelle étiologie de névrite optique
toxique: L'Amoproxan. Ann Oculist (Paris)
204:71, 1971 (Chapter 8)

Frank HR, Landers MB, Williams RJ, Sidbury JB: A
new dominant progressive foveal dystrophy. Am
J Ophthalmol 78:903–916, 1975 (Chapter 8)

Fraser GR: Estimation of the recombination fraction
between the protan and deutan loci. Am J Hum
Genet 21:593–599, 1969 (Chapter 7)

Fraser HB, Wallace DC: Sorsby's familial pseudo-
inflammatory macular dystrophy. Am J Ophthalmol 71:1216–1220, 1971 (Chapter 8)

Freeman E: An illuminant-stable color vision test. I. J
Opt Soc Am 38:532–538, 1948a (Chapter 5)

Freeman E: An illuminant-stable color vision test. II. J
Opt Soc Am 38:971–976, 1948b (Chapter 5)

Frey R: Welche pseudo-isochromatische Tafeln
sind für die Praxis am besten geeignet? Vergleichende Untersuchungen über die Ver-
wendbarkeit des Tafeln von Boström-Kugelberg,
Hardy-Rand-Rittler, Ishihara, Rabkin und Stilling. Graefes Arch Ophthalmol 160:301–320,
1958 (Chapter 5)

Frey RG: Die Trennschärfe einiger pseudoiso-
chromatischen Tafelproben. Graefes Arch
Ophthalmol 165:20–30, 1962 (Chapter 5)

Frey RG: Zur differentialdiagnose der angeborenen
Farbensinnstorüngen mit pseudoisochromatis-
chen Tafeln. Ophthalmologica 145:34–48, 1963
(Chapter 5)

Frey RG: Zur Wahl der geeigneten Beleuchtung für
die Farbensinnprüfung mit pseudoisochromatis-
chen Tafeln. Wien Klin Wochenschr 76:170–
172, 1964 (Chapter 5)

Frey RG: Schielamblyopie und Farbensinn. Ber 68
Zus Dtsch Ophthal Ges Heidelberg 1967. München, Bergmann, 1968 (Chapter 8)

Frey RG: Anforderungen an das Sehorgan des
Kraftfahrers. Osterr Arztez 28:16–18, 1973
(Chapter 9)

Frey RG: Zur Beurteilung der Kraftfahrtauglichkeit
bei mangelhaften Farbenunterscheidungsvermo-
gen. Osterr Arztez 30:691–695, 1975a (Chapter
9)

Frey RG: A railway accident a hundred years ago as
reason of systematic testing of colour vision.
Klin Mbl Augenh 167:125–127, 1975b (Chapter
9)

Frey RG: First experiences with the 25th edition of
Velhagen's "Tables for Examination of Colour-
Sense." Klin Mbl Augenh 166:830–831, 1975c
(Chapter 5)

Frisen L: A versatile color confrontation test for the central visual field, a comparison with quantitative perimetry. Arch Ophthalmol 89:1–9, 1973 *(Chapter 6)*

Früh D, Lauer HJ: Dominant vererbte Opticusatrophie mit Rot-Grünblindheit im Sinne einer erworbenen Deuterostörung. Bericht über die 71 zusammenkunft der Dtsch Ophthalmol Ges in Heidelberg, 1971, 517–522 *(Chapter 8)*

Frühauf A, Klein S, Ritter A: Farbsinnuntersuchungen mit dem Farnsworth-Munsell 100-hue-test bei Patienten mit Schielamblyopie und alternierendem Strabismus. Ophthalmologica 167:66–76, 1973 *(Chapter 8)*

Fujino T: Dark adaptation curves in amblyopic eyes. Jpn J Clin Ophthalmol 21:1289–1294, 1967 *(Chapter 8)*

Fuller D, Machemer R, Knighton RW: Retinal damage produced by intraocular fiber optic light. Am J Ophthalmol 85:519–537, 1978 *(Chapter 8)*

Gaillard G: Résultats Fonctionnels du Traitement Chirurgical du Décollement de la Rétine. Paris, Masson & Cie, 1962 *(Chapter 8)*

Galezowski X: Du Diagnostic des Maladies des Yeux par la Chromatoscopie Rétinienne. Paris, J. B. Baillierè & Fils, 1868 *(Chapter 8)*

Ganter H: Farbenfehlsichtige im Strassenverkehr. Zbl Verkehrsmed 1:7–18, 1955 *(Chapter 9)*

Gardiner P: A colour vision test for young children and the handicapped. Dev Med Child Neurol 15:437–440, 1973 *(Chapter 5)*

Gass JDM: Pathogenesis of disciform detachment of the neuro-epithelium. Am J Ophthalmol 63: 573–711, 1967 *(Chapter 8)*

Gass JDM, Norton EWD, Justice J: Serous detachment of retinal pigment epithelium. Trans Am Acad Ophthalmol Otolaryngol 70:990–1015, 1966 *(Chapter 8)*

Geeraets WJ, Williams RC, Chan G, Hamm WT, Gerry III D, Schmidt FH: The loss of light energy in retina and choroid. Arch Ophthalmol 64: 606–615, 1960 *(Chapter 8)*

Geiser EP, Falls HF: Hereditary retinoschisis. Am J Ophthalmol 51:1193–2000, 1961 *(Chapter 8)*

Gerde LS: Angioid streaks in sickel trait hemoglobinopathy. Am J Ophthalmol 77:462–464, 1974 *(Chapter 8)*

Gibson HC, Smith DM, Alpern M: π_5 Specificity in digitoxin toxicity. Arch Ophthalmol 74:154–158, 1965 *(Chapters 6 and 8)*

Gibson IM: Visual mechanisms in a cone-monochromat. J Physiol (London) 162:10P–11P, 1962 *(Chapter 7)*

Giessmann HG: Untersuchungen über die Pathophysiologie der Amblyopie. Thesis, Magdeburg, 1962 *(Chapter 8)*

Giessmann HG: Erworbene Farbsehstörungen. Proceedings of "Journées internationales de la couleur" 1.-4.6. 1965 Lucerne, 281–285, Göttingen, Musterschmidt Verlag, 1966 *(Chapter 8)*

Gilbert JG: Age changes in color matching. J Gerontol 12:210–215, 1957 *(Chapter 8)*

Gillespie L, Terry LL, Sjoerdsma A: The application of a monamine oxidase inhibitor 1-phenyl 2-hydrozinopropane (JB-516) to the treatment of primary hypertension. Am Heart J 58:1–12, 1959 *(Chapter 8)*

Girot D, Braum S: Un cas de névrite optique par intoxication à l'acétate de thallium. Rev Neurol 1:244–245, 1929 *(Chapter 8)*

Glickstein M, Heath GG: Receptors in the monochromat eye. Vision Res 15:633–636, 1975 *(Chapter 7)*

Goebel HH, Fix JD, Zeman W: The fine structure of the retina in neuronal ceroid lipofuscinosis. Am J Ophthalmol 77:25–39, 1974 *(Chapter 8)*

Goebel HH, Zeman W, Damaske E: An ultrastructural study of the retina in the Jansky-Bielschowsky type of neuronal ceroid-lipofuscinosis. Am J Ophthalmol 83:70–79, 1977 *(Chapter 8)*

Goldthwaite D, Lakowski R, Drance SM: A study of dark adaptation in ocular hypertensives. Can J Ophthalmol 11:55–60, 1976 *(Chapter 8)*

Goodeve CF, Lythgoe RJ, Schneider EE: The photosensitivity of visual purple solutions and the scotopic sensitivity of the eye in ultraviolet. Proc R Soc Edinb B 130:380–395, 1941 *(Chapter 8)*

Goodman G, Ripps H: Electro-retinography in the differential diagnosis of visual loss in children. Arch Opthalmol 64:221–235, 1960 *(Chapter 8)*

Goodman G, Ripps H, Siegel IM: Cone dysfunction syndromes. Arch Ophthalmol 70:214–231, 1963 *(Chapters 4, 7, and 8)*

Goodman G, Ripps H, Siegel IM: Sex-linked ocular disorders: Trait expressivity in males and carrier females. Arch Ophthalmol 73:387–398, 1965 *(Chapter 7)*

Gorn RA, Kuwabara T: Retinal damage by visible light. Arch Ophthalmol 77:115–118, 1967 *(Chapter 8)*

Gorrell GJ: A study of defective colour vision with the Ishihara test plates. Ann Hum Genet 31:39–43, 1967 *(Chapter 8)*

Göthlin G: Congenital red-green abnormality in colour-vision, and congenital total colour-blindness, from the point of view of heredity. Acta Ophthalmol 2:15–34, 1924 *(Chapter 7)*

Gouras P: Identification of cone mechanisms in monkey ganglion cells. J Physiol (London) 199:533–547, 1968 *(Chapter 3)*

Gouras P: Antidromic responses of orthodromically identified ganglion cells in monkey retina. J Physiol (London) 204:407–419, 1969 *(Chapters 3 and 6)*

Gouras P: Trichromatic mechanisms in single cortical neurons. Science 168:489–492, 1970 *(Chapter 6)*

Gowers WR: Medical Ophthalmology (ed 2). London, J & A Churchill, 1882 *(Chapter 8)*

Graham BV, Turner ME, Hurst DC: Derivation of wavelength discrimination from color naming. J Opt Soc Am 63:109–111, 1973 *(Chapter 6)*

Graham CH: Color mixture and color systems, in Graham CH (ed): Vision and Visual Perception. New York, John Wiley & Sons, 1965a *(Chapter 2)*

Graham CH: Color: Data and theories, in Graham CH (ed): Vision and Visual Perception. New York, John Wiley & Sons, 1965b *(Chapter 7)*

Graham CH, Brown JL: Color contrast and color appearances: Brightness constancy and color constancy, in Graham CH (ed): Vision and Visual Perception. New York, John Wiley & Sons, 1965 *(Chapter 2)*

Graham CH, Hsia Y: Luminosity losses in deuteranopes. Science 131:414, 1960 *(Chapter 7)*

Graham CH, Hsia Y: Some visual functions of a unilaterally dichromatic subject, in N. P. L. Symp. No. 8, "Visual Problems of Colour," U.S. ed. New York, Chemical Publishing Company, 1961, pp 279–295 *(Chapter 7)*

Graham CH, Hsia Y: Saturation and the foveal achromatic interval. J. Opt Soc Am 59:993–997, 1969 *(Chapter 6)*

Gramberg-Danielsen B: Farbenuntüchtigkeit und Strassenverkehr. Zentralbl Verkehrsmed 11:1–12, 1965 *(Chapter 9)*

Gramberg-Danielsen B: Sehen und Verkehr. Berlin, Springer-Verlag, 1967 *(Chapter 9)*

Gramberg-Danielsen B: Verkehrsophthalmologie, in Velhagen K: Der Augenarzt, vol II (ed 2). Leipzig, VEB Thieme, 1976, pp 286–369 *(Chapter 9)*

Grant WM: Toxicology of the Eye. Springfield, Ill., Charles C. Thomas, 1962 *(Chapter 8)*

Grassman H: Zur Theorie der Farbenmischung. Ann Phys Lpz 89:60–84, 1853 [English trans Philos Mag 7:254–264, 1854] *(Chapter 2)*

Green DG: Visual acuity in the blue cone monochromat. J Physiol (London) 222:419–426, 1972 *(Chapter 7)*

Greve ER, Verduin WM, Ledeboer M: Two-colour threshold in static perimetry. Mod Prob Ophthalmol 13:113–118, 1974 *(Chapter 6)*

Grignolo A, Orzalesi N, Castellazzo R, Vittone P: Retinal damage by visible light in albino rats. Ophthalmologica 157:43–59, 1969 *(Chapter 8)*

Groenouw A: Ueber die intoxicationsamblyopie. Arch Ophthalmol 38:1–70, 1892 *(Chapter 8)*

Grognot P, Perdriel G: Influence du bruit sur certaines fonctions visuelles. Vision Res 1:269–273, 1961 *(Chapter 8)*

de Groot SG, Gebhard JW: Pupil size as determined by adapting luminance. J Opt Soc Am 42:492–495, 1952 *(Chapter 2)*

Grützner P: Typische erworbene Farbensinnstörungen bei heredodegenerativen Maculaleiden. Graefes Arch Ophthalmol 163:99–116, 1961 *(Chapters 6 and 8)*

Grützner P: Maculäre Form der diffusen tapeto-retinalen Degeneration. Graefes Arch Ophthalmol 165:227–245, 1962 *(Chapter 6)*

Grützner P: Inter- und intrafamiliäre Variationen der infantilen, dominant vererbten Opticus-Atrophie. Sonderdruck aus: Bericht über die 8. Köln, Tagung der Deutschen Gesellschaft fur Anthropologie, 1963a *(Chapters 6 and 8)*

Grützner P: Über Diagnose und Funktionsstörungen bei der infantilen, dominant vererbten Opticusatrophie. Bericht über die 65 Zusammenkunft der Deutschen Opthalmologischen Gesellschaft in Heidelberg, 1963, München, Bergman, 1963b 268–273 *(Chapters 6 and 8)*

Grützner P: Über erworbene Farbeninnstorungen bei Sehnervenerkrankungen. Graefes Arch Klin Exp Ophthalmol 169:366–384, 1966 *(Chapters 6 and 8)*

Grützner P: Acquired color vision defects secondary to retinal drug toxicity. Ophthalmol Add 158:592–604, 1969a *(Chapter 8)*

Grützner P: Acquired color vision defects from drug intoxication of the retina. Color 69. Gottingen, Musterschmidt Verlag, 1969b, pp 107–114 *(Chapter 8)*

Grützner P: Funktionsstörungen bei Digitalisintoxikation. Klin Mbl Augenh 156:260, 1970 *(Chapter 8)*

Grützner P: Über Farbenanomalie, Farbenamblyopie und Farbenasthenopie. Klin Mbl Augenh 158:89–96, 1971 *(Chapters 6, 7, and 8)*

Grützner P: Acquired color vision defects, in Jameson D, Hurvich L (eds): Handbook of Sensory Physiology, vol VII/4, Visual Psychophysics. Berlin, Springer-Verlag, 1972 *(Chapter 6)*

Grützner P, Born G, Hemminger HJ: Coloured stimuli within the central visual field of carriers of dichromatism. Mod Prob Ophthalmol 17:147–150, 1976 *(Chapters 6 and 7)*

Grützner P, Schleicher S: Acquired color vision defects in glaucoma patients. Mod Prob Ophthalmol 11:136–140, 1972 *(Chapters 6 and 8)*

Grützner P, Schrapp A: Two different alleles for deuteranomaly within a family with Leber's optic atrophy. Mod Prob Ophthalmol 13:258–261, 1974 *(Chapters 7 and 8)*

Guild J: The colorimetric properties of the spectrum. Philos Trans R Soc Lond A 230:149–187, 1931 *(Chapter 2)*

Guillaumat L, Rouchy JP, Arrata M: Dégénérescence hyaloidéo-rétinienne de Wagner. Bull Soc Ophtalmol Fr 70:809–815, 1970 *(Chapter 8)*

Gunkel RD: Retinal profiles; A psychophysical test of rod and cone sensitivity. Arch Ophthalmol 77:22–25, 1967 *(Chapter 6)*

Gunkel RD, Cogan DG: Colorimetry by a new principle. Arch Ophthalmol 96:331–334, 1978 (Chapter 5)

Guth SL, Donley NJ, Marrocco RT: On luminance additivity and related topics. Vision Res 9:537–575, 1969 (Chapter 3)

Guth SL, Lodge HR: Heterochromatic additivity, foveal spectral sensitivity and a new color model. J Opt Soc Am 63:450–462, 1973 (Chapter 3)

Hager G: Das Sehorgan und das Unfallgeschehen im Strassenverkehr. Klin Mbl Augenh 142:427–433, 1963 (Chapter 9)

Halbertsma KTA: A History of the Theory of Colour. Amsterdam, Swets & Zeitlinger, 1949 (Chapter 4)

Hallden U: Nomogram för bestämning av grön-röd-Kvoten, ett proktiskt hjälpmodel vid anomaloskopundersökningen. Nord Med 61:244, 1959 (Chapter 5)

Halsey RM, Chapanis A: An experimental determination of some isochromaticity lines in color-deficient vision. J Opt Soc Am 42:722–739, 1952 (Chapter 7)

Hansen C: Factors causing uncertainty when conducting colour discrimination tests. Ann Inst Barraquer 4:250–292, 1963 (Chapter 5)

Hansen E: Colour vision defect after cranial trauma. Mod Prob Ophthalmol 11:160–164, 1972 (Chapter 8)

Hansen E: Chloroquine retinopathy evaluated with colour perimetry. Ann Ther Clin Ophthalmol 25:323–331, 1974a (Chapter 6)

Hansen E: The colour receptors studied by increment threshold measurements during chromatic adaptation in the Goldmann perimeter. Acta Ophthalmol (Kbh) 52:490–500, 1974b (Chapter 6)

Hansen E: The photoreceptors in cone dystrophies. Mod Prob Ophthalmol 13:318–327, 1974c (Chapters 6 and 8)

Hansen E: Static perimetry during chromatic adaptation. The method applied for investigation of amblyopia. Acta Ophthalmol (Kbh) (Suppl) 125:21–22, 1975 (Chapter 8)

Hansen E: Investigation of retinitis pigmentosa by use of specific quantitative perimetry. Doc Ophthalmol 14:461–472, 1977 (Chapter 6)

Hansen E, Larsen IF, Berg K: A familial syndrome of progressive cone dystrophy, degenerative liver disease, endocrine dysfunction and hearing defect. Acta Ophthalmol (Kbh) 54:129–144, 1976 (Chapters 6 and 8)

Hansson HA: A histochemical study of cellular reactions in rat retina transiently damaged by visible light. Exp Eye Res 12:270–274, 1971 (Chapter 8)

Hardy LH: Standard illuminants in relation to color-testing procedures. Arch Ophthalmol 34:278–282, 1945 (Chapter 5)

Hardy LH, Rand G, Rittler MC: Tests for the detection and analysis of color-blindness. I. The Ishihara test: An evaluation. J Opt Soc Am 35:268–275, 1945 (Chapter 5)

Hardy LH, Rand G, Rittler MC: The effect of quality of illumination on the results of the Ishihara test. J Opt Soc Am 36:86–94, 1946 (Chapter 5)

Hardy LH, Rand G, Rittler MC: The H-R-R polychromatic plates. J Opt Soc Am 44:509–523, 1954 (Chapters 5 and 7)

Harms H: Aufgaben der Deutschen Ophthalmologischen Gesellschaft im Bereich der Verkehrsmedizin. Ber Dtsch Ophthalmol Ges 62:525–529, 1961 (Chapter 9)

Harris GS, Yeung J: Maculopathy of sex-linked juvenile retinoschisis. Can J Ophthalmol 11:1–10, 1976 (Chapter 8)

Harrison R, Hoefnagel D, Hayward JN: Congenital total color blindness, a clinicopathological report. Arch Ophthalmol 64:685–692, 1960 (Chapter 7)

Hartung H: Ueber drei familiäre Fälle von Tritanomalie. Klin Mbl Augenh 76:229–240, 1926 (Chapter 7)

Hartung H: Untersuchungen über Farbenasthenopie. Klin Mbl Augenh 94:21–32, 1935 (Chapter 7)

Harwerth RS, Levi DM: Increment threshold spectral sensitivity in anisometropic amblyopia. Vision Res 17:585–590, 1977 (Chapters 6 and 8)

Harwerth RS, Sperling HG: Prolonged color blindness induced by intense spectral lights in rhesus monkeys. Science 174:520–523, 1971 (Chapter 8)

Haut J, Haye C, Legras M, Demailly P, Clay C: Troubles de la perception colorée après absorption d'acide nalixidique. Bull Soc Ophtalmol Fr 72:147–149, 1972 (Chapter 8)

Hayhoe MM, MacLeod DIA: A single anomalous photopigment? J Opt Soc Am 66:276–277, 1976 (Chapter 7)

Heath GG: Luminosity curves of normal and dichromatic observers. Science 128:775–776, 1958 (Chapter 7)

Heath GG: Luminosity losses in deuteranopes. Science 131:417–418, 1960 (Chapter 7)

Hecht S, Shlaer S: The color vision of dichromats. I. Wavelength discrimination, brightness distribution, and color mixture. J Gen Physiol 20:57–82, 1937a (Chapter 7)

Hecht S, Shlaer S: The color vision of dichromats. II. Saturation as the basis for wavelength discrimination and color mixture. J Gen Physiol 20:83–93, 1937b (Chapter 7)

Hecht S, Shlaer S, Smith EL, Haig C, Peskin JC: The visual functions of a completely colorblind person. Am J Physiol 123:94–95, 1938 (Chapter 7)

Hecht S, Shlaer S, Smith EL, Haig C, Peskin JC: The

visual functions of the complete colorblind. J Gen Physiol 31:459–472, 1948 *(Chapter 7)*

Hedin A: A study of the new series of Boström-Kugelberg pseudoisochromatic plates. Mod Prob Ophthalmol 136:64–66, 1974 *(Chapter 5)*

Heinsius E: Über die verschiedenen Formen der Trichromasie, sowie über die Grenze zwischen Farbentuchtigkeit und Farbenuntuchtigkeit. Klin Mbl Augenh 135:95–107, 1959 *(Chapter 7)*

Heinsius E: Über die Feststellung herabgesetzter Unterschiedsempfindlichkeit bei der Prüfung des Farbensinns. Klin Mbl Augenh 139:653–661, 1961 *(Chapter 7)*

Heinsius E: Beginn der Netzhautdegeneration mit Auswirkung auf Farbensinn und zentrale Sehschärfe. Aertzl Dienst DB 29:61, 1968 *(Chapter 8)*

Heinsius E: Effects of the beginning of macula degeneration on colour-vision tests. Mod Prob Ophthalmol 11:106–110, 1972 *(Chapter 8)*

Heinsius E, Grevsmuhl G: Untersuchungen über die Festellung der einzelnen Formen von Farbenfehlsichtigkeit mit Hilfe der Farbfleckverfahrens nach Trendelenburg. Klin Mbl Augenh · 118:269–282, 1951 *(Chapter 7)*

Helmbold R: Die erworbenen Farbensinnstörungen. Kurzes Handb Ophthalmol 2:320–331, 1932 *(Chapter 8)*

Helve J: A comparative study of several diagnostic tests of colour vision used for measuring types of degrees of congenital red-green defects. Acta Ophthalmol 115:1–64, 1972a *(Chapters 5 and 7)*

Helve J: Colour vision in X-chromosomal juvenile retinoschisis. Mod Prob Ophthalmol 11:122–129, 1972b *(Chapter 8)*

Helve J, Krause U: The influence of age on performance in the Panel D-15 colour vision test. Acta Ophthalmol (Kbh) 50:896–900, 1972 *(Chapter 8)*

Henkes HE: Oogafwijkingen ten Gevolge van Geneesmiddelengebruik. Leiden, Stafleu NV, 1968 *(Chapter 8)*

Henkes HE, Van Lith G, Canta LR: Indomethacin retinopathy. Am J Ophthalmol 73:846–856, 1972 *(Chapter 8)*

Henry GH, Cole BL, Nathan J: The inheritance of congenital tritanopia with the report of an extensive pedigree. Ann Hum Genet 27:219–231, 1964 *(Chapter 7)*

Hering E [Hurvich LM, Jameson D, trans]: Outlines of a Theory of the Light Sense. Cambridge, Mass., Harvard University Press, 1964 *(Chapter 3)*

Hermans G, Flerman LJR, Van Oye R, Watillon M, Robe-Van Wyck A, Dralands L, Garin P: Les effects nocifs des médications générales sur l'appareil visuel. Bull Soc Belge Ophtalmol 160:7–557, 1972 *(Chapter 8)*

Hess C: Über den Farbensinn bei indirekten Sehen.

Graefes Arch Ophthalmol 35:1–62, 1889 *(Chapter 6)*

Higgins KE, Knoblauch K: Validity of Pinckers' 100-hue version of the Panel D-15. Am J Opt Phys Opt 54:165–170, 1977 *(Chapter 5)*

Higgins KE, Moskowitz-Cook A, Knoblauch K: Color vision testing: An alternative "source" of illuminant C. Mod Prob Ophthalmol 19:113–121, 1978 *(Chapter 5)*

Hill AR, Connolly JE, Dundas J: An evaluation of the City Colour Vision Test. Mod Prob Ophthalmol 19:136–141, 1978 *(Chapter 5)*

Hokama H: A study on the determination of prognosis of amblyopia. Acta Soc Ophthalmol Jpn 72:2472–2522, 1968 *(Chapters 6 and 8)*

Hollows FC, Graham PA: The Ferndale glaucoma survey, in Hunt E: Glaucoma: Epidemiology, Early Diagnosis, and Some Aspects of Treatment. London, Livingstone, 1966 *(Chapter 8)*

Hollwich F: Apparition familiale d'un fundus flavimaculatus. Bull Soc Fr Ophtalmol 76:135–136, 1963 *(Chapter 8)*

Hommer K: Das Elektroretinogramm bei der zentralen Retinitis pigmentosa. Graefes Arch Ophthalmol 178:30–43, 1969 *(Chapter 8)*

Hommer K, Thaler A: ERG in dominant central retinopathia pigmentosa. Doc Ophthalmol 11:69–74, 1977 *(Chapter 8)*

Hong S: Types of acquired color-vision defects. Arch Ophthalmol 58:505–509, 1957 *(Chapter 8)*

Honig B, Ebrey TG: The structure and spectra of the chromophore of the visual pigments. Annu Rev Biophys Bioeng 3:151–177, 1974 *(Chapter 3)*

Horner JF: Die Erblichkeit des Daltonismus. Amtl Ber Verwalt Med Kantons Zurich, 1876 *(Chapter 7)*

Horner RG, Purslow ET: Dependence of anomaloscope matching on viewing distance or field size. Nature 160:23–24, 1947; 161:484, 1947 *(Chapter 6)*

Hsia Y, Graham CH: Spectral sensitivity of the cones in the dark adapted human eye. Proc Natl Acad Sci USA 38:80–85, 1952 *(Chapter 2)*

Hsia Y, Graham CH: Spectral luminosity curves for protanopic, deuteranopic and normal subjects. Proc Natl Acad Sci USA 43:1011–1019, 1957 *(Chapters 6 and 7)*

Hsia Y, Graham CH: Color blindness, in Graham CH (ed): Vision and Visual Perception. New York, John Wiley & Sons, 1965 *(Chapter 7)*

Hsieh RC, Fine BS, Lyons JS: Patterned dystrophies of the retinal pigment epithelium. Arch Ophthalmol 95:429–435, 1977 *(Chapter 8)*

Huber A: Eye Symptoms in Brain Tumors. St. Louis, C.V. Mosby Company, 1961 *(Chapter 8)*

Huddart JH: An account of persons who could not distinguish colours. Philos Trans R Soc Lond 67:260–265, 1777 *(Chapter 4)*

Hume EM, Krebs HA: Vitamin A Requirement in

Human Adults. London, MRC Special Report Service No. 264, 1949 *(Chapter 8)*

Huriez C: Optic neuritis with regression during dermomucosal reactions to mederel (amoproxan). Bull Soc Fr Dermatol Syph 78:11, 1971 *(Chapter 8)*

Hurvich LM: Color vision deficiencies, in Jameson D, Hurvich LM: Handbook of Sensory Physiology, vol VII/4: Visual Psychophysics. Berlin, Springer-Verlag, 1972, pp 582– 624 *(Chapters 5 and 7)*

Hurvich LM, Jameson D: Some quantitative aspects of an opponent-colors theory. II. Brightness, saturation, and hue in normal and dichromatic vision. J Opt Soc Am 45:602– 616, 1955 *(Chapter 3)*

Hurvich LM, Jameson D: An opponent-process theory of color vision. Psychol Rev 64:384– 404, 1957 *(Chapter 3)*

Hurvich LM, Jameson D: Color theory and abnormal red-green vision. Doc Ophthalmol 16:409– 422, 1962 *(Chapter 7)*

Hurvich LM, Jameson D: Does anomalous color vision imply color weakness? Psychol Sci 1:11– 12, 1964 *(Chapter 7)*

Hurvich LM, Jameson D: Quantum catches, color matches and discrimination failures. 50th Anniversary Spring Meeting, The Association for Research in Vision and Ophthalmology, Sarasota, Florida, 1978. Invest Ophthalmol Vis Sci 17 [Suppl]:197, 1978 *(Chapter 7)*

Ichikawa H, Hukami K, Majima A: Defective color vision and occupational adaptability, in François J (ed): Occupational and Medicative Hazards in Ophthalmology. Basel, Karger, 1969, pp 428– 433 *(Chapter 5)*

Ichikawa H, Hukami K, Tanabe S, Kawakami G: Standard Pseudoisochromatic Plates. Tokyo, Igaku-Shoin, 1978 *(Chapter 5)*

Ichikawa H, Majima A: Genealogical studies on interesting families of defective colour vision discovered by a mass examination in Japan and Formosa. Mod Prob Ophthalmol 13:265– 271, 1974 *(Chapter 7)*

Ikeda H, Ripps H: The electroretinogram of a conemonochromat. Arch Ophthalmol 75:513– 517, 1966 *(Chapter 7)*

Ikeda M, Hukami K, Urakubo M: Flicker photometry with chromatic adaptation and defective color vision. Am J Ophthalmol 73:270– 277, 1972 *(Chapters 6 and 7)*

Ikeda M, Urakubo M: Flicker HTRF as test of color vision. J Opt Soc Am 58:27– 31, 1968 *(Chapters 6 and 7)*

Imaizumi K: Electrophysiological study on retinitis pigmentosa. Acta Soc Ophthalmol Jpn 73: 2347– 2496, 1969 *(Chapter 8)*

Imaizumi K, Takahasi R, Mita K, Hoshi H: Clinical and electrophysiological findings of a case of fundus flavimaculatus. Doc Ophthalmol 10: 69– 76, 1976 *(Chapter 8)*

Imamura T: Long-term observations about color perception training of selective stimulating frequency currents for congenital defective color vision (5th report). Jpn J Clin Ophthalmol 29:363– 370, 1975 *(Chapter 8)*

Ingling Jr CR: The spectral sensitivity of the opponent-color channels. Vision Res 17:1083– 1090, 1977 *(Chapter 3)*

Ingling Jr CR: Luminance and opponent color contributions to visual detection and to temporal and spatial integration: Comment. J Opt Soc Am 68:1143-1146,1978 *(Chapter 3)*

Ingling Jr CR, Drum BA: Retinal receptive fields: Correlations between psychophysics and electrophysiology. Vision Res 13:1151– 1163, 1973 *(Chapter 3)*

Ingling Jr CR, Tsou BH: Orthogonal combination of the three visual channels. Vision Res 17:1075– 1082, 1977 *(Chapter 3)*

Ingling Jr CR, Tsou BH, Gast TJ, et al: The achromatic channel—I. The non-linearity of minimumborder and flicker matches. Vision Res 18:379– 390, 1978 *(Chapter 3)*

Ingram DJE: From radar to spectroscopy—New regions of the spectrum. Adv Sci 18:523– 536, 1962 *(Chapter 8)*

Israel A, Galan F: Perimetria coloreada. Arch Oftal Buen-Air 46:211– 217, 1971 *(Chapter 6)*

Israel A, Verriest G: Comparison in the central visual field of normal and amblyopic eyes of the increment thresholds for lights of short and long wavelengths. Mod Prob Ophthalmol 11:76– 81, 1972 *(Chapter 8)*

Israel A, Verriest G: Normal results of kinetic colour perimetry by means of the Goldmann perimeter. Doc Ophthalmol 14:435– 439, 1977 *(Chapter 6)*

Ivandic T: Sektorförmige tapetoretinale Degenerationen. Klin Mbl Augenh 160:98– 103, 1972 *(Chapter 8)*

Jaeger W: Systematische untersuchungen über "inkomplette" angeborene totale Farbenblindheit. (Eine "Zwischenform" zwischen angeborener totaler Farbenblindheit und Protanopie). Graefes Arch Ophthalmol 150:509– 528, 1950 *(Chapter 7)*

Jaeger W: Gibt es Kombinationsformen der verschiedenen Typen angeborener Farbensinnstörung? Graefes Arch Ophthalmol 151:229– 248, 1951 *(Chapter 7)*

Jaeger W: Typen der inkompletten Achromatopsie. Ber Dtsch Ophthalmol Ges 58:44– 47, 1953 *(Chapter 7)*

Jaeger W: Dominant vererbte Opticusatrophie (Unter besonderer Berücksichtigung der dabei vorhandenen Farbensinnstörung). Graefes Arch Ophthalmol 155:457–484, 1954 *(Chapter 8)*

Jaeger W: Tritoformen angeborener und erworbener Farbensinnstörungen. Farbe 4:197–215, 1955 *(Chapter 8)*

Jaeger W: Defective colour-vision caused by eye disease. Trans Ophthalmol Soc UK 76:477–489, 1956 *(Chapters 4 and 7)*

Jaeger W: Genetics of congenital deficiencies, in Jameson D, Hurvich LM: Handbook of Sensory Physiology, vol IV/4: Visual Psychophysics. Berlin, Springer-Verlag, 1972 *(Chapter 7)*

Jaeger W, Früh D, Lauer HJ: Types of acquired color deficiencies caused by autosomal-dominant infantile optic atrophy. Mod Prob Ophthalmol 11:145–147, 1972 *(Chapter 8)*

Jaeger W, Grützner P: Der Funktionsverfall bei progressiver tapetoretinale Degeneration (Choideremia). Ophthalmologica 143:305–311, 1962 *(Chapter 8)*

Jaeger W, Grützner P: Erworbene Farbensinnstorungen, in Sautter H (ed): Entwicklung und Fortschritt in der Augenheilkunde. Stuttgart, Enke, 1963, pp 591–614 *(Chapter 4)*

Jaeger W, Kroker K: Über das Verhalten der Protanopen und Deuteranopen bei grossen Rezflachen. Klin Mbl Augenh 121:445–449, 1952 *(Chapter 7)*

Jaeger W, Lauer HJ: Non-allelic compounds of protan and deutan deficiencies. Mod Prob Ophthalmol 17:121–130, 1976 *(Chapter 7)*

Jaeger W, Nover A: Störungen des Lichtsinns und Farbensinns bei Chorioretinitis centralis serosa. Graefes Arch Ophthalmol 152:111–120, 1951 *(Chapters 6 and 8)*

Jameson D: Theoretical issues of color vision, in Jameson D, Hurvich LM (eds): Visual Psychophysics. Berlin, Springer-Verlag, 1972, pp 381–412 *(Chapter 3)*

Jameson D, Hurvich LM: Some quantitative aspects of an opponent-colors theory. I. Chromatic responses and spectral saturation. J Opt Soc Am 45:546–552, 1955 *(Chapter 3)*

Jameson D, Hurvich LM: Theoretical analysis of anomalous trichromatic color vision. J Opt Soc Am 46:1075–1089, 1956 *(Chapter 7)*

Jameson D, Hurvich LM: Perceived color and its dependence on focal, surrounding, and preceding stimulus variables. J Opt Soc Am 49:890–898, 1959 *(Chapter 2)*

Jameson D, Hurvich LM: Color adaptation: sensitivity, contrast, after-images, in Jameson D, Hurvich LM (eds): Handbook of Sensory Physiology, vol VII/4, Visual Psychophysics. Berlin, Springer-Verlag, 1972 *(Chapter 2)*

Javal LE: Du strabisme dans ses applications à la physiologie de la vision. Thèse méd., Paris, Masson et Fils, 1868 *(Chapter 8)*

Javal LE: Du strabisme. Ann Oculist (Paris) 65:97–125, 66:197-221, 1871; 66:5-18, 66:113-117, 66:209-216, 1871 *(Chapter 8)*

Jayle GE, Ourgaud AG: La Vision Nocturne et ses Troubles. Paris, Masson & Cie, 1950, pp 705–713 *(Chapter 8)*

Jess A: Die Geschichte einer vergessenen retinotoxischen Substanz. Klin Mbl Augenh 152:649–654, 1968 *(Chapter 8)*

Joseph E, Berkmann H: Complications oculaires dues aux inhibiteurs de la monoamine-oxydase. Presse Med 73:1627–1629, 1965 *(Chapter 8)*

Judd DB: Facts of color-blindness. J Opt Soc Am 33:294–307, 1943 *(Chapters 4 and 7)*

Judd DB: Color perception of deuteranopic and protanopic observers. U.S. Dept of Commerce, Natl. Bureau of Standards Research Paper RP1922, J Res Natl Bur Stand 41:247–271, 1948 *(Chapter 7)*

Judd DB: Colorimetry and artificial daylight, in Technical Committee No. 7 Report of Secretariat United States Commission, International Commission on Illumination, Twelfth Session, Stockholm, 1951a, pp 1–60 *(Chapters 2 and 7)*

Judd DB: Basic correlates of the visual stimulus, in Stevens SS (ed): Handbook of Experimental Psychology. New York, John Wiley & Sons, 1951b *(Chapter 3)*

Judd DB: Relation between normal trichromatic vision and dichromatic vision representing a reduced form of normal vision. Acta Chromatica 1:89–92, 1964 *(Chapter 7)*

Judd DB, Plaza L, Farnsworth D: Tritanopia with abnormally heavy ocular pigmentation. J Opt Soc Am 40:835–841, 1950 *(Chapter 7)*

Judd DB, Wyszecki G: Color in Business, Science and Industry (ed 3). New York, John Wiley & Sons, 1975 *(Chapters 1 and 2)*

Just G: Zur Vererbung der Farbensinnstufe beim Menschen. Arch Mbl Augenh 96:406–418, 1925 *(Chapter 7)*

Kaiser PK: Luminance and brightness. Appl Opt 10:2768–2769, 1971 *(Chapter 3)*

Kaiser PK, Comerford JP, Bodinger DM: Saturation of spectral lights. J Opt Soc Am 66:818–826, 1976 *(Chapter 6)*

Kaiser PK, Herzberg PA, Boynton RM: Chromatic border distinctness and its relation to saturation. Vision Res 11:953–968, 1971 *(Chapters 2 and 3)*

Kaiser-Kupfer MI, Valle D, Del Valle IA: A specific enzyme defect in gyrate atrophy. Am J Ophthalmol 85:200–204, 1978 *(Chapter 8)*

Kalberer M: Ueber eine simulierte Farbensinnstörung

nach Schadel-Hirn-Verletsung. Klin Mbl Augenh 158:810–814, 1971a *(Chapter 5)*

Kalberer M: Zur Bedeutung von Farbensinnstörungen im Strassenverkehr. Ophthalmologica 163: 171–177, 1971b *(Chapter 9)*

Kalmus H: The familial distribution of congenital tritanopia with some remarks on some similar conditions. Ann Hum Genet 20:39–56, 1955 *(Chapter 7)*

Kalmus H: Distance and sequence of the loci for protan and deutan defects and for glucose-6-phosphate dehydrogenase deficiency. Nature 194:215, 1962 *(Chapter 7)*

Kalmus H, Luke I, Seedburgh D: Impairment of color vision in patients with ocular hypertension and glaucoma. Br J Ophthalmol 58:922–926, 1974 *(Chapter 8)*

Kapany NS, Peppers NA, Zweng HC, Flocks M: Retinal photocoagulation by lasers. Nature 199:146–149, 1963 *(Chapter 8)*

Karrantinos D: Étude clinique des troubles du sens chromatique pendant la maturation de la cataracte et après l'extraction du cristallin. Arch Ophtalmol (Paris) 31:235–244, 1971 *(Chapter 8)*

Katavisto M: Pseudo-isochromatic plates and artificial light. Acta Ophthalmol 39:377–390, 1961 *(Chapter 5)*

Keeping JA, Searle CW: Optic neuritis following isoniazid therapy. Lancet 2:278, 1955 *(Chapter 8)*

Kelecom J: Les dyschromatopsies acquises: Considérations sur 84 observations personnelles. Arch Ophtalmol (Paris) 23:15–25, 1963 *(Chapter 8)*

Kelly KL, Judd DB: The ISCC-NBS Method of Designating Colors and a Dictionary of Color Names. Washington D.C., U.S. Department of Commerce, National Bureau of Standards, Circular 553, 1955 *(Chapter 2)*

Kennedy H, Smith RJS: Eye signs in craniopharyngioma. Br J Ophthalmol 59:689–695, 1975 *(Chapter 8)*

Kherumian R, Pickford RW: Hérédité et Fréquence des Dyschromatopsies. Paris, Vigot Frères, 1959 *(Chapter 7)*

King-Smith PE: Visual detection analysed in terms of luminance and chromatic signals. Nature 255:69–70, 1975 *(Chapters 3 and 6)*

King-Smith PE, Carden D: Luminance and opponent-color contributions to visual detection and adaptation and to temporal and spatial integration. J Opt Soc Am 66:709–717, 1976 *(Chapters 3 and 6)*

King-Smith PE, Kranda K, Wood ICJ: An acquired color defect of the opponent-color system. Invest Ophthalmol 15:584–587, 1976 *(Chapters 3, 4, 6, and 8)*

Kingslake R (ed): Applied Optics and Optical Engineering, vol I. New York, Academic Press, 1965 *(Chapter 1)*

Kinnear PR: Proposals for scoring and assessing the 100 hue test. Vision Res 10:423–433, 1970 *(Chapter 5)*

Kinnear PR, Aspinall PA, Lakowski R: The diabetic eye and colour vision. Trans Ophthalmol Soc UK 92:69–78, 1972 *(Chapter 8)*

Kinsbourne M, Warrington EK: Observations on colour agnosia. J Neurol Neurosurg Psychiatr 27:296–299, 1964 *(Chapter 8)*

Kirkham TH, Ffytche TJ, Saunders MD: Placoid pigment epitheliopathy with retinal vasculitis and papillitis. Br J Ophthalmol 56:875–900, 1972 *(Chapter 8)*

Kitahara K, Ichikawa H: An approach to equalizing the energy and the number of photons of chromatic lights of the Tübingen perimeter. Acta Soc Ophthalmol Jpn 79:59–66, 1975 *(Chapter 6)*

Kittel V, Cornelius C: Sehnervenschädigung durch Chloramphenicol. Klin Mbl Augenh 155:83–87, 1969 *(Chapter 8)*

Kjer P: Infantile optic atrophy with dominant mode of inheritance. Acta Ophthalmol Suppl 54:1–146, 1959 *(Chapter 8)*

Klein S, Dressel H: Untersuchungen über den Farbsinn und die Dunkel adaptation bei Patienten mit chronischen Lebererkrankungen. Kongressber VII Kongr Ges Augenarzte DDR, 238, 1970 *(Chapter 8)*

Klien B, Krill AE: Fundus flavimaculatus; Clinical, functional and histopathological observations. Am J Ophthalmol 64:3–23, 1967 *(Chapter 8)*

Knight CL, Hoyt WF, Wilson CB: Syndrome of incipient prechiasmal optic nerve compression. Arch Ophthalmol 87:1–11, 1972 *(Chapter 8)*

Knowles A, Dartnall HJA: The photobiology of vision, in Davson H (ed): The Eye, vol IIB. New York, Academic Press, 1977, pp 321–533 *(Chapter 3)*

Kobrick JL: Effects of hypoxia and acetazolamide on colour sensitivity zones in the visual field. J Appl Physiol 28:741–747, 1970 *(Chapter 8)*

Köhler U: Farbsinnstörungen schielamblyoper. Klin Mbl Augenh 147:230–234, 1965 *(Chapter 8)*

Köhler U: Erworbene Farbsinnstörungen bei Erkrankungen des Sehnerven und der Makula mit dem Farbfleckverfahren nach Trendelenburg. Klin Mbl Augenh 152:578–584, 1968 *(Chapter 8)*

Kojima K, Matsubara H: Colour Vision Test Plates for the Infants. Tokyo, the Handaya Co., 1957 *(Chapter 5)*

Kok-van Alphen CC: A family with the dominant infantile form of optical atrophy. Acta Ophthalmol 38:675–685, 1960 *(Chapter 8)*

Kok-van Alphen CC: Four families with the dominant infantile form of optic nerve atrophy. Acta Ophthalmol 48:905–916, 1970 *(Chapter 8)*

Kok-van Alphen CC, Hagedoorn A: Peripheral melanoblastoma of choroid. Am J Ophthalmol 49:1406–1408, 1960 *(Chapter 8)*

Kolb H: Electro-oculogram findings in patients treated with antimalarial drugs. Br J Ophthalmol 49:573–590, 1965 *(Chapter 8)*

Koliopoulos JX: Acquired colour vision deficiency in open angle glaucoma. Proceedings 2nd International Glaucoma Congress, Miami, 1978 *(Chapter 8)*

Koliopoulos J, Chatzis P, Papgeoriou A: Acquired disturbances of color perception in vascular disease of the retina. Trans 5th Panhellen Ophthalmol Congr 238–254, 1971 *(Chapter 8)*

Koliopoulos J, Mangouritsas N, Andreanos D: Color vision disturbances in patients with chronic simple glaucoma. Bull Hell Ophthalmol Soc 43:99–109, 1975 *(Chapter 8)*

Koliopoulos J, Palimeris G: On acquired colour vision disturbances during treatment with ethambutol and indomethacin. Mod Prob Ophthalmol 11: 178–184, 1972 *(Chapter 8)*

Koliopoulos J, Theodosiasdis G: Retinal detachment and acquired colour vision disturbance. Mod Prob Ophthalmol 11:117–121, 1972 *(Chapter 8)*

Köllner H: Ueber das Gesichtsfeld bei der Typischen Pigmentdegeneration der Netzhaut. Z Augenheilkd 16:128–145, 1906 *(Chapter 8)*

Köllner H: Untersuchungen uber die Farbenstörung bei Netzhautablösung. Z Augenheilkd 17: 234–258, 1907a *(Chapter 8)*

Köllner H: Ueber den Einfluss der Refraktionsanomalien auf die Farbenwahrnehmung, besonders auf die Beurteilung spektraler Gleichungen. Z Augenheilkd 18:430–441, 1907b *(Chapter 8)*

Köllner H: Erwerbene Violettblindheit (Tritanopie) und ihre Verhalten gegenüber spectralen Mischungsgleichungen. Sinnesphysiol 42:281–296, 1908 *(Chapter 8)*

Köllner H: Die Störungen des Farbensinnes, Ihre Klinische Bedeutung und Ihre Diagnose. Berlin, Karger, 1912 *(Chapters 4, 6, and 8)*

Köllner H: Die Abweichungen des Farbensinnes (mit Nächtragen ab 1924 von Engelking E), in Behte A, et al: Handbuch der Normalen und Pathologischen Physiologie. Berlin, Springer-Verlag, 1929 *(Chapter 8)*

König A: Ueber Blaublindheit. Sitz Akad Wiss (Berlin) 718–731, 1897 *(Chapters 7 and 8)*

König A, Dieterici C: Die Grundempfindungen und ihre Intensitäts-Vertheilung im Spectrum. Sitz Akad Wiss (Berlin) 805–829, 1886 *(Chapters 3 and 7)*

König A, Dieterici C: Die Grundempfindungen in normalen und anomalen Farben Systemen und ihre Intensitäts-Verteilung im Spectrum. Z Psychol Physiol Sinnesorg 4:241–347, 1893 *(Chapters 3 and 7)*

Kranenburg EW: Craterlike holes in the optic disc and central serous retinopathy. Thesis, Amsterdam, 1959 *(Chapter 8)*

Kravkov SV: The influence of sound upon the light and colour sensibility of the eye. Acta Ophthalmol (Kbh) 14:348–360, 1936 *(Chapter 8)*

Krebs W, Hubbe J: Farbsinnuntersuchungen bei der Schielamblyopie. Albrecht Graefes Arch Klin Exp Ophthalmol 178:20–29, 1969 *(Chapter 8)*

von Kries J: Über Farbensysteme. Z Psychol Physiol Sinnesorg 13:241–324, 1897 *(Chapters 4, 6, and 7)*

von Kries J: Über die anomalen trichromatischen Farbensysteme. Z Sinnesphysiol 19:63–69, 1899 *(Chapter 7)*

von Kries J: Über einen Fall von einseitiger angeborener Deuteranomalie (Grunschwäche). Z Sinnesphysiol 50:137–152, 1919 *(Chapter 7)*

von Kries J: Normal and anomalous color systems, in von Helmholtz HLF: Treatise on Physiological Optics (ed 3), vol II [Trans by JPC Southall]. Rochester, Optical Society of America, 1924, pp 395–425 *(Chapter 7)*

Krill AE: The retinal disease of rubella. Arch Ophthalmol 77:445–449, 1967 *(Chapter 8)*

Krill AE: The electroretinogram in congenital color vision defects, in François J (ed): The Clinical Value of Electroretinography, ISCERG Symposium, Ghent. Basel, Karger, 1968 *(Chapter 7)*

Krill AE: Hereditary Retinal and Choroidal Diseases, vol I. Hagerstown, Harper & Row, 1972, pp 309–339 *(Chapter 4)*

Krill AE: Congenital color vision defects, in Krill AE, Archer DB (eds): Krill's Hereditary Retinal and Choroidal Diseases, vol II. Clinical Characteristics. Hagerstown, Harper & Row, 1977, pp 355–390 *(Chapter 7)*

Krill AE, Beutler E: The red-light absolute threshold in heterozygote protan carriers; possible genetic implications. Invest Ophthalmol 3:107–118, 1964 *(Chapter 7)*

Krill AE, Beutler E: Red-light thresholds in heterozygote carriers of protanopia: Genetic implications. Science 149:186–188, 1965 *(Chapter 7)*

Krill AE, Deutman AF: The various categories of juvenile macular degeneration. Trans Am Ophthalmol Soc 70:220–242, 1972a *(Chapter 8)*

Krill AE, Deutmann AF: Acute retinal pigment epitheliitis. Am J Ophthalmol 74:193–205, 1972b *(Chapter 8)*

Krill AE, Deutmann AF, Fishman M: The cone degenerations. Doc Ophthalmol 1:1–80, 1973 *(Chapter 8)*

Krill AE, Fishman GA: Acquired color vision defects. Trans Am Acad Ophthalmol Otolaryngol 75:1095–1112, 1971 *(Chapter 8)*

Krill AE, Klien BA, Archer DB: Precursors of angioid streaks. Am J Ophthalmol 76:875–879, 1973 *(Chapter 8)*

Krill AE, Lee GB: The electroretinogram in albinos and carriers of the ocular albino trait. Arch Ophthalmol 69:32–38, 1963 *(Chapter 8)*

Krill AE, Morse PA, Potts AM, Klien BA: Hereditary

vitelliruptive macular degeneration. Am J Ophthalmol 61:1405–1415, 1966 *(Chapter 8)*

Krill AE, Schneiderman A: A hue discrimination defect in so-called normal carriers of color vision defects. Invest Ophthalmol 3:445–450, 1964 *(Chapter 7)*

Krill AE, Schneiderman A: Retinal function studies, including the electroretinogram in an atypical monochromat, in: Clinical Electroretinography, Supplement to Vision Research, Proceedings of the Third International Symposium, October, 1964. Oxford, Pergamon Press, 1966, pp 351–361 *(Chapter 7)*

Krill AE, Smith VC, Pokorny J: Similarities between congenital tritan defects and dominant optic nerve atrophy: Coincidence or identity? J Opt Soc Am 60:1132–1139, 1970 *(Chapters 7 and 8)*

Krill AE, Smith VC, Pokorny J: Further studies supporting the identity of congenital tritanopia and hereditary dominant optic atrophy. Invest Ophthalmol 10:457–465, 1971 *(Chapters 7 and 8)*

Krümmel H: Klinische Beobachtungen zur Entwicklung der gefassahnlichen Streifen am Augenhintergrund. Graefes Arch Ophthalmol 151:167–178, 1950 *(Chapter 8)*

Kurata K: Study on the color discrimination of subjects with acquired anomalous color vision. Acta Soc Ophthalmol Jpn 69:1998–2006, 1965 *(Chapter 8)*

Kurata K: Study of color discrimination of subjects with acquired anomalous color vision. II. Color confusion in glaucomatous eyes due to fluctuations of brightness. Acta Soc Ophthalmol Jpn 71:223–229, 1967a *(Chapter 8)*

Kurata K: Study on the color discrimination of subjects with acquired anomalous color vision. III. Acta Soc Ophthalmol Jpn 71:336–344, 1967b *(Chapter 8)*

Kurstjens JH: Choroideremia and gyrate atrophy of the choroid and retina. Thesis, The Hague, W. Junk, 1965 *(Chapter 8)*

Kuwabara T: Retinal recovery from exposure to light. Am J Ophthalmol 70:187–198, 1970 *(Chapter 8)*

Kuwabara T, Gorn RA: Retinal damage by visible light. Arch Ophthalmol 79:69–78, 1968 *(Chapter 8)*

Laatikainen L, Erkkila H: Clinical and fluorescein angiographic findings of acute multifocal central subretinal inflammation. Acta Ophthalmol (Kbh) 51:645–655, 1973 *(Chapter 8)*

Lagerlöf O: Quantitative assessment of acquired colour vision deficiency in maculopathy. Mod Prob Ophthalmol 19:276–280, 1978 *(Chapter 5)*

Lakowski R: Age and color vision. Adv Sci 15:231–236, 1958 *(Chapters 5 and 8)*

Lakowski R: Is the deterioration of colour discrimination with age due to lens or retinal changes? Farbe 11:69–86, 1962 *(Chapters 4 and 8)*

Lakowski R: Testing of colour vision in prospective printers apprentices and the problems this presents in selection. Br J Physiol Opt 22:10–32, 1965a *(Chapters 5 and 7)*

Lakowski R: Colorimetric and photometric data for the 10th edition of the Ishihara plates. Br J Physiol Opt 22:195–207, 1965b *(Chapters 5 and 7)*

Lakowski R: A critical evaluation of colour vision tests. Br J Physiol Opt 23:186–209, 1966 *(Chapters 5 and 7)*

Lakowski R: The Farnsworth-Munsell 100 Hue test. Ophthalmol Optician 81:862–872, 1968a *(Chapter 5)*

Lakowski R: Colour-matching ability: Can it be measured? J Soc Dyers Colourists 84:3–9, 1968b *(Chapter 5)*

Lakowski R: Theory and practice of colour vision testing. A review. Part 1. Br J Industr Med 26:173–189, 1969a *(Chapter 5)*

Lakowski R: Theory and practice of colour vision testing. A review. Part 2. Br J Industr Med 26:265–288, 1969b *(Chapter 7)*

Lakowski R: Calibration, validation, and population norms for the Pickford-Nicolson anomaloscope. Br J Physiol Opt 26:166–182, 1971 *(Chapters 5, 6, and 7)*

Lakowski R: The Pickford-Nicolson anomaloscope as a test for acquired dyschromatopsias. Mod Prob Ophthalmol 11:25–33, 1972 *(Chapters 5, 6, and 8)*

Lakowski R: Effects of age on the 100-hue scores of red-green deficient subjects. Mod Prob Ophthalmol 13:124–129, 1974 *(Chapter 4)*

Lakowski R: Objective analysis of the Stilling tables. Mod Prob Ophthalmol 17:166–171, 1976 *(Chapters 5 and 7)*

Lakowski R, Aspinall PA, Kinnear PR: Association between colour vision losses and diabetes mellitus. Ophthalmol Res 4:145–159, 1973 *(Chapter 8)*

Lakowski R, Begg I: Acquired dyschromatopsia in carotid occlusive disease and chronic central retinal vein obstruction: A comparison with diabetic retinopathy, in Cant JS (ed): Vision and Circulation, 3rd William McKenzie Symposium. London, Kimpton, 1976 *(Chapter 8)*

Lakowski R, Bryett J, Drance SM: A study of color vision in ocular hypertensives. Can J Ophthalmol 7:86–95, 1972 *(Chapter 8)*

Lakowski R, Creighton D: Foveal chromatic dark adaptation functions of red-green deficient subjects. Mod Prob Ophthalmol 17:41–45, 1976 *(Chapter 6)*

Lakowski R, Davenport M: The effect of

chloroquine-therapy on 100 hue test results. Preprints of the Second Scott Symposium on Colour, Edinburgh, 1968 *(Chapter 8)*

Lakowski R, Drance SM: Acquired dyschromatopsias: The earliest functional losses in glaucoma. Doc Ophthalmol Proc Ser 19:159–165, 1979 *(Chapter 8)*

Lakowski R, Drance SM, Goldthwaite D: Chromatic extrafoveal dark adaptation function in normal and glaucomatous eyes. Mod Prob Ophthalmol 17:304–310, 1976 *(Chapter 6)*

Lakowski R, Oliver K: Effect of pupil diameter on color vision test performance. Mod Prob Ophthalmol 13:307–311, 1974 *(Chapter 8)*

Lakowski R, Oliver K: Diamond grading by the colour deficient. Mod Prob Ophthalmol 19:97–100, 1978 *(Chapter 9)*

Lakowski R, Wright WD, Oliver K: High luminance chromatic Goldmann perimeter. Doc Ophthalmol Proc Ser 14:441–443, 1977 *(Chapter 6)*

Lanthony P: Etude de la saturation au cours des dyschromatopsies acquises au moyen de l'album de Munsell. Ann Oculist (Paris) 207:741–751, 1974a *(Chapter 5)*

Lanthony P: Le Test Panel D-15 Désaturé Selon Farnsworth-Munsell. Paris, Luneau, 1974b *(Chapter 5)*

Lanthony P: New Color Test de Lanthony Selon Munsell. Paris, Luneau, 1975a *(Chapter 5)*

Lanthony P: Applications cliniques du New Color Test. Bull Soc Ophtalmol Fr 75:1055, 1975b *(Chapter 5)*

Lanthony P: Quantitative study of the neutral zone in color vision defectiveness. Mod Prob Ophthalmol 19:122–124, 1978a *(Chapter 5)*

Lanthony, P: The desaturated Panel D-15. Doc Ophthalmol 46:185-189, 1978b *(Chapter 5)*

Lanthony P: The New Color Test. Doc Ophthalmol 46:191-199, 1978c *(Chapter 5)*

Lanthony P, Dubois-Poulsen A: Le Farnsworth-15 désaturé. Bull Soc Ophtalmol Fr 73:861, 1973 *(Chapter 5)*

Larimer J, Krantz DH, Cicerone CM: Opponent-process additivity—I. Red/green equilibria. Vision Res 14:1127–1140, 1974 *(Chapter 3)*

Larimer J, Krantz DH, Cicerone CM: Opponent process additivity—II. Yellow/blue equilibria and nonlinear models. Vision Res 15:723–731, 1975 *(Chapter 3)*

Laroche J: Modifications de la vision des couleurs chez l'homme sous l'action de certaines substances médicamenteuses. Ann Oculist 200: 275–286, 1967 *(Chapter 8)*

Laroche J, Laroche C: Action de quelques antibiotiques sur la vision des couleurs. Ann Pharmacol Fr 28:333–341, 1970 *(Chapter 8)*

Laroche J, Laroche C: Modification de la vision des couleurs sous l'action de quelques antibiotiques et vitamines. Therapie 25:671–685, 1971 *(Chapter 8)*

Laroche J, Laroche C: Modifications de la vision des couleurs apportées par l'usage, à dose thérapeutique normale, de quelques médicaments. Ann Pharmacol Fr 30:433–444, 1972 *(Chapter 8)*

Larsen H: Demonstration microscopischer Präparate von einem monochromatischen Auge. Klin Mbl Augenh 67:301–302, 1921 *(Chapter 7)*

Larsen H: Hemeralopie und Akyanopsie (Blaublindheit). Acta Ophthalmol (Kbh) 1:177–184, 1923 *(Chapter 8)*

Lasagni F, De Molfetta V, Miglior M: Il comportamento del senso cromatico e del campo visivo centrale nella ambliopia strabica. Atti Soc Oftalmol Ital 22:192–195, 1964 *(Chapter 8)*

Laszczyk WA, Szubinska H: Colour discrimination prognosis of amblyopia treatment in squinting children. Klin Oczna 43:1147–1150, 1973 *(Chapter 8)*

Laties A, Enoch JM: An analysis of retinal receptor orientation. I. Angular relationship of neighboring photoreceptors. Invest Ophthalmol 10: 69–77, 1971 *(Chapter 6)*

Latte B, Filippi G, Siniscalco M: Genetica della cecità per I colori (Daltonismo): Un secondo caso di ricombinzaione tra I loci deutan e protan. Atti Assoc Genet Ital 10:282–294, 1965 *(Chapter 7)*

La Vail MM: Rod outer segment disc shedding in rat retina: Relationship to cyclic lighting. Science 194:1071–1074, 1976 *(Chapter 8)*

Leber T: Ueber hereditare und congenital-angelegte Schnervenleiden. Graefes Arch Ophthalmol 17:249–291, 1871a *(Chapter 8)*

Leber T: Über anormale Formen der Retinitis pigmentosa. Graefes Arch Ophthalmol 17:325–332, 1871b *(Chapter 8)*

Leber T: Ueber die Theorie der Farbenblindheit und über die Art und Weise, wie gewisse, der Untersuchung von Farbenblinden entnommene Einwärde gegen die Young-Helmholtz'sche Theorie sich mit derselben vereinigen lassen. Klin Mbl Augenh 11:467–473, 1873 *(Chapter 7)*

Le Grand Y: Light, Colour and Vision (ed 2). London, Chapman & Hall, 1968 *(Chapter 2)*

Le Grand Y: About the photopigments of colour vision. Mod Prob Ophthalmol 11:185–192, 1972 *(Chapter 8)*

Legras M, Coscas G: Edematous maculopathies and colour sense. Mod Prob Ophthalmol 11:111–116, 1972 *(Chapters 5 and 8)*

Legros J: Contribution a l'étude chromatique dans le glaucome chronique. Thesis, University of Bordeaux, 1966 *(Chapter 8)*

Letourneau JE, Zeidel NS: The effect of sound on the perception of color. Am J Opt Arch Opt 48:133–137, 1971 *(Chapter 8)*

Levinson JM: The birth control pill and its ophthalmologic side effects. Delaware Med J 41:118–120, 1969 *(Chapter 8)*

Levy NS, Toskes PP: Fundus albipunctatus and vitamin A deficiency. Am J Ophthalmol 78:926–929, 1975 *(Chapter 8)*

Lewis RA, Lee GB, Martonyi CL, Barnett JM, Falls HF: Familial Foveal retinoschisis. Arch Ophthalmol 95:1190–1196, 1977 *(Chapter 8)*

Lewis SD, Mandelbaum J: Achromatopsia. Arch Ophthalmol 30:225, 1943 *(Chapter 7)*

Liebman PA: Microspectrophotometry of photoreceptors, in Dartnall HJA (ed): Photochemistry of Vision. Berlin, Springer-Verlag, 1972, pp 481–528 *(Chapter 3)*

Lindstein J, Fraccaro M, Polani PE, Hamerton JL, Sanger R, Race RR: Evidence that the Xg blood-group genes are on the short arm of the X chromosome. Nature 197:648–649, 1963 *(Chapter 7)*

Linksz A: An Essay on Color Vision and Clinical Color-Vision Tests. New York, Grune & Stratton, 1964 *(Chapter 5)*

Linksz A: The Farnsworth Panel D-15 test. Am J Ophthalmol 62:27–37, 1966 *(Chapter 5)*

Litwin MS, Glew DH: The biological effects of laser radiation. JAMA 187:842–847, 1964 *(Chapter 8)*

Liuzzi L, Bartoli F: La perimetria con luce laser, in Grignolo A, Tagliasco V, Zingirian M: L'esame del campo visivo. Roma, Soc Optal Ital, 1975, pp 223–238 *(Chapter 6)*

Lizzi FL, Coleman DJ, Driller J, Franzen LA, Jakabiec FA: Experimental ultrasonically induced lesions in the retina, choroid and sclera. Invest Ophthalmol Vis Sci 17:350–360, 1978 *(Chapter 8)*

Llermitte F, Chain F, Aron D, Leblanc M, Souty O: Les troubles de la vision des couleurs dans les lésions postérieures de cerveau. Rev Neurol 121:5–29, 1969 *(Chapter 8)*

Lobanova NV, Speranskaya NI: The spectral sensitivity of the retinal elements of anomalous trichromats. Biophysics 6:71–78, 1961 *(Chapter 7)*

London ID: Research on sensory interaction in the Soviet Union. Psychol Bull 51:531–568, 1954 *(Chapter 8)*

Lort M: An account of a remarkable imperfection of sight in a letter from J. Scott to the Rev. Mr. Whisson of Trinity College, Cambridge. Philos Trans R Soc Lond 68:611–614, 1778 *(Chapter 4)*

Lövsund P, Nilsson SE, Öberg PA: The influence of low-frequency magnetic fields on visual perception. Proceedings of the 2nd World Congress of Ergophthalmology, 1978 (in press) *(Chapter 8)*

Ludvigh E, McCarthy EF: Absorption of visible light by refractive media of the human eye. Arch Ophthalmol 20:37-51, 1938 *(Chapter 3)*

Lukaszewicz B, Wysocki J, Wozmy J: Disturbances of colour discrimination in the visual field of patients with acute hepatitis. Klin Oczna 42:617–620, 1972 *(Chapter 8)*

Lumbroso BD, Proto F: Le anomalie del senso cromatico nei soggetti ambliopici con fissazione eccentrica. Boll Oculist 42:699–718, 1963 *(Chapter 8)*

Lumbroso BD, Proto F: Le anomalie del senso cromatico nei soggetti ambliopici con fissazione eccentrica. Cit Zentralbl Ophthalmol 93:182, 1965 *(Chapter 8)*

Lundsgaard R: Leber's disease. A genealogic, genetic and clinical study of 101 cases of retrobulbar optic neuritis in 20 Danish families. Acta Ophthalmol Suppl 21:1–306, 1944 *(Chapter 8)*

Luria SM: Color-name as a function of stimulus-intensity and duration. Am J Psychol 80:14–27, 1967 *(Chapter 7)*

Lyle WM: Drugs and disease conditions which may affect color vision. J Am Optom Assoc 45:47–60, 173–182, 1974 *(Chapter 8)*

Lyon MF: Gene action in the X-chromosome of the mouse (Mus musculus L). Nature 190:372–373, 1961 *(Chapter 7)*

MacAdam DL: Visual sensitivities to color differences in daylight. J Opt Soc Am 32:247–274, 1942 *(Chapter 6)*

MacAdam DL: Uniform color scales. J Opt Soc Am 64:1691–1702, 1974 *(Chapter 2)*

MacAdam DL: Colorimetric data for samples of OSA uniform color scales. J Opt Soc Am 68:121–130, 1978 *(Chapter 2)*

MacCulloch C: Choroideremia: A clinical and pathological review. Trans Am Ophthalmol Soc 57:142–191, 1969 *(Chapter 8)*

MacLeod DIA: Visual sensitivity. Annu Rev Psychol 29:613–645, 1978 *(Chapter 3)*

MacLeod DIA, Hayhoe MM: Three pigments in normal and anomalous color vision. J Opt Soc Am 64:92–96, 1974 *(Chapter 7)*

MacLeod DIA, Lennie P: A unilateral defect resembling deuteranopia. Mod Prob Ophthalmol 13:130–134, 1974 *(Chapter 7)*

MacLeod DIA, Lennie P: Red-green blindness confined to one eye. Vision Res 16:691–702, 1976 *(Chapter 8)*

Mailáth L: The AN-59 anomaloscope in the research of acquired colour vision deficiencies. Mod Prob Ophthalmol 11:34–39, 1972 *(Chapter 5)*

Maione M, Carta F: Statistical investigations on the achromatic isopters in normal individuals. Atti Fond G Ronchi 22:635–638, 1967 *(Chapter 6)*

Maione M, Carta F: The visibility of the Goldmann's perimeter coloured targets in the ageing and in retrobulbar neuritis. Mod Prob Ophthalmol 11:72–75, 1972 *(Chapter 6)*

Maione M, Carta F, Barberini E, Scoccianti L. Achromatic isopters and coloured backgound in some acquired colour vision deficiencies. Mod Prob Ophthalmol 17:86–93, 1976 *(Chapter 8)*

Majima A: Studies on Farnsworth dichotomous test Panel D-15 for congenital color vision defectives. Acta Soc Ophthalmol Jpn 73:224–232, 1969 *(Chapter 5)*

Mandelbaum J, Mintz EU: The sensitivities of the color receptors as measured by dark adaptation. Am J Ophthalmol 24:1241–1254, 1941 *(Chapter 6)*

Marks WB, Dobelle WH, MacNichol EF: Visual pigments of single primate cones. Science 143: 1181–1183, 1964 *(Chapter 3)*

Marmion VJ: The results of a comparison between the hundred hue test and static colour perimetry. Doc Ophthalmol Proc Ser 14:473–474, 1977 *(Chapter 6)*

Marmion VJ: The colour vision deficiency in open angle glaucoma. Mod Prob Ophthalmol 19: 305–307, 1978 *(Chapter 8)*

Marmor MF, Byers B: Pattern dystrophy of the pigment epithelium. Am J Ophthalmol 84:32–44, 1977 *(Chapter 8)*

Marré E, Marré M: The influence of the three color vision mechanisms on the spectral sensitivity of the fovea. Mod Prob Ophthalmol 11:219–223, 1972 *(Chapter 6)*

Marré M: Eine quantitative Analyse erworbener Farbensehstörungen. Thesis, Magdeburg, 1969 *(Chapters 6 and 8)*

Marré M: Die darstellung von drei Farbseh-Mechanismen bei erwobenen Farbenssehstörungen. Colour 69, Göttingen, Musterschmidt Verlag, 1970, pp 97–104 *(Chapters 6 and 8)*

Marré M: Clinical examination of the three color vision mechanisms in acquired color vision defects. Mod Prob Ophthalmol 11:224–227, 1972a *(Chapter 6)*

Marré M: Das Farbensehen bei Schielamblyopie. Klin Mbl Augenh 160:734–735, 1972b *(Chapter 8)*

Marré M: The investigation of acquired colour vision deficiencies, in Colour 73, London, A Hilger 1973, pp 99–135 *(Chapters 4, 6, and 8)*

Marré M: The role of congenital colour deficiencies in the practice of traffic (analysis of 2000 traffic accidents). Regional IRGCVD Symposium, Dresden, September 5–6, 1978 *(Chapter 9)*

Marré M, Marré E: Colour vision in squint amblyopia. Mod Prob Ophthalmol 19:308–313, 1978a *(Chapter 8)*

Marré M, Marré E: Different types of acquired colour vision deficiencies on the base of CVM patterns in dependence upon the fixation mode of the diseased eye. Mod Prob Ophthalmol 19: 248–252, 1978b *(Chapter 8)*

Marré M, Marré E: Das Farbensehen bei Schielamblyopie. Graefes Arch 1979 (in press) *(Chapter 8)*

Marré M, Nemetz U, Neubauer O: Colour vision and the "pill." Mod Prob Ophthalmol 13:345–348, 1974 *(Chapter 8)*

Marriott FHC: The two-colour threshold technique of Stiles, in Davson H (ed): The Eye, vol 2A. New York, Academic Press, 1976 *(Chapter 6)*

Marshall J, Ansell PL: Membranous inclusions in the retinal pigment epithelium: Phagosomes and myeloid bodies. J Anat (Lond) 110:91–104, 1971 *(Chapter 8)*

Martin M, Menezo JC, Lopez H: Alterations in colour vision in patients operated on for retinal detachment. Arch Soc Zsp Oftalmol 32:793–808, 1972 *(Chapter 8)*

Massof RW, Finkelstein D: Rod sensitivity relative to cone sensitivity in retinitis pigmentosa. Invest Ophthalmol & Vis Sci 18:263–272, 1979 *(Chapters 6 and 8)*

Massof RW, Finkelstein D, Starr SJ, Kenyon KR, Fleischman JA, Maumenee IH: Bilateral symmetry of vision disorders in typical retinitis pigmentosa. Brit J Ophthalmol 63:90–96, 1979 *(Chapter 8)*

Massof RW, Guth SL: Central and peripheral achromatic points in protanopes and deuteranopes. Mod Prob Ophthalmol 17:75–78, 1976 *(Chapter 7)*

Matsuo H, Ohta Y, Endo N, Kato H: Studies on the new central scotometric plates. Acta Soc Ophthalmol Jpn 76:1336–1343, 1972 *(Chapter 6)*

Matsuo K, Okabe S, Ueno H, Takabatake M, Maeta K: Studies on acquired anomalous colour vision in patients with subacute myelo-opticoneuropathy. Folia Ophthalmol Jpn 22:158–166, 1971 *(Chapter 8)*

De Mattiello MLF, Gonella A: Size and desaturation scales in test for diagnosis of color vision deficiencies. Mod Prob Ophthalmol 17:185–192, 1976 *(Chapter 8)*

Mauthner L: Uber Farbige Schatten, Farbenproben und Erworbene Erythrochloropsie (Blaugeblindheit). Wien Med Wochenschr 31:38–39, 1881 *(Chapter 8)*

McCree KJ: Small-field tritanopia and the effects of voluntary fixation. Opt Acta 7:317–323, 1960 *(Chapter 6)*

McCullogh C, Marliss EB: Gyrate atrophy of the choroid and retina with hyperornithinemia. Am J Ophthalmol 80:1047–1057, 1975 *(Chapter 8)*

McKeon WM, Wright WD: The characteristics of protanomalous vision. Proc Physiol Soc Lond 52:464–479, 1940 *(Chapter 7)*

McNaught EI, Rennie A, McClure E, Chisholm IA: Pattern of visual damage after acute angle closure glaucoma. Trans Ophthalmol Soc UK 94:406–415, 1974 *(Chapter 8)*

Meadows JC: Disturbed perception of colours associated with localized cerebral lesions. Brain 97:615–632, 1974 *(Chapters 4 and 8)*

Meier-Ruge W: Zur Aethiologie von Retinaekrankungen durch Arzneimittel. Verh Dtsch Ges Pathol 56:338– 340, 1972a *(Chapter 8)*

Meier-Ruge W: Toxicology: Review and prospect. Proc Eur Soc Drug Toxicity 14:133– 145, 1972b *(Chapter 8)*

Meier-Ruge W: Zur Aethiologie und Pathogenese toxischer Arzneimittelnebenwirkungen and der Netzhaut. Klin Mbl Augenh 163:155– 172, 1973 *(Chapter 8)*

Merin S, Auerbach E: The central and peripheral retina in macular degeneration. Arch Ophthalmol 84:710– 718, 1970 *(Chapter 8)*

Metge P, Jayle GE, Vola J, Fonta D, Aurran Y: Corrélations anatomiques et fonctionelles dans les chorio-rétinopathies séreuses centrales en période d'activité. Bull Mem Soc Ophtalmol Fr 85:255– 266, 1972 *(Chapter 8)*

Meyer F: Über einen atypische Fall von Retinitis punctat albescens. Klin Mbl Augenh 107:526– 528, 1941 *(Chapter 8)*

Meyer-Schwickerath G: Light coagulation (tr. S.M. Drance, London, Kimpton, 1960) Klin Mbl Augenh Suppl 33:1– 114, 1959 *(Chapter 8)*

Miglior M, Spinelli D, Castellani F: La rétinopathie pigmentaire péricentrale. Ann Oculist 202: 447– 456, 1969 *(Chapter 8)*

Miller SA: Multifocal Best's vitelliform dystrophy. Arch Ophthalmol 95:984– 990, 1977 *(Chapter 8)*

Miller SA, Bresnick GH, Chandra SR: Choroidal neovascular membrane in Best's vitelliform macular dystrophy. Am J Ophthalmol 82:252– 255, 1976 *(Chapter 8)*

Miller SS: Psychophysical estimates of visual pigment densities in red-green dichromats. J Physiol ′(London) 223:89– 107, 1972 *(Chapter 7)*

Mitchell DE, Rushton WAH: Visual pigments in dichromats. Vision Res 11:1033– 1044, 1971a *(Chapter 7)*

Mitchell DE, Rushton WAH: The red/green pigments of normal vision. Vision Res 11:1045– 1056, 1971b *(Chapters 6 and 7)*

Möller– Ladekarl P: Über Farbendistinktion bei Normalen und Farbenblinden. Acta Ophthalmol Suppl 3:1– 128, 1934 *(Chapter 7)*

Moon P: The Scientific Basis of Illuminating Engineering. New York, Dover, 1961 *(Chapter 1)*

Moore T: Systemic action of vitamin A. Exp Eye Res 3:305– 315, 1964 *(Chapter 8)*

Morax V: Sur quelques symptomes de début du sarcome de la choroide. Bull Soc Ophtalmol (Paris):552– 556, 1925 *(Chapter 8)*

Moreland JD: The effect of inert ocular pigments on anomaloscope matches and its reduction. Mod Prob Ophthalmol 11:12– 18, 1972 *(Chapters 5 and 7)*

Moreland JD: Temporal variation in anomaloscope equations. Mod Prob Ophthalmol 19:167– 172, 1978 *(Chapter 5)*

Moreland JD, Cruz A: Colour perception with the peripheral retina. Opt Acta 6:117– 151, 1959 *(Chapter 2)*

Moreland JD, Kerr J: Optimization of stimuli for trit-anomaloscopy. Mod Prob Ophthalmol 19:162– 166, 1978 *(Chapters 5 and 7)*

Moreland JD, Maione M, Carta F, Barberini E, Scoccianti L, Lettieri S: The clinical assessment of chromatic mechanisms of the retinal periphery. Doc Ophthalmol Proc Ser 14:413– 421, 1977 *(Chapter 6)*

Moreland JD, Young WB: A new anomaloscope employing interference filters. Mod Prob Ophthalmol 13:47– 55, 1974 *(Chapters 5 and 7)*

Morgan TH: Sex-limited inheritance in Drosophila. Science 32:120– 122, 1910 *(Chapter 7)*

Müller GE: Darstellung and Erklärung der verschiedenen Typen der Farbenblindheit, etc. Göttingen, Vandenhoed & Ruprecht, 1924 *(Chapter 4)*

Münchow W: Verkehrsophthalmologische Untersuchungen. II. Epidemiologische Untersuchungen zum Problem Strassenverkehrunfall und Sehorgan. Klin Mbl Augenh 151:566– 575, 1967 *(Chapter 9)*

Mustonen E, Varonen T: Congenital pit of the optic nerve head associated with serous detachment of the macula. Acta Ophthalmol (Kbh) 50:689– 698, 1972 *(Chapter 8)*

Nagel WA: Die Diagnose der anomalen trichromatischen Systeme. Klin Mbl Augenh 42:366– 370, 1904 *(Chapter 7)*

Nagel WA: Dichromatische Fovea, trichomatische Peripherie. Z Psychol Physiol Sinnesorg 39: 93– 101, 1905 *(Chapter 7)*

Nagel WA: Neue Erfahrungen über das Farbensehen der Dichromaten auf grossem Felde. Z Sinnesphysiol 41:319– 337, 1907a *(Chapter 7)*

Nagel WA: Zwei Apparate für die augenärztliche Funktionsprüfung: Adaptometer und kleines Spektralphotometer (Anomaloskop). Atschr Augenh 17:201, 1907b *(Chapter 5)*

Nathan J, Henry GH, Cole BL: Recognition of colored road traffic light signals by normal and color-vision-defective observers. J Opt Soc Am 54:1041– 1045, 1964 *(Chapter 9)*

Naumann G, Lüllwitz W: Allgemeine Pathologie der Makulaerkrankungen. Proc Dtsch Ophthalmol Ges 73:44– 45, 1975 *(Chapter 8)*

Nelson JH: Anomalous trichromatism and its relation to normal trichromatism. Physiol Soc Lond 50:661– 702, 1938 *(Chapter 7)*

Neubauer O: Farbsinnstörungen bei langerer Verwendung von Oculationshemmern. Klin Mbl Augenheilkd 162:803– 806, 1973 *(Chapter 8)*

Neubauer O, Dittrich H: Farbsehstörungen und

Lebererkrankungen. Kongressber VII Kongr Ges Augenarzte DDR, 229–237, 1970 *(Chapter 8)*

Neubauer O, Harrer S: Tritan defects found by using Velhagens pseudoisochromatic plates 24th edition. Mod Prob Ophthalmol 17:172–174, 1976 *(Chapter 5)*

Neubauer O, Harrer S, Marré M, Verriest G: Colour vision deficiencies in road traffic. Mod Prob Ophthalmol 19:77–81, 1978 *(Chapter 9)*

Neuhann T, Kalmus H, Jaeger W: Ophthalmological findings in the tritans, described by Wright and Kalmus. Mod Prob Ophthalmol 17:135–142, 1976 *(Chapter 7)*

Nickerson D: History of the Munsell Color System, Company, and Foundation. Color Res Appl 1:7–10, 69–77, 121–130, 1976 *(Chapter 2)*

Nickerson D: History of the OSA Committee on Uniform Color Scales. Opt News, 8–17, Winter 1977 *(Chapter 2)*

Nikoskelainen E: Symptoms, signs and early course of optic neuritis. Acta Ophthalmol 53:254–271, 1975 *(Chapter 8)*

Nikoskelainen E, Sogg RL, Rosenthal AR, Fribert TR, Dorfman LJ: The early phase in Leber hereditary optic atrophy. Arch Ophthalmol 95:969–978, 1977 *(Chapter 8)*

Nimeroff I: Deuteranopic convergence point. J Opt Soc Am 60:966–969, 1970 *(Chapter 7)*

Noble KG: Central areolar choroidal dystrophy. Am J Ophthalmol 84:310–318, 1977 *(Chapter 8)*

Noble KG, Carr RE, Siegel IM: Familial foveal retinoschisis associated with a rod-cone dystrophy. Am J Ophthalmol 85:551–557, 1978 *(Chapter 8)*

Noell WK, Walker VS, Kang BS, Berman S: Retinal damage by light in rats. Invest Ophthalmol 5:450–473, 1966 *(Chapter 8)*

Nolte W: Bestimmung achromatischer Schnellen für verschiedene Spektrallichter. Thesis, Tübingen, 1962 *(Chapter 6)*

Norren DV, Vos JJ: Spectral transmission of the human ocular media. Vision Res 14:1237–1244, 1974 *(Chapter 3)*

Notting JGA, Pinckers AJLG: Dominant cystoid macular dystrophy. Am J Ophthalmol 83:234–241, 1977 *(Chapter 8)*

Notting JGA, Pinckers AJLG: Diagnostic problems in Stargardt's macular dystrophy and fundus flavimaculatus. Doc Ophthalmol Proc Ser 17:307–312, 1978 *(Chapter 8)*

Ohta Y: The improvement of 40 hue test. Acta Soc Ophthalmol Jpn 70:798–801, 1966 *(Chapter 5)*

Ohta Y: Studies on the acquired anomalous color vision. Color sense anomalies in patients with subacute myelo-optico-neuropathy (SMON). Acta Soc Ophthalmol Jpn 72:1551–1560, 1968 *(Chapter 8)*

Ohta Y: One case of slight hemeralopia with tritanopia. Acta Chromat 2:42–47, 1969 *(Chapter 8)*

Ohta Y: Studies on the acquired anomalous colour vision. Colour vision anomalies in patients with lesions of the retina, optic chiasma, and post-occipital centre. Color 69, Gottingen, Musterschmidt Verlag, 1970, pp 88–96 *(Chapters 4 and 8)*

Ohta Y: Central scotometric plates (Umazume-Ohta) utilizing color confusion resulting from an acquired anomalous colour vision. Mod Prob Ophthalmol 11:40–48, 1972 *(Chapters 6 and 8)*

Ohta Y, Kato H: Colour perception changes with age. Test results by P-N anomaloscope. Mod Prob Ophthalmol 17:345–352, 1976 *(Chapter 8)*

Ohta Y, Kogure S, Izutsu Y, Miyamota T, Nagai I: Clinical analysis on colour vision deficiencies with the City University test. Mod Prob Ophthalmol 19:126–130, 1978 *(Chapter 5)*

Ohta Y, Kogure S, Yamaguchi T: Clinical experience with the Lovibond colour vision analyser. Mod Prob Ophthalmol 19:145–159, 1978 *(Chapter 5)*

Ohtani K, Ohta Y, Kogure S, Seki R: Screening of congenital colour defects by Farnsworth's tritan plate. Jpn J Clin Ophthalmol 28:1217–1222, 1975 *(Chapter 5)*

Okuma T, Masuda H, Kawada C, Shinjo U: Ishihara-Okuma's new test plates for colour defectives. Acta Soc Ophthalmol Jpn 77:1359–1365, 1973 *(Chapter 5)*

Oppel O: Vergleichende Farbsinnuntersuchungen zwischen normalen und schielamblyopen Augen. Albrecht Graefes Arch Ophthalmol 165:387–391, 1963 *(Chapter 8)*

Oppel O, Kranke D: Vergleichende Untersuchungen über das Verhalten der Dunkeladaptation normaler und schielamblyoper Augen. Albrecht Graefes Arch Ophthalmol 159:486–501, 1958 *(Chapter 8)*

Orou F, Sideroff G, Schabel F: Frequenzuntersuchung von Opticus-Erkrankungen im Rahmen der MyambutolR-Behandlung. Klin Mbl Augenh 161:601–603, 1972 *(Chapter 8)*

Ourgaud AG, Etienne R: L'exploration Fonctionnelle de L'oeil Glaucomateux. Paris, Masson & Cie, 1961 *(Chapters 4 and 8)*

Ourgaud A, Vola J, Cornu L: Intérêt des examens de la vision des couleurs sous éclairment élevé. Bull Soc Ophtalmol Fr 73:209–215, 1973 *(Chapter 8)*

Ourgaud A, Vola J, Jayle G, Daud C: A study on the influence of the illumination level of pupillary diameter on chromatic discrimination in glaucomatous patients. Mod Prob Ophthalmol 11:141–144, 1972 *(Chapter 8)*

Oxbury JM, Oxbury SM, Humphrey NK: Varieties of colour anomia. Brain 92:847–860, 1969 *(Chapter 8)*

Padmos P, van Norren D, Faijer JW: Blue cone function in a family with an inherited tritan defect, tested with electroretinography and psychophysics. Invest Ophthalmol & Visual Science 17:436–441, 1978 *(Chapter 7)*

Pajor R, Medgyaszay A: Color sensitivity of eyes with squint amblyopia. Am J Ophthalmol 59:493–494, 1965 *(Chapter 8)*

Palimeris G, Koliopoulos J, Velissaropoulos P: Ocular side effects of indomethacin. Ophthalmologica 164:339–353, 1972 *(Chapter 8)*

Pallis CA: Impaired identification of faces and places with agnosia for colour. J Neurol Neurosurg Psychiat 18:218–224, 1955 *(Chapter 8)*

Palmer CAL: Toxic amblyopia due to pheniprazine. Br Med J 1:38, 1963 *(Chapter 8)*

Palmer CAL: Toxic amblyopia from Ibuprofen. Br Med J 2:765, 1972 *(Chapter 8)*

Pameyer JK, Waardenburg PJ, Henkes HE: Choroideremia. Br J Ophthalmol 44:724–738, 1960 *(Chapter 8)*

Parinaud H: Le Strabisme et son Traitement. Paris, Doin, 1899 *(Chapter 8)*

Paulson HM: Colour vision testing, in Pierce JR, Levene JR (eds): Visual Science. Bloomington, Indiana University Press, 1968, pp 164–176 *(Chapter 5)*

Paulson HM: Comparison of color vision tests used by the Armed Forces, in Committee on Vision, Division of Behavioral Sciences, National Research Council: Color Vision, Symposium conducted at the Spring Meeting, 1971. Washington, D.C. National Academy of Sciences, 1973 *(Chapter 5)*

Paulson HM: Congenital color deficiencies. Mod Prob Ophthalmol 13:363–368, 1974 *(Chapter 5)*

Pearlman JT, Kamin DF, Kopelow SM, Saxton J: Pigmented paravenous, retinochoroidal atrophy. Am J Ophthalmol 80:630–635, 1975 *(Chapter 8)*

Pearlman JT, Owen WG, Brounley DW, Sheppard JJ: Cone dystrophy with dominant inheritance. Am J Ophthalmol 77:293–303, 1974 *(Chapters 6 and 8)*

Pearlman JT, Saxton J, Hoffman G: Unilateral retinitis pigmentosa sine pigmento. Br J Ophthalmol 60:354–360, 1976 *(Chapter 8)*

Pears MA, Pickering GW: Changes in the fundus oculi after hemorrhage. Q J Med 29:153–178, 1960 *(Chapter 8)*

Perdriel G: Le test de Farnsworth 100 Hue. Ann Oculist 195:120–130, 1962 *(Chapter 5)*

Perdriel G: A propos d'un nouveau cas de nevrite optique due au disulfiram. Bull Soc Ophtalmol Fr 66:159–165, 1966 *(Chapter 8)*

Perdriel G: Explorations fonctionnelles et électrophysiologiques au cours des dégénérescences maculaires séniles. Arch Ophtalmol (Paris) 29:877–880, 1970 *(Chapter 8)*

Perdriel G: Oeil et vitamines. Med Trop 32:376–383, 1972 *(Chapter 8)*

Perdriel G, Chevaleraud J, Delpuget J, Bourgeois H: L'exploration fonctionnelle dans les dégénérescences maculaires séniles. Bull Mem Soc Fr Ophtalmol 82:458–463, 1970 *(Chapter 8)*

Perdriel G, Lanthony Pl, Chevaleraud J: Pathologie du sens chromatique. Diagnostic pratique. Intérêt clinique et applications socio-professionelles. Bull Soc Ophtalmol Fr (rapport annuel, numéro spécial) pp 1–280, 1975 *(Chapter 5 and 8)*

Perez LJ: General blood pressure and pressure of the ophthalmic artery and its relation to evaluation of chronic glaucoma. Arch Soc Oftalmol Hisp-Am 23:966–969, 1963 *(Chapter 8)*

Peters GA: A colour-blindness test for use in vocational guidance. Personnel Guidance J 34:572–575, 1956 *(Chapter 5)*

Piantanida TP: Phenotypic diagnosis of protan and deutan heterozygosity. Invest Ophthalmol 10:979–984, 1971 *(Chapter 7)*

Piantanida TP: A replacement model of X-linked recessive colour vision defects. Ann Hum Genet 37:393–404, 1974 *(Chapter 7)*

Piantanida TP: A portable filter anomaloscope. Opt Eng 15:325–327, 1976 *(Chapter 5)*

Piantanida TP, Bruch TA, Latch M, Varner FD: Detection of quantum flux modulation by single photopigments in human observers. Vision Res 16:1029–1034, 1976 *(Chapters 3 and 7)*

Piantanida TP, Sperling HG: Isolation of a third chromatic mechanism in the protanomalous observer. Vision Res 13:2033–2047, 1973a *(Chapter 7)*

Piantanida TP, Sperling HG: Isolation of a third chromatic mechanism in the deuteranomalous observer. Vision Res 13:2049–2058, 1973b *(Chapter 7)*

Pickard R: The photochromatic interval in glaucoma and cavernous atrophy. Br J Ophthalmol 22:391–400, 1938 *(Chapter 8)*

Pickford RW: Three pedigrees for colour blindness. Nature 165:82, 1950 *(Chapter 7)*

Pickford RW: Individual Differences in Colour Vision. London, Routledge and Kegan Paul, 1951 *(Chapter 7)*

Pickford RW: Weak and anomalous colour vision in industry and the need for adequate tests. Occup Psychol 29:182–192, 1955 *(Chapter 9)*

Pickford RW: A practical anomaloscope for testing colour vision and colour blindness. Br J Physiol Opt 14:2–26, 1957 *(Chapters 5 and 7)*

Pickford RW: A review of some problems of colour vision and colour blindness. Adv Sci 15:104–117, 1958a *(Chapter 7)*

Pickford RW: Colour vision of three albinos. Nature 181:361–362, 1958b *(Chapter 8)*

Pickford RW: Compound hemizygotes for red-green colour vision defects. Vision Res 2:245–252, 1962 *(Chapter 7)*

Pickford RW: Variability and consistency in the manifestation of red-green colour vision defects. Vision Res 7:65–77, 1967 *(Chapter 7)*

Pickford RW: Colour vision research in Scotland in the first part of the 20th century. Second Scottish Symposium on Colour, Scottish Section of the Colour Group and the Visual Laboratory, Department of Psychology, University of Edinburgh, September 1968 *(Chapter 5)*

Pickford RW: A case of hysterical colour blindness reconsidered. Mod Prob Ophthalmol 11:165–167, 1972 *(Chapter 5)*

Pickford RW, Lakowski R: The Pickford-Nicolson anomalsocope. Br J Physiol Opt 17:131–150, 1960 *(Chapters 5 and 7)*

Pickford RW, Taylor WOG: Colour vision of two albinos. Br J Ophthalmol 52:640–641, 1968 *(Chapter 8)*

Pierce WOD: The Selection of the Colour Workers. London, Sir Isaac Pitman and Sons, 1934 *(Chapters 5 and 8)*

Pinckers A: Le syndrome de Wagner: Électrooculographie et sens chromatique. Ann Oculist (Paris) 203:569–578, 1970a *(Chapter 8)*

Pinckers A: Portée du 100 Hue test de Farnsworth-Munsell dans les examens follow-up. Ann Oculist (Paris) 203:811–820, 1970b *(Chapter 8)*

Pinckers A: Verworven stoornissen van de kleurzin. Eeen Klinisch anderzock. Thesis, Nijmegen, 1971a *(Chapter 8)*

Pinckers A: La maladie de Stargardt. Ann Oculist 204:1331–1346, 1971b *(Chapter 8)*

Pinckers A: Combined Panel D-15 and 100 hue recording. Ophthalmologica 163:232–234, 1971c *(Chapter 5)*

Pinckers A: Achromatopsie congénitale. Ann Oculist (Paris) 205:821–834, 1972a *(Chapters 4 and 7)*

Pinckers A: An analysis of colour vision in 314 patients. Mod Prob Ophthalmol 11:94–97, 1972b *(Chapter 8)*

Pinckers A: The Farnsworth tritan plate. Ophthalmologica 164:137–142, 1972c *(Chapter 5)*

Pinckers A: Dyschromatopsies acquises d'axe bleu-jaune. Ann Oculist (Paris) 208:659–666, 1975a *(Chapters 4, 5, and 8)*

Pinckers A: Toxische neuropathie van de nervus opticus. Medikon 4:18–27, 1975b *(Chapter 8)*

Pinckers A: The Umazume-Ohta test. Mod Prob Ophthalmol 17:175–178, 1976a *(Chapters 6 and 8)*

Pinckers A: An analysis of acquired disorders of color vision with a view to distinction from hereditary ocular anomalies. Ophthalmologica 173:221–226, 1976b *(Chapter 4)*

Pinckers A: Lanthony's New Color Test—Part I. Ophthalmologica 177:284–291, 1978a *(Chapter 5)*

Pinckers A: Lanthony's New Color Test—Part II. Clinical evaluation. Ophthalmologica 177:311–316, 1978b *(Chapter 5)*

Pinckers A: Lanthony's New Color Test—Part III. The neutral zone. Int Ophthalmol (in press, b) *(Chapter 5)*

Pinckers A, Baron J: Clinical evalution of Lanthony's New Color Test and Desaturated 15-hue. Mod Prob Ophthalmol 19:144, 1978 *(Chapter 5)*

Pinckers A, Bolmers D: Neuronal ceroid lipofuscinosis. Ann Oculist 207:523–529, 1974 *(Chapter 8)*

Pinckers A, Deutman AF: Peripheral cone disease. Ophthalmologica 174:145–150, 1977 *(Chapter 8)*

Pinckers A, Deutman AF, Notting JGA: Retinal functions in dominant cystoid macular dystrophy (D.C.M.D.). Acta Ophthalmol (Kbh) 54:579–590, 1976 *(Chapter 8)*

Pinckers A, Hopee RLE: Neuronal ceroid lipofuscinosis in the Netherlands. (Vth International Congress of Neurogen and Neuro-Ophthal) Doc Ophthalmol Proc Ser 377–382, 1978 *(Chapter 8)*

Pinckers A, Jansen LMAA: Wagner's syndrome. Doc Ophthalmol 37:245–259, 1974 *(Chapter 8)*

Pinckers A, Nabbe B, Bogaard PVD: Le test 15-hue désaturé de Lanthony. Ann Oculist 209:731–738, 1976 *(Chapters 5 and 8)*

Pinckers A, Nabbe B, Bogaard PVD: Lanthony's New Color Test. Mod Prob Ophtalmol 19:125, 1978 *(Chapter 5)*

Pinckers A, Notting JGA, Lion F: Dégénérescence maculaire cystoide dominante. J Fr Ophthalmol 1:107–110, 1978 *(Chapter 8)*

Pinckers A, Thijssen JM: Absent cone function. Doc Ophthalmol Proc Ser (XIth ISCERG Symposium) 107–111, 1974 *(Chapter 8)*

Pinckers A, Van Der Eerden J: La polyarthrite thumatismale et les antipaludéens de synthèse. Ann Oculist 206:305–309, 1973 *(Chapter 8)*

Pitt FHG: Characteristics of Dichromatic Vision. London, Medical Research Council, 1935, pp 5–58 *(Chapter 7)*

Pitt FHG: Monochromatism. Nature 154:466–468, 1944 *(Chapter 7)*

Pokorny J, Moreland JD, Smith VC: Photopigments in anomalous trichromats. J Opt Soc Am 65:1522–1524, 1975 *(Chapters 5 and 7)*

Pokorny J, Smith VC: Wavelength discrimination in the presence of added chromatic fields. J Opt Soc Am 60:562–569, 1970 *(Chapter 7)*

Pokorny J, Smith VC: Luminosity and CFF in deuteranopes and protanopes. J Opt Soc Am 62:111–117, 1972 *(Chapter 7)*

Pokorny J, Smith VC: Effect of field size on red-green color mixture equations. J Opt Soc Am 66:705–708, 1976 *(Chapters 2, 6, and 7)*

Pokorny J, Smith VC: Evaluation of single-pigment shift model of anomalous trichromacy. J Opt Soc Am 67:1196–1209, 1977 *(Chapters 6 and 7)*

Pokorny J, Smith VC, Ernest JT: Macular color defects: Specialized psychophysical testing in acquired and hereditary chorioretinal diseases, in Sokol S (ed): Electrophysiology and Psychophysics: Their Use in Ophthalmic Diagnosis. International Ophthalmology Clinics. Boston, Little, Brown & Company (in press) *(Chapters 4 and 6)*

Pokorny J, Smith VC, Johnston PB: Photoreceptor misalignment accompanying a fibrous scar. Arch Ophthalmol 97:867–869, 1979 *(Chapters 4 and 6)*

Pokorny J, Smith VC, Katz I: Derivation of the photopigment absorption spectra in anomalous trichromats. J Opt Soc Am 63:232–237, 1973 *(Chapters 6 and 7)*

Pokorny J, Smith VC, Lund D: Technical characteristics of "color-test glasses." Mod Prob Ophthalmol 19:110–112, 1978 *(Chapter 5)*

Pokorny J, Smith VC, Starr SJ: Variability of color mixture data—II. The effect of viewing field size on the unit coordinates. Vision Res 16:1095–1098, 1976 *(Chapters 3 and 7)*

Pokorny J, Smith VC, Swartley R: Threshold measurements of spectral sensitivity in a blue monocone monochromat. Invest Ophthalmol 9:807–813, 1970 *(Chapter 7)*

Pokorny J, Smith VC, Trimble J: A new technique for proper illumination for color vision tests. Am J Ophthalmol 83:429, 1977 *(Chapter 5)*

Post RH: Population differences in red and green color vision deficiency: A review, and a query on selection relaxation. Eugenics Q 9:131–146, 1962 *(Chapter 7)*

Potts AM, Johnson LV: Studies on the visual toxicity of methanol. Am J Ophthalmol 35:107–113, 1952 *(Chapter 8)*

Priest IG, Brickwedde FG: Minimum perceptible colorimetric purity as a function of dominant wavelength. J Res Natl Bur Stand 20:673–682, 1938 *(Chapter 6)*

Pugh Jr EN, Sigel C: Evaluation of the candidacy of the π-mechanisms of Stiles for color-matching fundamentals. Vision Res 18:317–330, 1978 *(Chapter 3)*

Purdy DM: The Bezold-Brucke phenomenon and contours for contrast hue. Am J Psychol 49:313–315, 1937 *(Chapter 2)*

Raudrant-Mathian C: Contribution a l'étude des verrucosités hyalines de la macula. Thesis, Lyon, 1972 *(Chapter 8)*

Rautian GN: A new anomaloscope and the classification of color vision forms. Visual Problems of Color, Vol II, NPL Symposium No 8. New York, Chemical Publishing Co. 1961, pp 121–130 *(Chapter 5)*

Lord Rayleigh: Experiments on colour. Nature 25:64–66, 1881 *(Chapters 5 and 7)*

Reddy V, Vijayalaxmi: Colour vision in vitamin A deficiency. Br Med J 1:81, 1977 *(Chapter 8)*

Reed JD: The effect of illumination in changing the stimuli in pseudoisochromatic plates. J Opt Soc Am 34:350, 1944 *(Chapter 5)*

Remky H: La rétinopathie de la dystrophy myotonique (Steinert). Bull Mem Soc Fr Ophtalmol 85:500–502, 1972 *(Chapter 8)*

Remky H, Kolbl I: Multiple vitelliforme Zysten. Klin Mbl Augenh 159:322–330, 1971 *(Chapter 8)*

Remky H, Rix J, Klier HF: Dominant-autosomale Makuladegeneration mit zystischen und vitelliforme Stadien. Klin Mbl Augenh 146:473–497, 1965 *(Chapter 8)*

Renard G, Morax PV: Névrite optique au cours des traitements antituberculeux. Ann Oculist (Paris) 210:53–61, 1977 *(Chapter 8)*

Rey-Kokott U: Ueber erworbene Farbensinnstörungen bei Glaukom. Thesis, University of Heidelberg, 1964 *(Chapter 8)*

Ricci A: Clinique et transmission génétique des différentes formes de dégénérescences vitréorétiniennes. Ophthalmologica 139:338–343, 1960 *(Chapter 8)*

Richards OW, Tack TO, Thomé C: Fluorescent lights for color vision testing. Am J Opt Arch Am Acad Optom 48:747–753, 1971 *(Chapter 5)*

Riddell WJB: The early stages of tobacco amblyopia. Glas Med J 75:268–275, 1936 *(Chapter 8)*

Riffenburgh RS, Shea JF: Lack of association between colour blindness and alcoholism. Eye Ear Nose Throat Mon 49:240–242, 1970 *(Chapter 8)*

Ripps H: Night blindness and the retinal mechanisms of visual adaptation. Ann R Col Surg Eng 58:222–232, 1976 *(Chapter 7)*

Ripps H, Weale RA: The physiology of vertebrate colour vision, in Giese AC (ed): Photophysiology, vol 5. New York, Academic Press, 1970, pp 127–168 *(Chapter 3)*

Ripps H, Weale RA: The visual stimulus, in Davson M (ed): The Eye, vol 2A. London, Academic Press, 1976, pp 43–49 *(Chapter 3)*

Robertson DM, Hollenhorst RW, Callahan JH: Ocular manifestations of digitalis toxicity. Arch Ophthalmol 76:640–645, 1966a *(Chapter 8)*

Robertson DM, Hollenhorst RW, Callahan JH: Receptor function in digitalis therapy. Arch Ophthalmol 76:852–857, 1966b *(Chapter 8)*

Rodieck RW: Ganglion cells: Receptive fields, in Rodieck RW: The Vertebrate Retina, Principles of Structure and Function. San Francisco, W.H. Freeman & Company, 1973, pp 559–645 *(Chapter 3)*

Røe O: Methanol poisoning. Acta Med Scand 126 Suppl 182:1–253, 1946 *(Chapter 8)*

Romanchuk KG, Pollak V, Schneider RJ: Retinal burn from a welding arc. Can J Ophthalmol 13:120–122, 1978 *(Chapter 8)*

Romeskie M: Chromatic opponent-response functions of anomalous trichromats. Vision Res 18:1521–1532, 1978 *(Chapter 7)*

Romeskie M, Yager D: Psychophysical measures and theoretical analysis of dichromatic opponent-response functions. Mod Prob Ophthalmol 19:212–217, 1978 *(Chapter 7)*

Rondont P, Tzavaras A, Garcin R: Sur un cas de prosopagnosie persistant depuis quinze ans. Rev Neurol 117:424–428, 1967 *(Chapter 8)*

Rönne H: Gesichtsfeldstudien über das Verhältnis zwischen der peripheren Sehscharfe und dem Farbensinn, speziell die Bedeutung derselben fur die Prognose der Sehnervenatrophie. Klin Mbl Augenh 49:154–184, 1911 *(Chapters 6 and 8)*

Rosmanit J: Anleitung zur Feststellung der Farbentüchtigkeit. Leipzig, Deuticke, 1914 *(Chapter 7)*

Roth A: Le sens chromatique dans l'amblyopie fonctionelle. Doc Ophthalmol 24:113–200, 1968 *(Chapter 8)*

Roth A, Renaud JC, Vienot JC: Prototype of a direct observation anomaloscope. A preliminary note. Mod Prob Ophthalmol 13:31–35, 1974 *(Chapter 5)*

Rothstein TB, Shapiro MW, Sacks JG, Weis MJ: Dyschromatopsia with hepatic cirrhosis: Relation to serum B12 and folic acid. Am J Ophthalmol 75:859–895, 1973 *(Chapter 8)*

Rowland LS: Daylight fluorescent lamp as a source of illumination in tests of color perception with pseudo-isochromatic plates. Project 130, Report 1. Randolph Field, School of Aviation Medicine, 1943 *(Chapter 5)*

Rubin ML: Spectral hue loci of normal and anomalous trichromats. Am J Ophthalmol 52:166–172, 1961 *(Chapter 7)*

Ruddock KH: The effects of age upon colour vision. I. Response in the receptoral system of the human eye. Vision Res 5:37–45, 1965a *(Chapter 8)*

Ruddock KH: The effect of age upon colour vision. II. Changes with age in light transmission of the ocular media. Vision Res 5:47–58, 1965b *(Chapters 3 and 8)*

Ruddock KH: Parafoveal colour vision responses of four dichromats. Vision Res 11:143–156, 1971 *(Chapter 7)*

Ruddock KH, Naghshineh S: Mechanisms of red-green anomalous trichromacy: Hypothesis and analysis. Mod Prob Ophthalmol 13:210–214, 1974 *(Chapter 7)*

Rushton WAH: Pigments in anomalous colour vision. Br Med Bull 26:179–181, 1970 *(Chapter 7)*

Rushton WAH: Visual pigments in man, in Dartnall HJA (ed): Handbook of Sensory Physiology, vol VII/1. Berlin, Springer-Verlag, 1972, pp 364–394 *(Chapter 3)*

Rushton WAH, Baker HD: Red/green sensitivity in normal vision. Vision Res 4:75–85, 1964 *(Chapter 6)*

Rushton WAH, Powell DS, White KD: Pigments in anomalous trichromats. Vision Res 13:2017–2031, 1973 *(Chapter 7)*

Sachensenreger R, Nothaas E: Eine Analyse von 4011 Verkehrsunfällen aus augenarztlicher Sicht. Dtsch Gesundheitswesen 16:868–872, 1961 *(Chapter 9)*

Saebo J: Atrophia gyrata chorioideae et retinae. Br J Ophthalmol 32:824–847, 1948 *(Chapter 8)*

Safir A, Hyams L: Distribution of cone orientations as an explanation of the Stiles-Crawford effect. J Opt Soc Am 59:757–765, 1969 *(Chapter 6)*

Safir A, Kulikowski AA, Kuo MI, Edgerton F: An extraordinarily eccentric Stiles-Crawford effect. Presented at the Association for Research in Vision and Ophthalmology, Sarasota, Fl., April 25, 1972 *(Chapter 6)*

Said FS, Weale RA: The variation with age of the spectral transmissivity of the living human crystalline lens. Gerontologia 3:213–231, 1959 *(Chapter 3)*

Sakuma Y: Studies on color vision anomalies in subjects with alcoholism. Ann Ophthalmol 5:1277–1292, 1973 *(Chapter 8)*

Salvia J: Four tests of color vision: A study of diagnostic accuracy with the mentally retarded. Am J Ment Defic 74:421–427, 1969 *(Chapter 5)*

Salvia J, Ysseldyke J: An analysis of the reliability and validity of the Ishihara color plates with mentally retarded males. Percept Mot Skills 33:243–246, 1971a *(Chapter 5)*

Salvia JA, Ysseldyke JE: Validity and reliability of the red-green AO H-R-R pseudoisochromatic plates with mentally retarded children. Percept Mot Skills 33:1071–1074, 1971b *(Chapter 5)*

Sandberg MA, Berson EL: Blue and green cone mechanisms in retinitis pigmentosa. Invest Ophthalmol 16:149–157, 1977 *(Chapter 6)*

Sandberg MA, Rosen JB, Berson EL: Cone and rod function in vitamin A deficiency with chronic alcoholism and in retinitis pigmentosa. Am J Ophthalmol 84:658–665, 1977 *(Chapter 6)*

Saraux H: Les anomalies du sens coloré comme étiologie de certaines amblyopies relatives de l'enfant. Bull Mem Soc Fr Ophtalmol 76:115–121, 1963 *(Chapter 8)*

Saraux H: Névrite optique par amoproxan. Ann Oculist 204:71, 1971 *(Chapter 8)*

Saraux H: Les affections oculaires induites par les médications générales. Ann Oculist 208:257–266, 1975 *(Chapter 8)*

Saraux H, Bechetoille A, Offret H, Nou B: La dégénérescence choriorétinienne paraveineuse pigmentée. Ann Oculist 207:643–649, 1974 *(Chapter 8)*

Saraux H, Biais B: Névrite optique par le disulfirame. Ann Oculist 203:769–774, 1970 *(Chapter 8)*

Saraux H, Labet R, Biais B: Aspects actuels de la névrite optique de l'ethylique. Ann Oculist 199:943–954, 1966 *(Chapter 8)*

Sassoon HF, Wise JB, Watson JJ: Alcoholism and colour-vision: Are there familial links? Lancet 2:367–368, 1970 *(Chapter 8)*

Scharf PT: Filters, in Kingslake R (ed): Applied Optics and Optical Engineering, vol 1. New York, Academic Press, 1965, pp 111–125 *(Chapter 1)*

Scheibner H, Boynton RM: Residual red-green discrimination in dichromats. J Opt Soc Am 58:1151–1158, 1968 *(Chapter 7)*

Scheibner H, Thranberend C: Colour vision in a case of neuritis retrobulbaris. Mod Prob Ophthalmol 13:339–344, 1974 *(Chapters 6 and 8)*

von Schelling H: A method for calculating the effect of filters on color vision. J Opt Soc Am 40:419–423, 1950 *(Chapter 7)*

Schepens CL: Inflammation of the 'ora serrata' region and its sequelae. Bull Mem Soc Fr Ophtalmol 63:113–125, 1950 *(Chapter 8)*

Schiffer H-P, Busse P: Beitrag zum Krankheitsbild des Fundus Flavimaculatus mit Makuladegeneration. Klin Mbl Augenh 166:365–368, 1975 *(Chapter 8)*

Schmidt I: Ueber manifeste Heterozygotie bei Konduktorinnen für Farbensinnstörungen. Klin Mbl Augenh 92:456–467, 1934 *(Chapter 7)*

Schmidt I: Ueber "Ermüdbarkeit" des Farbensystems bei normalen Trichromaten. Klin Mbl Augenh 94:433–442, 1935 *(Chapter 7)*

Schmidt I: Ueber zwei Falle von angeborener Blaügelbsehstörung. Klin Mbl Augenh 109:635–652, 1942 *(Chapter 7)*

Schmidt I: Effect of illumination in testing color vision with pseudoisochromatic plates. J Opt Soc Am 42:951–955, 1952 *(Chapter 5)*

Schmidt I: A sign of manifest heterozygosity in carriers of color deficiency. Am J Optom 32:404–408, 1955a *(Chapter 7)*

Schmidt I: Some problems related to testing color vision with the Nagel anomaloscope. J Opt Soc Am 45:514–522, 1955b *(Chapters 5 and 7)*

Schmidt I: On congenital tritanomaly. Vision Res 10:717–743, 1970 *(Chapter 7)*

Schmidt I: Visual aids for correction of red-green color deficiencies. Can J Optom 38:38–47, 1976 *(Chapter 9)*

Schober H: Die physiologischen Anforderungen an die Augen des Kraftfahrers und Hilfsmittel zur Verbesserung des Sehens. Z Verkehrssichereit 9:9–34, 1963 *(Chapter 9)*

Schuurmans RP, Van Lith GHM, Oosterhuis JA: Photocoagulation and the electroretinogram. Doc Ophtamol Proc Ser 15:297–301, 1978 *(Chapter 8)*

Scotti G, Spinnler H: Colour imperception in unilateral hemisphere damaged patients. J Neurol Neurosurg Psychiat 33:22–28, 1970 *(Chapter 8)*

Scuderi G, Recupero SM, Valvo A: Acute posterior multifocal placoid pigment epitheliopathy. Ann Ophthalmol 9:189–194, 1977 *(Chapter 8)*

Sebestyén J, Gálfi I: Retinal function in Niemann-Pick lipidosis. Ophthalmologica 157:349–356, 1969 *(Chapter 8)*

Seebeck A: Ueber den bei manchen Personen vorkommenden Mangel an Farbesinn. Pogg Ann Phys Chem 42:177–233, 1837 *(Chapter 7)*

Seki R: The experience in the xanthopsia by latent icterus. Ganka-Rinsyo-Iho 48:316–318, 1954 *(Chapter 8)*

van Senus AHC: Leber's disease in the Netherlands. Doc Ophthalmol 17:1–162, 1963 *(Chapter 8)*

Siegel IM, Bruno B: Determination of fixation in the dark-adapted eye by means of fundus photography. Arch Ophthalmol 72:670–671, 1964 *(Chapters 4 and 7)*

Siegel IM, Graham CH, Ripps H, Hsia Y: Analysis of photopic and scotopic function in an incomplete achromat. J Opt Soc Am 56:699–704, 1966 *(Chapter 7)*

Siegel IM, Smith BF: Acquired cone dysfunction. Arch Ophthalmol 77:8–13, 1967 *(Chapter 8)*

Simon R: Über typische Violettblindheit bei Retinitis Albuminurica. Zentralbl Prakt Augenheilkd 18:132–139, 1894 *(Chapter 8)*

Singerman LJ, Berkow JW, Patz A: Dominant slowly progressive macular dystrophy. Am J Ophthalmol 83:680–693, 1977 *(Chapter 8)*

Siniscalco M, Filippi G, Latte B: Recombination between protan and deutan genes; Data on their relative positions in respect to the G6PD locus. Nature 204:1062–1064, 1964 *(Chapter 7)*

Sjögren H: Dystrophia reticularis laminae pigmentosae retinae. Arch Ophthalmol (Kbh) 28:279–295, 1950 *(Chapter 8)*

Sliney DH: The development of laser safety criteria—biological considerations, in Wolbarsht ML (ed): Laser Applications in Medicine or Biology. New York, Plenum Press, 1971, pp 163–238 *(Chapter 8)*

Sloan LL: The use of pseudo-isochromatic charts in detecting central scotomas due to lesions in the conducting pathways. Am J Ophthalmol 25:1352–1356, 1942 *(Chapter 8)*

Sloan LL: A quantitative test for measuring degree of red-green color deficiency. Am J Ophthalmol 27:941–949, 1944 *(Chapter 5)*

Sloan LL: An improved screening test for red-green color deficiency composed of available pseudo-isochromatic plates. J Opt Soc Am 35:761–766, 1945 *(Chapter 5)*

Sloan LL: A case of atypical achromatopsia. Am J Ophthalmol 29:290–294, 1946 *(Chapter 7)*

Sloan LL: Congenital achromatopsia: A report of 19 cases. J Opt Soc Am 44:117–128, 1954 *(Chapters 5, 6, and 7)*

Sloan LL: The photopic retinal receptors of the typical achromat. Am J Ophthalmol 46:81–86, 1958 *(Chapters 6 and 7)*

Sloan LL: Evaluation of the Tokyo Medical College color vision test. Am J Ophthalmol 52:650–659, 1961 *(Chapter 5)*

Sloan LL, Feiock K: Selective impairment of cone function, perimetric techniques for its detection. Mod Prob Ophthalmol 11:50–62, 1972 *(Chapter 6)*

Sloan LL, Gilger AP: Visual effects of tridione. Am J Ophthalmol 30:1387–1405, 1947 *(Chapter 8)*

Sloan LL, Habel A: Tests for color deficiency based on the pseudoisochromatic principle. Arch Ophthalmol 55:229–239, 1956 *(Chapter 5)*

Sloan LL, Newhall SM: Comparison of cases of atypical and typical achromatopsia. Am J Ophthalmol 25:945–961, 1942 *(Chapter 7)*

Sloan LL, Wollach L: A case of unilateral deuteranopia. J Opt Soc Am 38:502–509, 1948 *(Chapter 7)*

Smith BF, Ripps HA, Goodman G: Retinitis punctata albescens; A functional and diagnostic evalation. Arch Ophthalmol 61:93–101, 1959 *(Chapter 8)*

Smith DP: Derivation of wavelength discrimination from colour-naming data. Vision Res 11:739–742, 1971 *(Chapter 6)*

Smith DP: The assessment of acquired dyschromatopsia and clinical investigation of the acquired tritan defect in dominantly inherited juvenile atrophy. Am J Optom Arch Am Acad Optom 49:574–588, 1972a *(Chapter 8)*

Smith DP: Diagnostic criteria in dominantly inherited juvenile optic atrophy. A report of three new families. Am J Optom Arch Am Acad Optom 49:183–200, 1972b *(Chapter 8)*

Smith DP: The clinical detection of optic atrophy with special reference to the temporal form in dominantly inherited juvenile optic atrophy. Aust J Optom 55:195–205, 1972c *(Chapter 8)*

Smith DP: Color naming and hue discrimination in congenital tritanopia and tritanomaly. Vision Res 13:209–218, 1973 *(Chapters 6 and 7)*

Smith DP, Cole BL, Isaacs A: Congenital tritanopia without neuroretinal disease. Invest Ophthalmol 12:608–617, 1973 *(Chapters 6, 7, and 8)*

Smith JW, Brinton GA: Color vision defects in alcoholism. Q J Stud Alcohol 32:41–44, 1971 *(Chapter 8)*

Smith RJS: Visual fields in supra-sellar lesions. Trans Ophthalmol Soc UK 84:697–711, 1964 *(Chapter 8)*

Smith VC, Ernest JT, Pokorny J: Effect of hypoxia on FM 100 hue test performance. Mod Prob Ophthalmol 17:248–256, 1976 *(Chapter 8)*

Smith VC, Pokorny J: Spectral sensitivity of color-blind observers and the cone photopigments. Vision Res 12:2059–2071, 1972 *(Chapters 3 and 7)*

Smith VC, Pokorny J: Letter to the Editors. Psychophysical estimates of optical density in human cones. Vision Res 13:1199–1202, 1973a *(Chapter 7)*

Smith VC, Pokorny J: Letter to the Editor. Autosomal dominant tritanopia. Invest Ophthalmol 13:706–707, 1973b *(Chapter 7)*

Smith VC, Pokorny J: Spectral sensitivity of the foveal cone photopigments between 400 and 500 nm. Vision Res 15:161–171, 1975 *(Chapters 3 and 7)*

Smith VC, Pokorny J: Large-field trichromacy in protanopes and deuteranopes. J Opt Soc Am 67:213–220, 1977 *(Chapters 5 and 7)*

Smith VC, Pokorny J, Diddie KR: Color matching and Stiles-Crawford effect in central serous choriodopathy. mod Prob Ophthalmol 19:284–295, 1978 *(Chapters 3, 4, 5, 6, and 8)*

Smith VC, Pokorny J, Ernest JT, Starr SJ: Visual function in acute posterior multifocal placoid pigment epitheliopathy. Am J Ophthalmol 85:192–199, 1978 *(Chapters 4, 6, and 8)*

Smith VC, Pokorny J, Newell FW: Autosomal recessive incomplete achromatopsia with protan luminosity. Ophthalmologica 177:197–207, 1978 *(Chapter 6)*

Smith VC, Pokorny J, Newell FW: Autosomal recessive incomplete achromatopsia with deutan luminosity. Am J Ophthalmol 87:393–402, 1979 *(Chapter 7)*

Smith VC, Pokorny J, Starr SJ: Variability of color mixture data—I. Interobserver variability in the unit coordinates. Vision Res 16:1087–1094, 1976 *(Chapters 3 and 7)*

Smith VC, Pokorny J, Swartley R: Continuous hue estimation of brief flashes by deuteranomalous observers. Am J Psychol 86:115–131, 1973 *(Chapters 6 and 7)*

Sorsby A, Joll Mason ME, Gardener N: A fundus dystrophy with unusual features. Br J Ophthalmol 33:67–97, 1949 *(Chapter 8)*

Sorsby A, Savory M, Davey JB, Fraser RJL: Macular cysts. A dominantly inherited affection with a progressive course. Br J Ophthalmol 40:144–158, 1956 *(Chapter 8)*

Speelman RG, Krauskopf J: Effects of chromatic adaptation on normal and dichromatic red-green brightness matches. J Opt Soc Am 53:1103–1107, 1963 *(Chapter 7)*

Speranskaya NI: Determination of spectrum color coordinates for twenty-seven normal observers. Opt Spectrosc 7:424–428, 1959 *(Chapter 2)*

Speranskaya NI: Methods of determination of the co-ordinates of spectrum colours, in: Visual

Problems of Colour, vol I, pp 319–325. NPL Symposium No 8. New York, Chemical Publishing Co., 1961 *(Chapter 2)*

Sperling HG: Case of congenital tritanopia with implications for a trichromatic model of color reception. J Opt Soc Am 50:156–163, 1960 *(Chapter 7)*

Sperling HG: An experimental investigation of the relationship between colour mixture and luminous efficiency, in: Visual Problems of Colour, vol I, pp 251-279. NPL Symposium No 8. New York, Chemical Publishing Co., 1961 *(Chapter 2)*

Sperling HG, Harwerth RS: Red-green cone interaction in the increment-threshold spectral sensitivity of primates. Science 172:180–184, 1971 *(Chapters 3, 4, and 6)*

Sperling HG, Johnson C: Histological findings in the receptor layer of primate retina associated with light-induced dichromacy. Mod Prob Ophthalmol 13:291–298, 1973 *(Chapter 8)*

Sperling HG, Piantanida TP: Isolation of the third chromatic mechanisms in simple anomalous trichromats. Mod Prob Ophthalmol 13:145–164, 1974 *(Chapter 7)*

Sperling HG, Piantanida TP, Garrett DS: An atypical color deficiency with extreme loss of sensitivity in the yellow region of the spectrum. Mod Prob Ophthalmol 17:338–344, 1976 *(Chapters 4, 6, and 8)*

Spiecker HD: Praktische Untersuchungen über das Verhalten Farbsinngestörter im Strassenverkehr. Ber Dtsch Ophthalmol Ges 66:186–190, 1965. *(Chapter 9)*

Spiecker HD: Neue Gesichtspunkte bei der augenärztlichen Begutachtung. Wien Med Wochenschr 117:804, 1967 *(Chapter 9)*

Spitznas M: Der normale ophthalmoskopische und histologische Befund der Maculazone und seine Varianten. Ber 73 Zus Dtsch Ophthalmol Ges, Heidelberg 1973, München, Bergmann, 1975 *(Chapter 8)*

Spivey BE: The X-linked recessive inheritance of atypical monochromatism. Arch Ophthalmol 74:327–333, 1965 *(Chapter 7)*

Spivey BE, Pearlman JT, Burian HM: Electroretinogaphic findings (including flicker) in carriers of congential X-linked achromatopsia. Doc Ophthalmol 18:367–375, 1964 *(Chapter 7)*

Stams A: Widersprechende Ergebnisse bei der Farbsinnprüfung unter Anwendung gebrauchlicher Methode. Klin Mbl Augenh 147:261–264, 1965 *(Chapter 7)*

Stanescu B, Michiels J: Electroretinography and temporal aspects in macular dystrophy. Ophthalmologica 172:367–378, 1976 *(Chapter 8)*

Stargardt K: Uber familiäre, progressive Degeneration in der Makulagegend des Auges. Graefes Arch Ophthalmol 71:534–550, 1909 *(Chapter 8)*

Starr SJ: Effect of luminance and wavelength on the Stiles-Crawford effect in dichromats. Ph.D. Dissertation, The University of Chicago, 1977 *(Chapters 3 and 6)*

Steindler O: Die Farbenempfindlichkeit des normalen und farbenblinden Auges. Sitz Ber Akad Wien, Math-Natur Klasse 115:39–62 (Abt 2A), 1906 *(Chapter 7)*

Steiner C: Un cas d'intoxication par P.A.S. et produits analogues. Ann Oculist. 184:637, 1951 *(Chapter 8)*

Steinmetz RD, Ogle KK, Rucker CW: Some physiological considerations of hereditary macular degeneration. Am J Ophthalmol 42:304–317, 1956 *(Chapter 8)*

Stengel E: The syndrome of visual alexia and colour agnosia. J Ment Sci 94:46–58, 1948 *(Chapter 8)*

Stenstrom S: Investigation of the variation and the correlation of the optical elements of human eyes. Am J Optom 25 (monograph), 1948 *(Chapter 8)*

Sternheim CE, Boynton RM: Uniqueness of perceived hues investigated with a continuous judgmental technique. J Exp Psychol 72:770–776, 1966 *(Chapter 6)*

Stiles WS: Increment thresholds and the mechanisms of colour vision. Doc Ophthalmol 3:138–165, 1939a *(Chapter 7)*

Stiles WS: The directional sensitivity of the retina and the spectral sensitivities of the rods and cones. Proc R Soc Lond 127:64–105, 1939b *(Chapters 3 and 6)*

Stiles WS: Further studies of visual mechanisms by the two-colour threshold method. Cologuio Sobre Problemas Opticas de la Vision, Madrid. Union Int Phys Pure Appl 1:65–103, 1953 *(Chapter 3)*

Stiles WS: Interim report to the Commission internationale de l'Éclairage, Zurich, 1955, on the National Physical Laboratory's investigation of color-matching (1955) with an appendix by W.S. Stiles and J.M. Burch. Opt Acta 2:168–181, 1955 *(Chapter 2)*

Stiles WS: Color vision: The approach through increment threshold sensitivity. Proc Natl Acad Sci USA 45:100–114, 1959 *(Chapters 3 and 6)*

Stiles WS: The directional sensitivity of the retina. Ann R Coll Surg Engl 30:73–101, 1962 *(Chapter 6)*

Stiles WS, Burch JM: NPL colour-matching investigation: Final report. Opt Acta 6:1–26, 1959 *(Chapters 2 and 3)*

Stiles WS, Crawford BH: The luminous efficiency of the rays entering the eye pupil at different points. Proc R Soc Lond B 112:428, 1933 *(Chapter 6)*

Svaetichin G, Negichi K, Fatehchand R: Cellular mechanisms of Young-Hering visual system, in De Rouck AVS, Knight J (eds): CIBA Foundation Symposium: Colour Vision. Boston, Little,

Brown & Company, 1965, pp 178–207 *(Chapter 3)*

Swinson RP: Colour vision defects in alcoholism. Br J Physiol Opt 27:43–50, 1972 *(Chapter 8)*

Szucs S: Perception chromatique et coefficients de sommation en vision centrale et paracentrale chez les normaux et chez les amblyopes. Excerpta Med 1:584–586, 1966 *(Chapter 8)*

Takki K: Gyrate atrophy of the choroid and retina associated with hyperornithinaemia. Br J Ophthalmol 58:3–23, 1974a *(Chapter 8)*

Takki K: Differential diagnosis between the primary total choroidal vascular atrophies. Br J Ophthalmol 58:24–35, 1974b *(Chapter 8)*

Tamai A, Setogawa T, Kandori F: Electroretinographic studies on retinitis punctata albescens. Am J Ophthalmol 62:125–131, 1966 *(Chapter 8)*

Tan KEWP: Vision in the ultraviolet. Thesis, Utrecht, 1971 *(Chapter 3)*

Tansley BW, Boynton RM: A line, not a space, represents visual distinctness of borders formed by different colors. Science 191:954–957, 1976 *(Chapter 2)*

Tansley BW, Glushko RJ: Spectral sensitivity of long-wavelength-sensitive photoreceptors in dichromats determined by elimination of border percepts. Vision Res 18:699–706, 1978 *(Chapter 7)*

Taylor WOG: Screening red-green blindness. Ann Ophthalmol 2:184–194, 1970 *(Chapter 5)*

Taylor WOG: The effects on employment of defects in colour vision. Br J Ophthalmol 55:753–760, 1971 *(Chapter 9)*

Taylor WOG: Problems in performance and interpretation of Farnsworth's 100 hue test. Mod Prob Ophthalmol 13:73–78, 1974 *(Chapter 5)*

Taylor WOG: Constructing your own P.I.C. test. Br J Physiol Opt 30:22–24, 1975 *(Chapter 5)*

Taylor WOG: Albinism and colour defects. Mod Probl Ophthalmol 17:292–298, 1976 *(Chapter 8)*

Taylor WOG, Donaldson GB: Recent developments in Farnsworth's color vision tests. Trans Ophthalmol Soc UK 96:262–264, 1976 *(Chapter 5)*

Teele RP: Photometry, in Kingslake R (ed): Applied Optics and Optical Engineering, vol I. New York, Academic Press, 1965, pp 1–42 *(Chapters 1 and 2)*

Thaler A, Heilig P, Heiss W-D, Lessel MR: Toxische Schädigung des Nervus opticus durch Ethambutol. Klin Mbl Augenheilkd 165:660–664, 1974 *(Chapter 8)*

Thaler A, Heilig P, Slezak H: Kombination einer angeborenen Achromatopsie mit sektorförmigen Degeneratio pigmentosa retinae. Graefes Arch Augenh 183:310–316, 1972 *(Chapter 8)*

Thomson LC, Wright WD: The colour sensitivity of the retina within the central fovea of man. J Physiol (Lond) 105:316-331, 1947 *(Chapter 2)*

Thomson LC, Wright WD: The convergence of the tritanopic confusion loci and the derivation of the fundamental response functions. J Opt Soc Am 43:890–894, 1953 *(Chapters 2 and 7)*

Thornton WA: Colour discrimination enhancement by the illuminant. Mod Prob Ophthalmol 13:312–313, 1974 *(Chapter 9)*

Thuline HC: Inheritance of alcoholism. Lancet 1:274–275, 1967 *(Chapter 8)*

Thurn G: Beitrag zur Neurotoxizität der Oxychinoline. Klin Mbl Augenh 163:760–762, 1973 *(Chapter 8)*

Tiffin J, Kuhn NS: Color discrimination in industry. Arch Ophthalmol 28:851–859, 1942 *(Chapter 9)*

Traquair HM: An Introduction to Clinical Perimetry, 6th ed. London, Henry Kimpton, 1949 *(Chapter 8)*

Trendelenburg W: Zur Diagnostik des abnormen Farbensinnes. Klin Mbl Augenh 83:721–732, 1929 *(Chapters 5 and 7)*

Trendelenburg W: Verfahren zur feststellung der Formen von abweichendem Farbensinn mittels Farbflecker. Klin Mbl Augenh 104:473, 1940 *(Chapter 8)*

Trendelenburg W: Ein Anomaloskop zur Untersuchung von Tritoformen der Farbenfehlsichtigkeit mit spektraler Blaugleichung. Klin Mbl Augenh 106:537–546, 1941a *(Chapter 5)*

Trendelenburg W: Ueber Vererbung bei einem Fall von anomalem Farbensinn des einen und normalem Farbensinn des anderen Auges beim Mann. Klin Mbl Augenh 107:280–292, 1941b *(Chapter 7)*

Trendelenburg W: Der Gesichtsinn, Grundzüg der physiologischen Optik. Berlin, Springer-Verlag, 1943 [revised by Monjé M, Schmidt I, Schultz E: Berlin, Springer-Verlag, 1961] *(Chapter 7)*

Trendelenburg W, Schmidt I: Untersuchungen über Vererbung von angeborener Farbenfehlsichtigkeit. Berl Acad Sitz: 13-81, 1935 *(Chapter 5)*

Trevor-Roper P: The World Through Blunted Sight. Indianapolis, Bobbs-Merrill Company, 1970 *(Chapter 4)*

Trusiewicz D: Farnsworth 100 Hue-test in diagnosis of ethambutol-induced damage to the optic nerve. Ophthalmologica 171:425–431, 1975 *(Chapter 8)*

Trusov MS: Disturbances in color vision in hypertensive disease and atherosclerosis. Oftalmol Ab 27:19–22, 1972 *(Chapter 8)*

T'so MOM, Robbins DO, Zimmermann LE: Photic maculopathy: A study of functional and pathologic correlation. Mod Prob Ophthalmol 12:220–228, 1974 *(Chapter 8)*

Turut P: La dégénérescence vitelliforme de la macula. Thesis, Lille, 1972 *(Chapter 8)*

Turut P, Hache JC, François P: L'alteration précoce de la fonction maculaire dans la dégénérescence vitelliforme de la macula. Bull Soc Ophtalmol Fr 72:1121–1124, 1972 *(Chapter 8)*

Umazume K: Studies on colour sensation and clinical use. Jpn J Ophthalmol 2:6–12, 1958 *(Chapter 5)*

Umazume K, Seki R, Obi S: Trial manufacture of a new colour vision test plates. Acta Soc Ophthalmol Jpn 58:732–735, 1954 *(Chapter 5)*

Umazume K, Seki R, Obi S: Studies in trial make of new colour vision test plates. Acta Soc Ophthalmol Jpn 60:1780–1782, 1956 *(Chapter 5)*

Umazume K, Seki R, Obi S, Shimizu K: Studies in trial make of new colour vision test plates. Acta Soc Ophthalmol Jpn 59:765–766, 1955 *(Chapter 5)*

Vainio-Mattila BA, Eriksson AW, Forsius H: X-chromosomal recessive retinoschisis in the region of Pori. Acta Ophthalmol 47:1135–1148, 1969 *(Chapter 8)*

Valberg A, Tansley BW: Tritanopic purity-difference function to describe the properties of minimally distinct borders. J Opt Soc Am 67:1330–1336, 1977 *(Chapter 2)*

Vanderdonck R, Verriest G: Femme protanomale et hétérozygote mixte ayant deux fils deutéranopes, un fils protanomale et deux fils normaux. Biotypologie 21:110–120, 1960 *(Chapter 7)*

Van Lith GHM: General cone dysfunction without achromatopsia. Doc Ophthalmol Proc Ser (10th ISCERG Symposium) 175–180, 1973 *(Chapter 8)*

Van Loo Jr JA, Enoch JM: The scotopic Stiles-Crawford effect. Vision Res 15:1005–1009, 1975 *(Chapter 6)*

Vannas S, Setala M: On atypical night blindness. Acta Ophthalmol (Kbh) 36:849–859, 1958 *(Chapter 8)*

Varela A, Rivera L, Mardomes J, Cruz-Coke R: Colour vision defects in non-alcoholic relatives of alcoholic patients. Br J Addict 64:67–73, 1969 *(Chapter 8)*

Verduyn Lunel HFE, Crone RA: Static perimetry with purely chromatic stimuli. Mod Prob Ophthalmol 13:103–108, 1974 *(Chapter 6)*

Verduyn Lunel HFE, Crone RA: Determination of peripheral spectral sensitivity and saturation discrimination characteristics with a modified Goldmann perimeter. Mod Prob Ophthalmol 19:181–186, 1978 *(Chapter 6)*

Vérin P, Pesme D, Yacoubi M, Morax S: Toxicité oculaire de l'éthambutol. Arch Ophtalmol (Paris) 31:669–686, 1971 *(Chapter 8)*

Verrey A: Variation du sens chromatique dans les dyschromatopsias acquises. Arch Ophtalmol (Paris) 43:612–623, 1926 *(Chapter 8)*

Verriest G: Contribution à l'étude de la corrélation entre la quotient d'anomalie et l'étendue des confusions colorimétriques dans les systèmes trichromatiques anormaux. Rev Opt (Paris) 39:467–471, 1960a *(Chapter 5)*

Verriest G (ed): A Study of the Achromatic Visual Functions in the Congenital Sensory Abnormalities of the Human Eye and in Some Amphibians and Reptiles. The Hague, W. Junk, 1960b *(Chapters 6 and 7)*

Verriest G: Further studies on acquired deficiency of color discrimination. J Opt Soc Am 53:185–195, 1963 *(Chapters 4, 5, 6, 7, and 8)*

Verriest G: Les déficiences acquises de la discrimination chromatique. Mem Acad R Med Belg II/IV:5, 1964 *(Chapters 4 and 8)*

Verriest G: Etude comparative des efficiences de quelques test pour la reconnaissance des anomalies de la vision des couleurs. Arch Mal Profess Med Travail Sec Soc (Paris) 29:293–314, 1968 *(Chapters 5 and 7)*

Verriest G: La variation de la courbe spectrale photopique d'efficacité lumineuse relative chez les sujets normaux. Nouv Rev Opt Appl 1:107–126, 1970a *(Chapters 6 and 8)*

Verriest G: The spectral curve of relative luminous efficiency in acquired colour-vision deficiency. Color 69, Göttingen, Musterschmidt Verlag, 1970b, pp 115–130 *(Chapters 6 and 8)*

Verriest G: Les courbes spectrales photopiques d'éfficacité lumineuse dans les déficiences congénitales de la vision des couleurs. Vision Res 11:1407–1434, 1971a *(Chapter 7)*

Verriest G: L'influence de l'âge sur les fonctions visuelles de l'homme. Bull Acad R Med Belg VII/XI/8:527–577, 1971b *(Chapter 8)*

Verriest G: Chromaticity discrimination in protan and deutan heterozygotes. Farbe 21:7–16, 1972a *(Chapter 7)*

Verriest G: The relative spectral luminous efficiency in different age groups of aphakic eyes. Farbe 21:17–25, 1972b *(Chapter 8)*

Verriest G: Recent advances in the study of the acquired deficiencies of colour vision. Fondazione Giorgio Ronchi XXIV. Florence, Baccini & Chiappi, 1974a, pp 1–80 *(Chapter 8)*

Verriest G: The spectral curve of relative luminous efficiency in different age groups of aphakic eyes. Mod Prob Ophthalmol 13:314–317, 1974b *(Chapters 3 and 8)*

Verriest G: Chairman's report on the answers and comments on the third questionnaire issued by the IPS RG on colour perimetry. IPS document, 1978 *(Chapter 6)*

Verriest G, Buyssens A, Vanderdonck R: Etude quantitative de l'effet qu'exerce sur les résultats de quelques tests de la discrimination chromatique une diminution non sélective du niveau d'un éclairage C. Rev Opt (Paris) 42:105, 1963 *(Chapters 5 and 7)*

Verriest G, Caluwaerts MR: An evaluation of three new colour vision tests. Mod Prob Ophthalmol 19:131– 135, 1978 *(Chapter 5)*

Verriest G, Gonella A: An attempt at clinical determination by means of surface colours of the convergence points in congenital and acquired defects of colour vision. Mod Prob Ophthalmol 11:205– 212, 1972 *(Chapter 7)*

Verriest G, Hermans G: Les aptitudes visuelles professionnelle. Bull Soc Belge Ophtalmol 169:1– 552, 1975 *(Chapters 5 and 9)*

Verriest G, Israel A: Application du périmètre statique de Goldmann au relevé topographique des seuils différentiels de luminance pour de petits objets colorés projetés sur un fond blanc. Vision Res 5:151– 174, 341– 359, 1965 *(Chapter 6)*

Verriest G, Kandemir M: Normal spectral increment thresholds on a white background. Farbe 23:3– 16, 1974 *(Chapter 6)*

Verriest G, Laplasse D: New data concerning the influence of ethyl alcohol on human visual thresholds. Exp Eye Res 4:95– 101, 1965 *(Chapter 8)*

Verriest G, Metsälä P: Résultats en vision latérale de quelques tests de la discrimination chromatique maculaire. Rev Opt (Paris) 42:391– 400, 1963 *(Chapter 6)*

Verriest G, Neubauer O, Uvijls A, Sintobin W: An experimental study comparing the visual performances of normal and congenitally colour defective drivers in the recognition of road safety targets. Second International Ergophthalmology Symposium, Nagoya, 1978 *(Chapter 9)*

Verriest G, Padmos P, Greve EL: Calibration of the Tübinger perimeter for colour perimetry. Mod Prob Ophthalmol 13:109– 112, 1974 *(Chapter 6)*

Verriest G, Popescu MP: 'Umstimmung' of normal subjects at the Nagel anomaloscope. Mod Prob Ophthalmol 13:26– 30, 1974 *(Chapter 7)*

Verriest G, Seki R: Nouveaux cartons pseudo-isochromatiques destinés à la reconnaissance d'une vision de type scotopique. Tagungsbericht Int Farbtagung Luzern 1, Göttingen, Musterschmidt Verlag, 1965, pp 229– 239 *(Chapter 5)*

Verriest G, Uvijls A: Spectral increment thresholds on a white background in different age groups of normal subjects and in acquired ocular diseases. Doc Ophthalmol 43:217– 248, 1977a *(Chapters 4, 6, and 8)*

Verriest G, Uvijls A: Central and peripheral increment thresholds for white and spectral lights on a white background in different kinds of congenitally defective colour vision. Atti Fond G Ronchi 32:213– 254, 1977b *(Chapters 4, 6, and 7)*

Verriest G, Van De Velde R, Vanderdonck R: Etude quantitative de l'effet qu'exerce sur la discrimination chromatique une absorption sélective de la partie froide du spectre visible. Rev Opt (Paris) 41:109– 118, 1962 *(Chapter 8)*

Verriest G, Vandevyvere R, Vanderdonck R: Nouvelles recherches se rapportant à l'influence du sexe et de l'âge sur la discrimination chromatique, ainsi qu'à la signification pratique du test 100 hue de Farnsworth-Munsell. Rev Opt (Paris) 41:499– 509, 1962 *(Chapter 8)*

Vierling O: Die Farbensinnprufung bei der deutschen Reichsbahn. Melsungen, Verlag Bernecker, 1935 *(Chapter 7)*

Vints LA: The effect of lead on the visual organ. Vestn Oftalmol 1:74– 75, 1975 *(Chapter 8)*

Vogt G: Aufstellung von Spektralwerkfunktionen aus einer Folge von Farbgleichheitseinstellungen für Spektrallichter verschiedener Wellenlängen von Personen mit angeborener anomaler Trichromasie und Dichromasie. Farbe 23:51– 107, 1974 *(Chapter 7)*

Volk D, Fry GA: Effect of quality of illumination and distance of observation upon performance in the Ishihara test. Am J Optom Arch Am Acad Optom 24:99– 122, 1947 *(Chapter 5)*

Voke J: Stiles-Crawford chromatic effect in congenital colour defective observers. Mod Prob Ophthalmol 13:140– 144, 1974 *(Chapter 7)*

Voke J: The industrial consequences of deficiencies of colour vision. Thesis, London, 1976 *(Chapter 9)*

Voke J: Industrial requirements and testing of colour vision. Mod Prob Ophthalmol 19:82– 87, 1978 *(Chapters 5 and 9)*

Vola JL, Leprince G, Cornu L, Saracco JB: The 100 hue at mesopic level. Mod Prob Ophthalmol 19:67– 70, 1978 *(Chapter 8)*

Vola J, Leprince G, Langle D, Cornu L, Saracco JB: Preliminary results on the clinical interpretation of Stiles two-colour thresholds method. Mod Prob Ophthalmol 19:266– 269, 1978 *(Chapter 6)*

Vola JL, Riss M, Jayle GE, Gosset A, Tassy A: Acquired deficiency of colour vision in lateral homonymous hemianopia. Mod Prob Ophthalmol 11:150– 159, 1972 *(Chapter 8)*

Völker-Dieben HF, van Lith GHM, Went LN, Klawer JW, Staal H, de Vries-de Mol EC: A family with sex linked optic atrophy (ophthalmological and neurological aspects). Doc Ophthalmol 37:307– 326, 1974 *(Chapter 8)*

Vos JJ: A new apparatus to measure the Stiles-Crawford effect all over the pupil. Rep No IZF 1959-14 and annex. Soesterberg, Institute for Perception, RVO-TNO, 1960 *(Chapter 6)*

Vos JJ: Twenty-five years Stiles-Crawford effect. Adv Ophthalmol 10:32– 48, 1969 *(Chapter 6)*

Vos JJ: Literature review of human macular absorption in the visible and its consequences for the cone receptor primaries. Soesterberg, Rep Inst Percept, TNO Report 1972-17, 1972 *(Chapter 3)*

Vos JJ, Huigen A: A clinical Stiles-Crawford apparatus. Am J Optom Arch Am Acad Optom 39:68–76, 1962 *(Chapter 6)*

Vos JJ, Walraven PL: On the derivation of the foveal receptor primaries. Vision Res 11:799–818, 1971 *(Chapters 3 and 7)*

Vos JJ, Verkaik W, Boogaard J: Kleurenzien-tests. Evaluatie van enige kleurzien-tests ten behoeve van standaardisatie van testmethoden en procedures. Ujd Soc Geneesk [Suppl 2] 49:1–12, 1971 *(Chapter 5)*

Vos JJ, Verkaik W, Boogaard J: The significance of the TMC and HRR color vision tests as to red-green defectiveness. Am J Optom Arch Am Acad Optom 49:847–859, 1972 *(Chapter 5)*

Vos JJ, van Os FL: The effect of lens density on the Stiles-Crawford effect. Vision Res 15:749–775, 1975 *(Chapter 6)*

De Vries-de Mol EC: Een Studie Over Erfelijke Afwijkingen Van Het Kleurenzien. Pijnacker, Dutch Efficiency Bureau, 1977 *(Chapters 6 and 7)*

De Vries-de Mol EC, Went LN: Unilateral colour vision disturbance. A family study. Clin Genet 2:15–27, 1971 *(Chapter 7)*

De Vries-de Mol EC, Went LN, Van Norren D, Pols LCW: Increment spectral sensitivity of hemizygotes and heterozygotes for different classes of colour vision. Mod Prob Ophthalmol 19:224–228, 1978 *(Chapters 6 and 7)*

De Vries-de Mol EC, Went LN, Völker-Dieben HJ: Farnsworth-Munsell 100 hue results in a series of patients with longstanding therapeutic carotinaemia. Mod Prob Ophthalmol 13:349–352, 1974 *(Chapter 8)*

De Vries HL: The heredity of the relative numbers of red and green receptors in the human eye. Genetica 24:199–212, 1947 *(Chapters 6 and 7)*

De Vries HL: The luminosity curve of the eye as determined by measurements with the flicker-photometer. Physica 14:319-348, 1948a *(Chapter 7)*

De Vries HL: The fundamental response curves of normal and abnormal dichromatic and trichromatic eyes. Physica 14:367–380, 1948b *(Chapter 7)*

Waaler GHM: Über die Erblichkeitsverhältnisse der verschiedenen Arten von angeborener Rotgrünblindheit. Z Abst Vererbungslehre 45:279–333, 1927 *(Chapter 7)*

Waardenburg PJ: Atrophie congénitale du nerf optique avec troubles du sens des couleurs, caractère héréditaire récessif. J Genet Hum 5:99–105, 1956 *(Chapter 8)*

Waardenburg PJ: Different types of hereditary optic atrophy. Acta Genet 7:287–290, 1957 *(Chapter 8)*

Waardenburg PJ: Achromatopsia congenita, in Waardenburg PJ, Franceschetti A, Klein D: Genetics and Ophthalmology, vol II. Assen, Netherlands, Royal Van Gorcum, 1963a, pp 1695–1718 *(Chapter 7)*

Waardenburg PJ: Colour sense and dyschromatopsia, in Waardenburg PJ, Franceschetti A, Klein D: Genetics and Ophthalmology, vol II. Assen, Netherlands, Royal Van Gorcum, 1963b, pp 1425–1566 *(Chapter 7)*

Wagner G, Boynton RM: Comparison of four methods of heterochromatic photometry. J Opt Soc Am 62:1508–1515, 1972 *(Chapters 2 and 3)*

Wald G: Photo-labile pigments of the chicken retina. Nature 140:545–546, 1937 *(Chapter 3)*

Wald G: Human vision and spectrum. Science 101:653–658, 1945 *(Chapter 3)*

Wald G: Analysis of retinal function by a two-filter method. J Opt Soc Am 50:633–641, 1960 *(Chapter 6)*

Wald G: The receptors of human color vision. Science 145:1007–1017, 1964 *(Chapters 3 and 6)*

Wald G: Defective color vision and its inheritance. Proc Natl Acad Sci USA 55:1347–1363, 1966 *(Chapter 7)*

Wald G, Brown K: Human color vision and color blindness. Cold Spring Harbor Symp Quant Biol 30:345–361, 1965 *(Chapter 6)*

Wald G, Brown PK, Smith PH: Iodopsin. J Gen Physiol 38:623–681, 1955 *(Chapter 3)*

Wald G, Burian HM: The dissociation of form, vision and light perception in strabismic amblyopia. Am J Ophthalmol 27:950–963, 1944 *(Chapter 8)*

Walls GL: How good is the H-R-R test for colour blindness? Am J Optom 36:169–193, 1959a *(Chapter 5)*

Walls GL: Peculiar color blindness in peculiar people. Arch Ophthalmol 62:13–32, 1959b *(Chapter 7)*

Walls GL: Notes on four tritanopes. Vision Res 4:3–16, 1964 *(Chapter 7)*

Walls GL, Heath GG: Typical total color blindness reinterpreted. Acta Ophthalmol 32:253–278, 279–297, 1954 *(Chapter 7)*

Walls GL, Heath GG: Neutral points in 138 protanopes and deuteranopes. J Opt Soc Am 46:640–649, 1956 *(Chapter 7)*

Walls GL, Matthews RW: New Means of Studying Color Blindness and Normal Foveal Color Vision. Berkeley, University of California Press, 1952 *(Chapter 7)*

Walraven PL: A closer look at the tritanopic convergence point. Vision Res 14:1339–1343, 1974 *(Chapter 7)*

Walraven PL: Basic mechanisms of defective color vision. Mod Prob Ophthalmol 17:2–16, 1976 *(Chapters 3 and 7)*

Walraven PL, Leebeek HL: Recognition of color code

by normals and color defectives at several illumination levels; An evaluation study of the H.R.R. plates. Am J Optom 37:82–92, 1960 *(Chapter 5)*

Walraven PL, Leebeek HJ: Chromatic Stiles-Crawford effect of anomalous trichromats. J Opt Soc Am 52:836, 1962 *(Chapter 7)*

Walraven PL, van Hout AMJ, Leebeek HJ: Fundamental response curves of a normal and a deuteranomalous observer derived from chromatic adaptation data. J Opt Soc Am 56:125–127, 1966 *(Chapter 7)*

Walsh FB, Hoyt WF: Clinical Neuro-Ophthalmology, vol 3. Baltimore, Williams & Wilkens, 1969, p 2606 *(Chapter 8)*

Walsh JWT: Photometry (3rd ed), London, Constable, 1958 *(Chapter 2)*

Watkins RD: Foveal increment thresholds in normal and deutan observers. Vision Res 9:1185–1196, 1969a *(Chapter 7)*

Watkins RD: Foveal increment thresholds in protan observers. Vision Res 9:1197–1204, 1969b *(Chapter 7)*

Weale RA: Hue-discrimination in paracentral parts of the human retina measured at different luminance levels. J Physiol (London) 113:115–122, 1951 *(Chapter 6)*

Weale RA: Cone-monochromatism. J Physiol (London) 121:548–569, 1953 *(Chapter 7)*

Weale RA: Light absorption by the lens of the human eye. Optica Acta 1:107-110, 1954 *(Chapter 3)*

Weale RA: Trichromatic ideas in the seventeenth and eighteenth centuries. Nature 179:648–651, 1957 *(Chapter 3)*

Weale RA: Photo-sensitive reactions in foveae of normal and cone-monochromatic observers. Opt Acta 6:158–174, 1959 *(Chapter 7)*

Weale RA: Notes on the photometric significance of the human crystalline lens. Vision Res 1:183–191, 1961 *(Chapters 3, 6, and 8)*

Weale RA: The Aging Eye. London, H.K. Lewis, 1963 *(Chapter 8)*

Weale RA: Vision and fundus reflectometry: A review. Photochem Photobiol 4:67–87, 1965a *(Chapter 3)*

Weale RA: Vision and fundus reflectometry. Doc Ophthalmol 19:252–286, 1965b *(Chapter 3)*

De Weerdt CJ, Went LN: Neurological studies in families with Leber's optic atrophy. Acta Neurol Scand 47:541–554, 1971 *(Chapter 8)*

Weitzman DO, Kinney JS: Appearance of color for small, brief, spectral stimuli in the central fovea. J Opt Soc Am 57:665–670, 1967 *(Chapter 7)*

Went LN: Leber disease and variants, in Vinken PJ, Bruyn GW (eds): Handbook of Clinical Neurology, vol 13. Amsterdam, North-Holland Publishing Company, 1972, pp 94–110 *(Chapter 8)*

Went LN, Völker-Dieben H, de Vries-de Mol EC: Colour vision, ophthalmological and linkage studies in a pedigree with a tritan defect. Mod Prob Ophthalmol 13:272–276, 1974 *(Chapter 7)*

Went LN, de Vries-de Mol EC: Genetics of colour vision. Mod Prob Ophthalmol 17:96–107, 1976 *(Chapter 7)*

Went LN, de Vries-de Mol EC, Völker-Dieben HJ: A family with apparently sex-linked optic atrophy. J Med Genet 12:94–98, 1975 *(Chapter 8)*

Wentworth MA: A quantitative study of achromatic and chromatic sensitivity from center to periphery of the visual field. Psychol Monogr 40:183–375, 1930 *(Chapter 6)*

Wessely K: Ueber die Bedeutung der Farbenperimetrie beim Glaukom. Klin Mbl Augenh 79:811–812, 1927 *(Chapter 8)*

Whitehead TP, Clarke CA, Whitfield AGW: Biochemical and haematological markers of alcohol intake. Lancet 1:978–981, 1978 *(Chapter 8)*

Wiedman M: New ocular research in the Everest mountain. Bull Mem Soc Fr Ophtalmol 86:201–207, 1973 *(Chapter 8)*

Wienke R: Refractive error and the green/red ratio. J Opt Soc Am 50:341–342, 1960 *(Chapter 8)*

Wiesel T, Hubel DH: Spatial and chromatic interactions in the lateral geniculate body of the rhesus monkey. J Neurophysiol 29:1115–1156, 1966 *(Chapter 3)*

Wijngaard W, Van Kruysbergen J: The function of the nonguided light in some explanations of the Stiles-Crawford effects, in Snyder AW, Menzed R (eds): Photo Receptor Optics. Berlin, Springer-Verlag, 1975, pp 175–183 *(Chapter 6)*

Wilbrand H: Ophthalmiatrische Beiträge zur Diagnostik der Gehirn-Krankheiten. Wiesbaden, J.F. Bergmann, 1884 *(Chapter 8)*

Wilbrand H, Saenger A: Die Neurologie des Auges. Wiesbaden, J.F. Bergmann, 1913 *(Chapter 6)*

Wilberger HGH, van Lith GHM: Color vision and visual evoked response (VECP) in the recovery period of optic neuritis. Mod Prob Ophthalmol 17:320–324, 1976 *(Chapter 8)*

Willis MP, Farnsworth D: Comparative evaluation of anomaloscopes. Medical Research Laboratory Report No. 190, Bureau of Medicine and Surgery, Navy Department Project NM 003 041.26.01, 1952 *(Chapters 5 and 7)*

Willmer EN: Colour vision in the central fovea. Doc Ophthalmol 3:194–213, 1949 *(Chapter 7)*

Wilson AS: The unity of matter: A dialogue on the relation between the various forms of matter which affect the senses. London, Samuel Highley, 1855 *(Chapter 8)*

Wilson EB: The sex chromosomes. Arch Mikrosk Anat 77:249–271, 1911 *(Chapter 7)*

Wright WD: A re-determination of the trichromatic coefficients of the spectral colours. Trans Ophthalmol Soc UK 30:141–164, 1929 *(Chapter 2)*

Wright WD: The sensitivity of the eye to small colour

differences. Proc Phys Soc Lond 53:93–112, 1941 *(Chapter 6)*

Wright WD: Researches in Normal and Defective Colour Vision. London, Kimpton, 1946 *(Chapters 6 and 7)*

Wright WD: The characteristics of tritanopia. J Opt Soc Am 42:509–520, 1952 *(Chapter 7)*

Wyszecki G: Color matching at moderate to high levels of retinal illuminance. Invest Ophthalmol Vis Sci 17(Suppl):197, 1978 *(Chapter 2)*

Wyszecki G, Fielder GH: New color-matching ellipses. J Opt Soc Am 61:1135–1152, 1971 *(Chapter 6)*

Wyszecki G, Stiles WS: Color Science—Concepts and Methods, Quantitative Data and Formulas. New York, John Wiley and Sons, 1967 *(Chapters 1, 2, 3, 5, and 7)*

Yee RD, Herbert PN, Bergsma DR: Atypical retinitis pigmentosa in familial hypobetalipoproteinemia. Am J Ophthalmol 82:64–71, 1976 *(Chapter 8)*

Yokoi T: Color critical fusion frequency in the Bjerrum area; The basic condition for its measure. Acta Soc Ophthalmol Jpn 75:2243–2248, 1971 *(Chapter 6)*

Yokoi T: Color critical fusion frequency in the Bjerrum area; Comparison experiment of glaucoma with other cases. Acta Soc Ophthalmol Jpn 76:219–238, 1972 *(Chapter 6)*

Yonemura D, Aoki T, Tsuzuki K: Electroretinogram in diabetic retinopathy. Arch Ophthalmol 68: 19–24, 1962 *(Chapter 8)*

Young T: On the theory of light and colours. Philos Trans R Soc Lond 92:12–48, 1802 *(Chapter 3)*

Zanen J: Les connexions du phénomène de Troxler. Bull Soc Belge Ophtalmol 99:509–515, 1951 *(Chapter 8)*

Zanen J: Introduction a l'étude des dyschromatopsies rétiniennes centrales acquises. Bull Soc Belge Ophtalmol 103:7–148, 1953 *(Chapters 6 and 8)*

Zanen J: L'intervalle photochromatique en pathologie oculaire. Bull Mem Soc Fr Ophtalmol 72:498, 1959 *(Chapter 8)*

Zanen J: Discussion du rapport sur les ambliopies. Bull Soc Belge Ophtalmol 151:309, 1969 *(Chapter 8)*

Zanen J: La méthode des seuils en pathologie oculaire. 21 Conc Ophthalmol Acta 2:1750–1756, 1971 *(Chapter 8)*

Zanen J: The foveal spectral thresholds in acquired dyschromatopsia. Mod Prob Ophthalmol 11:213–218, 1972 *(Chapter 6)*

Zanen J: Foveal spectral thresholds in ambiguous dyschromatopsia. Mod Prob Ophthalmol 13:176–179, 1974 *(Chapter 6)*

Zanen J, Meunier A: La perception colorée et les seuils absolus et chromatiques dans la rétinopathie séreuse centrale. Bull Soc Belge Ophtalmol 140:359–396, 1965 *(Chapter 8)*

Zanen J, Meunier A: La méthode des seuils dans les dégénérescences maculaires non séniles. Bull Mem Soc Fr Ophtalmol 82:466–476, 1969 *(Chapter 8)*

Zanen J, Rausin G: Kyste vitelliforme congénital de la macula. Bull Soc Belge Ophtalmol 96:544–549, 1950 *(Chapter 8)*

Zanen J, Rausin G: Kyste vitelliforme congénital de la macula. Bull Soc Belge Ophtalmol 98:400–401, 1951 *(Chapter 8)*

Zanen J, Szucs S: Les seuils achromatiques et chromatiques en vision centrale dans l'amblyopie strabique. Bull Soc Belge Ophtalmol 112: 193–206, 1956 *(Chapter 8)*

Zanen J, Szucs S, Pirart J: Les seuils achromatiques et chromatiques dans le diabete. Bull Soc Belge Ophtalmol 115:210–218, 1957 *(Chapter 8)*

Zanen J, Vazquez R: Contribution à l'étude des valeurs énergétiques absolues des seuils achromatiques fovéaux. Vision Res 2:477–494, 1962 *(Chapter 6)*

Zehnder E: Die bewährung farbensinngestörter Motorfahrzeuglenker im Verkehr. Schweiz Med Wochenschr 101:530–537, 1971 *(Chapter 9)*

Zeki SM: Colour coding in rhesus monkey prestriate cortex. Brain Res 53:422–427, 1973 *(Chapter 8)*

Zigmann S, Vaughan T: Near-ultraviolet light effects on the lenses and retinae of mice. Invest Ophthalmol 13:462–465, 1974 *(Chapter 8)*

Zimmermann U: Farbinnstörungen bei Glaukom. Klin Mbl Augenh 148:845–850, 1966 *(Chapter 8)*

Zisman F, Bhargava SK, King-Smith PE: Spectral sensitivities of acquired colour defectives analysed in terms of opponent colour theory. Mod Prob Ophthalmol 19:254–257, 1978 *(Chapters 4, 6, and 8)*

Zuege P, Drance SM: Studies of dark adaptation of discrete paracentral retinal areas in glaucomatous subjects. Am J Ophthalmol 64:56–63, 1967 *(Chapter 8)*

Zwick H, Beatrice ED: Long-term changes in spectral sensitivity after low level laser (514 nm) exposure. Mod Prob Ophthalmol 19:319–325, 1978 *(Chapter 8)*

Zwick H, Bedell RB, Bloom K: Spectral and visual deficits associated with laser irradiation. Mod Prob Ophthalmol 13:299–306, 1974 *(Chapter 8)*

British Standards Institution, London: Specification for artifical daylight for the assessment of colour. Part 1. Illuminant for colour matching and colour appraisal. BS 950:Part 1:1–11, 1967 *(Chapter 5)*

Colors of light signals, Publication CIE No. 2.2 (TC-1.6) 1975. Paris, 1975 *(Chapter 9)*

Colour vision requirements in different operational roles (NATO Advisory Group for Aerospace Research and Development). AGARD Conference Proceedings, 1972, p 86 *(Chapter 9)*

Commission Internationale de D'eclairage, Committee TC-1.4 "Vision:" Light as a true visual quantity: Principles of measurement. 1977, pp 1–64 *(Chapter 2)*

Statistical studies on the blind population of Canada registered with the C.N.I.B. Toronto, Canadian National Institute for the Blind, 1977 *(Chapter 8)*

Index